D0898151

Criminal Justice and Mental Health

Jada Hector • David Khey

Criminal Justice and Mental Health

An Overview for Students

Second Edition

 Springer

Jada Hector
Criminal Justice
University of Louisiana at Lafayette
Lafayette, LA, USA

David Khey
Criminal Justice
University of Louisiana at Lafayette
Lafayette, LA, USA

ISBN 978-3-031-15337-2   ISBN 978-3-031-15338-9   (eBook)
https://doi.org/10.1007/978-3-031-15338-9

This Springer imprint is published by the registered company Springer Nature Switzerland AG
The registered company address is: Gewerbestrasse 11, 6330 Cham, Switzerland

Preface

As with many "great" ideas, this text was borne from a casual conversation. The lead author – Jada Hector – had developed a course for criminal justice students on the intersectionality of mental health and criminal justice using her experience as a mental health professional embedded in Louisiana. In a spontaneous conversation with a Springer content manager, Jada conveyed that her students were responding positively to an insider's perspective on "the struggles" of the entrenched problems inherent in the system for individuals living with mental illness. A simple response – write a book about that – certainly was not something Jada was expecting to hear, but that is what occurred on that fateful day.

Just over 5 years has passed, and the following represents the second edition of this effort in collaboration with Dave Khey. Dave is a criminologist with expertise in drug use and abuse, criminal justice programming, and aligning evidence-based programs, services, and curricula to address the needs of the people to live successful lives. For a decade, Jada and Dave have teamed up to help criminal justice systems adopt programs and policies to help communities – and the people within them – to heal, thrive, and minimize the use of the system.

This text presents core material for all students with aspirations of aiding justice-involved populations at high risk of developing or those living with mental illness. While not exhaustive, such fields include emergency medicine, probation and parole, court and legal services, policing, corrections, mental health professionals, vulnerable population services (e.g., domestic violence, at-risk youth, and underserved populations), and beyond. The material is presented in a way that would lead anyone interested in these fields to have meaningful knowledge about the state of mental health services in the field, the types of programming that have made substantial progress in helping people, and the areas that continue to require improvement. While the text focuses on the criminal justice system in the United States, it also explores commonalities of the problems facing justice-involved people across the globe.

This text is organized in a way that allows for the study of mental health concerns at each stage of criminal justice processing – in the community, upon arrest and transfer to a jail, at court hearings and in attempts to care for individuals in the least restrictive setting possible, and if prison terms are unavoidable, in custody and into reentry back to communities. In addition, the text explores broad trends in mental health awareness to help students understand the current arc of change. That is, we seem to live in a different era – compared to previous attempts to "cure the system" of the entrenched problems described in the chapter on history of mental health treatment, and the incremental changes being made to the system now may prove to be successful.

In this edition, the text seeks to explicitly address stigma in much greater detail. This aligns with a recent recognition and awareness in popular culture of the harm stigma can produce in people's lives. Stigma can alter lives, and if left unaddressed, can produce unintended poor outcomes that are lasting and durable for those directly stigmatized and those in proximity. Stigma research is not new – yet a renewed interest from a wider array of disciplines continues to expand in recent years. Jada and Dave explore some of these recent trends to situate students into the important findings from this line of inquiry.

Lastly, data elements have all been updated to be as recent as possible while acknowledging that many of these estimates are already outdated given vast disruptions caused by the COVID-19 pandemic. The lasting impact of the pandemic will continue to put outsized pressure on both the criminal justice and public health (to include mental health) systems that were already under considerable stress before the public health emergency. One key impact is on the "helper professionals" – shortages in staffing among police, emergency medical services, corrections officers, health professionals (including mental health), and beyond are ongoing while mental health indicators are suggesting that we are entering a time of increased need for care and services. In addition, while violence is not a common feature of mental illnesses or for people with a mental illness, various interests are suggesting (perhaps, pushing) a link between increasing rates of violence across cities across the world and floundering mental health indicators. No such link exists when critically examined – this text dives into the trends to give students a better understanding of the current realities in the field.

Lafayette, LA, USA   Jada Hector
                                                                                                David Khey

Contents

Chapter 1
Mental Illness, Then and Now

Of all the calamities to which humanity is subject, none is so dreadful as insanity.... All experience shows that insanity seasonably treated is as certainly curable as a cold or a fever. –

Dorothea Dix

Mental illness impacts millions of people as well as their loved ones. It can take many forms; it can ebb and flow throughout the life course; it can be the root of a life of suffering; yet, in most cases, it does not have to be a life sentence of misery. The intersection of *crime* and *mental health* has been a long-standing issue spanning across many decades, even centuries. In more recent times, professionals in the United States have begun to detail the "cracks" within the criminal justice system with better precision, especially in relation to inmates with mental health concerns. Unfortunately, despite the recognition of these cracks and their potential "fixes," the implementation of change continues to be a struggle. The federal system, state system, and local county/parish jail system each have their own obstacles to overcome. These systems do not always work together for the common cause of public health for various reasons, and integrating fragmented mental health systems with the highly bureaucratized criminal justice system can seem impossible. Yet, the capacity for coordinated change has never been more possible. This text serves to educate students – the current and future stakeholders of change – on the current intersection of criminal justice and mental health with a laser focus on the fragmentation and weak spots in care for justice-involved individuals. Also, this text offers empirically driven recommendations and reviews innovations in localities across the world as well as breakthroughs in broader systems of care at greater units of analysis (e.g., counties, states, regions, and nations). Many answers to the most entrenched problems remain, yet the impetus for change is on the horizon for those with mental illness in the criminal justice system. The hopes of change begin with discussion on the problems, particularly in a historical context. This text seeks to be that vehicle for change in the future to ensure the care and safety of justice-involved individuals with mental illness.

© The Author(s), under exclusive license to Springer Nature Switzerland AG 2022
J. Hector, D. Khey, *Criminal Justice and Mental Health*,
https://doi.org/10.1007/978-3-031-15338-9_1

1.1 A Brief History

Most detailed histories of American mental health care begin with a discussion of the vast abuses and subhuman conditions endured by those with mental illnesses in the pre-Civil War era. The plight of this vulnerable class came to light in the mid-nineteenth century primarily due to the tenacity of a woman named Dorothea Dix. In fact, it is her words that first underscore the issues of the "idiots" and the "insane," which were the most productive terms for people with mental illness available in the mid-1800s. Margaret Muckenhoupt's (2003) biography of Dix aptly describes how she "single-handedly created most of the 19th-century public institutions east of the Mississippi River that served people with mental illness" by being "unyielding and effective, a symbol of women's good works" (pg. 7). In an era when most women spent their time homemaking and serving a family, Dix never fit that mold; this, in part, allowed her to be an effective advocate for change.

1.1.1 The First Impetus for Change: Dorothea Dix

A brief explanation of Dix's life begins with a child born into a complicated family. The Dix family ascended into Bostonian wealth beginning with her grandfather, Elijah. Her father, Joseph, was the misfit of a rich family – a Harvard dropout and alcoholic with a temper who ended up marrying a woman from a less well-to-do family. This meant that Dorothea's branch of the family tree was considered a stain and an embarrassment, to say the least – quite plainly, they were "the black sheep" of the family. After Elijah Dix died, he left his son Joseph with nothing while leaving Dorothea an annuity that would provide an income for her until she married (Muckenhoupt, 2004). It was this source of funds that would allow for her to run away from her parents and seek help from her grandmother, Dorothy. Madame Dix would eventually arrange for Dorothea to live with one of her well-to-do cousins. She would live there as a very independent teenager, and when she came of age, Dorothea became an educator and operated her own schoolhouse. Ironically, she never had attended school in her life. She would also go on to write successfully, bringing additional income to support her independent lifestyle. Yet, it seemed Dorothea always wanted something more, just not a husband or a traditional female role. She would end up travelling Europe, turning her mind on to social justice, and bringing that passion back to America (Fig. 1.1).

The quintessential "spark" for Dix's advocacy for mental illness occurred by happenstance in the Spring of 1841. Back in Boston, Dix was offered a position to take over a Sunday school class at a local jail, the Middlesex County House of Correction (Muckenhoupt, 2004). It was here where Dix saw the suffering of "public drunks, poor men paying their debts by making shoes, and people who were mentally ill" (p. 42). She observed all these men cramped in cold rooms without access to heat or fire. Dix first reported this issue to the warden who refused to build

Fig. 1.1 Portrait of
Dorothea Dix. (Courtesy of
the U.S. National Library
of Medicine)

a fire as it would be dangerous. Besides, he claimed, it did not seem necessary. Dix would then go to court on this matter. At the time, there was a state law requiring "a suitable and convenient apartment or receptacle for idiots and lunatic or insane persons, not furiously mad," (p. 42) which Dix would cite in her arguments for more humane treatment of inmates at the jail. The courts sided with Dix and ordered the warden to heat the cells. Quickly, she singlehandedly created change, and this changed her life; this gave her a spark of inspiration and a taste for and reward of successful advocacy. Over the next few years, Dix would travel across the state visiting jails and prisons, cataloging what she witnessed. This culminated in a defining moment as an advocate for social justice for those with mental illness, *Memorial to the Legislature of Massachusetts,* testimony delivered on January 19th, 1843:

> About two years since leisure afforded opportunity and duty prompted me to visit several prisons and almshouses in the vicinity of this metropolis. I found, near Boston, in the jails and asylums for the poor, a numerous class brought into unsuitable connection with criminals and the general mass of paupers. I refer to idiots and insane persons, dwelling in circumstances not only adverse to their own physical and moral improvement, but productive of extreme disadvantages to all other persons brought into association with them....I shall be obliged to speak with great plainness, and to reveal many things revolting to the taste, and from which my woman's nature shrinks with peculiar sensitiveness.... *I tell what I have seen* - painful and shocking as the details often are - that from them you may feel more deeply the imperative obligation which lies upon you to prevent the possibility of a repetition or continuance of such outrages upon humanity.
>
> I proceed, gentlemen, briefly to call your attention to the *present* state of insane persons confined within this Commonwealth, in *cages, closets, cellars, stalls, pens! Chained, naked, beaten with rods,* and *lashed into obedience.*
>
> ...[F]ound the mistress, and was conducted to the place, which was called "*the home*" of the *forlorn* maniac, a young woman, exhibiting a condition of neglect and misery blotting out the faintest idea of the comfort, and outraging every sentiment of decency. She had

been, I learnt, "a respectable person, industrious and worthy. Disappointments and trials shook her mind, and, finally, laid prostrate reason and self-control. She became a maniac for life. She had been at Worcester Hospital for a considerable time, and had been returned as incurable." …[T]here she stood with naked arms and disheveled hair; the unwashed frame invested with fragments of unclean garments, the air so extremely offensive, though ventilation was afforded on all sides save one, that it was possible to remain beyond a few moments without retreating for recovery to the outward air. Irritation of body, produced by utter filth and exposure, incited her to the horrid process of tearing off her skin by inches; her face, neck, and person, were thus disfigured to hideousness; she held up a fragment just rent off; to my exclamation of horror, the mistress replied, "oh, we can't help it; half the skin is off sometimes; we can do nothing with her; and it makes no difference what she eats, for she consumes her own filth as readily as food which is brought to her."

These words would soon culminate in the increased capacity of the Massachusetts state insane asylum in Worcester (Worcester State Hospital) as authorized through state legislation, with broad support by the state legislators. Importantly, the new laws shifted the care of the idiots, lunatics, and insane persons, not furiously mad, from local "caretakers" to state specialists with the hopes that this would lead to "moral treatment" and humane conditions. Dix would continue on to petition other state governments: New Jersey would open an asylum as ordered by the legislature in 1845, Illinois – its first – ordered in 1847, and North Carolina ordered in 1849. All of this eventually surmounted into the Bill for the Benefit of the Indigent Insane, a Federal bill that would earmark over 12 million acres of Federal land and resources to address the "newly" identified problem. U.S. Congress would passionately shepherd it through the legislation process, only to have then President Franklin Pierce veto the bill, demanding this issue be relegated to individual states. Dix would end up traveling abroad after this defeat, continuing her efforts in other countries (Fig. 1.2).

Fig. 1.2 Portrait of Horace Mann. (Courtesy of the U.S. Library of Congress. Historian Gerald Grob discovered Mann was a founder of the Worcester State Hospital. Interestingly, some historians note that there is scant historical reflection on Mann's body of work)

1.1.2 Moral Treatment Thrives and Declines

Yet, the momentum spearheaded by Dix and other activists of the era – such as Horace Mann – was beyond reproach. Even in their absence, broad reform continued to develop. Dedicated institutions for individuals with mental illness blossomed in the post-Dix era, particularly those that offered forms of "moral treatment," an early progressive treatment modality developed in the Enlightenment in Europe. Historian Gerald Grob (1983) noted that by the 1880s, nearly 140 public and private mental hospitals were brought into service, caring for just about 41,000 patients. Many of these facilities favored and practiced moral treatment.

The American concept of *moral treatment* was championed by Benjamin Rush, a prominent medical doctor in Philadelphia (Trent Jr., 2017). Rush argued that the root of mental illness was chaos of a modern life that, theoretically, could be treated in a hospital setting mainly by withdrawing someone from all of life's stressors under supervised medical care. While Rush used some provocative procedures – blood-letting and prolonged restraint in a "tranquilizer chair" (that he invented) being two of the more controversial – moral treatment was grounded in medical interventions seeking to soothe a patient in a comfortable setting, engage in exercise and conversation, and explore the individual needs of each individual under care (Fig. 1.3).

Fig. 1.3 A negative of Benjamin Rush's tranquilizer chair (left), and an image of Benjamin Rush (right). (Courtesy of the National Library of Medicine. A note from the NLM catalog regarding the tranquilizer chair: "A patent sitting in a chair; his body is immobilized by straps at the shoulders, arms, waist, and feet; a box-like apparatus is used to confine the head. There is a bucket attached beneath the seat")

Even with this progressive modality – which would eventually become a mainstay in the mental health care of the rich and powerful as it became perfected – the sciences of psychiatry and psychology were far too nascent to offer substantial care for this population. Grob noted that the first generation of mental hospitals that came about in the 1830s and 1840s rode high on perceived successes in outcomes and public support. This was, in part, due to the relatively small patient census of these early years. As the industry grew in the mid-1800s and drew professionals into the field, patient outcomes became abysmal, with breakthroughs few and far between. The growing body of mental health research reinforced a sense of pessimism, which starkly contrasts with the vast sense of optimism shared among the superintendents of the first-generation mental hospitals. In context with the progress of discovery in the broader medical sciences, this stagnation may start to make sense. It helps to consider that medical science figured out that surgical complications and deaths can be drastically reduced by sterilizing operator's hands in 1846 (Ignaz Semmelweis), the American Medical Association was established in 1847, crude medicines like morphine began to show marked medical utility in the mid-1850s, and the first modern American medical school (Johns Hopkins University Medical School) opened its doors in 1893 (Carter & Carter, 1994; Haller, 1981; Packard, 1901). But, while medicine continued to progress and grow rapidly, treatment for mental illness was stymied.

Muckenhoupt (2004) suggests that the progress Dix helped to influence hit a turning point when Pliny Earle – a founding member of the Association of Medical Superintendents of American Institutions for the Insane – published his research on the lack of success of mental health treatment. In doing so, Earle only affirmed what most medical professionals of the era already had suspected. Nothing was working. Earle discovered that patients who were discharged and formally cleared as "sane" were consistently readmitted, casting doubt on the true number of "recoveries." Meanwhile, these readmittances bogged down institutions in their ability to care for the broader population in need, critically at a time when this population appeared to be growing (Grob, 1983). Specifically:

> Earle charged that the reports of recoveries were grossly exaggerated: the proportion of cures represented the ratio of recoveries to cases discharged rather than to cases admitted; readmissions had been disregarded; and many individuals had "recovered" on more than one occasion. He concluded that the older claims of high curability rates were not sustained by the evidence, and that the percentage of reported recoveries was declining because of the increase of cases in the chronic and degenerate category (Grob, 1983: 39).

This failure is just one reason states began to divest in mental hospitals, layered with the consistent underlying and persistent stigma and lack of understanding of mental illness. Asylums gradually became overcrowded, dilapidated, and disorderly. Public support had already waned. For professionals, working in these state institutions never gained the prestige as did being a professional in the other medical sciences – *any* other medical science. Thus, the administrators of these facilities were not typically the best and brightest. Beyond these forces, scientific advances in understanding heredity entered the void in psychiatry presented by not yet understanding the etiology of mental illness. Genetic predisposition and determinism, while not fully embraced by psychiatrists of the era, only served to amplify the pessimism of the 1880s.

One can easily argue that this is the point where America has simply replicated the manner it treats the idiots and lunatics or insane persons and that policy simply changed the setting in which "treatment" was given – from jails and prisons to prison-like asylums. "Moreover, discussions about social policy generally took place within a framework dominated by the conviction of pauperism, crime, and degeneracy were all related" (Grob, 1983: 40). Further, these prison-like asylums, or "hospitals," concentrated stigma and rapidly became a place for a "new" class of people. It would not be a stretch of the imagination to conceive that this concentration of the problem of the mentally ill in these ghastly institutions only helped the eugenics movement of the early twentieth century to target this class of people for sterilization or complete elimination from the gene pool. Thankfully, this is not the path history takes us. The twentieth century would bring waves of change in psychiatry, in line with the broader currents of American social forces. Camps within psychiatry would form and compete to define our understanding of mental illness. Perhaps more important, the profession would begin to decouple from mental hospitals and "institutional practice," laying the groundwork for the modern era.

1.1.3   The Miracle Drugs

Finally, over a hundred years into this American story, a breakthrough occurred; research on chlorpromazine, known for its trade name Thorazine®, began to surface in the 1950s. The drug launched quickly from laboratory to trial use, and on to widespread use, all during that same decade. Physicians quickly knew Thorazine® as a wonder drug for its abilities to breakthrough psychotic symptoms, so much that when they saw marked improvements in their patients, mental hospital doctors would release them in droves – even without knowing the long-term efficacy or potential pitfall of these decisions. Just think, Thorazine® was first produced in a laboratory in 1950, showed significant promise in animal studies in early 1951, was released to physicians as a research drug in the late spring of 1951, and was documented to produce dramatic improvement in psychotic symptoms by the end of the year (Healy, 2009). By late 1957, psychiatrists Kris and Carmichael (1957) observed that "modern drug therapy has brought about a considerable increase in the number of patients returning to the community" in their follow-up study of 160 patients released from the New York metro area hospitals.

This New York study, as many others like it, vetted the viability of using drug therapy to treat diagnoses such as schizophrenia, "manic-depressive" or "manic disorders," alcohol psychosis, and "involutional psychosis." The prognosis seemed positive with the following caveats: (1) patients must be re-evaluated by professionals often "not only in order to avoid unpleasant complications, but also to vary the dosage according to individual needs, taking into account increased stress situations which (sic) have to be faced by these patients outside the hospital," (2) patients with "enduring" conditions (e.g., chronic and severe mental illness) must receive maintenance dosages of Thorazine® to prevent recurrence of symptoms once the drug is discontinued, (3) physicians must ensure compliance with doctor's orders (particularly with taking the correct dose at the recommended intervals), and (4) physicians must evaluate the social situations that may trigger a return to the hospital. The last point they make is interesting regarding the social situations that may trigger relapse; Kris and Carmichael go on to suggest that Thorazine® may be the most potent and valuable "weapon" against mental illness, yet they want to make clear that when it fails to treat someone effectively, social factors should be to blame, not the drug (Fig. 1.4).

Drugs like Thorazine® thrived in this scientific environment so eager for a breakthrough after decades of slow progress, signaling a dawn of effective treatments for diseases that we were only beginning to understand. In fact, the drug revolution brought a renaissance of psychiatric treatment of mental illness, helping to vastly expand our knowledge of the topic at a quickened pace. In his history of therapeutic medicines, Healy noted, "the 1955 meeting of the American Psychiatric Association (APA) should have been dominated by Thorazine®. But while

Fig. 1.4 Thorazine® advertisement in the *Journal of American Psychiatry* in 1980. (Courtesy of Glaxo Smith Kline)

Thorazine® was on stage, the whispers in the wings were of an even newer drug, Miltown® (meprobamate) which was launched in the second half of 1955....By any reckoning, therefore, while Miltown® might never have made a splash elsewhere (outside of the United States), Thorazine's time at the center stage in American psychiatry should have been short. The fact that it survived the inroads of Miltown® and remained at the center of the scientific stage is compelling testimony to the recognition that chlorpromazine truly was a different drug" (98–99). He goes on to describe the amazement some experts had with Thorazine®. For example, one professional was so impressed that he took equity out of his house to buy stock in the pharmaceutical company manufacturing the drug.

Thus, Thorazine® exploded onto therapeutic use in the United States, and American practitioners were more eager than their European counterparts to push the limits of the drug, increase dosage, and begin pursuing advancing outpatient care in the community now that severe symptoms were being significantly allayed. And while there were many success stories, it truly took science over 40 years to understand the psychopharmacology of what would be known as a broader class of drugs – the antipsychotics.

1.1.4   Deinstitutionalization

Thorazine® and the first-generation antipsychotic family of drugs – called the phenothiazines – thus sparked the *deinstitutionalization* movement. Plainly, deinstitutionalization refers to the shift of caring for individuals with severe mental illness in state mental hospitals to community centers and outpatient services from the 1950s arguably through the date of this writing. E. Fuller Torrey (1997) calls this shift "one of the largest social experiments in American history," as he opines over the sheer magnitude this change as demonstrated by the numbers of patients residing in state mental hospitals from the 1950s. Torrey cites that in 1955, state hospitals had a population of 558,239 persons; yet, by 1994, this population was reduced to 71,619 nationwide. The exact numbers often vary in the literature; however, three key sources have reliably documented the dramatic changes over this period – the National Institute of Mental Health, the Center for Mental Health Services, and individual states. A summary of CMHS data can be found in Fig. 1.5. Likely, these data will be updated through 2020 in the near future.

Further, psychiatry had progressed as a science enough to broadly define the types of diseases facing this population: roughly half had a diagnosis of schizophrenia, about 10–15% were diagnosed with manic depression (now, bipolar disorder) or "severe" depression, another 10–15% had mental health issues due to organic brain disease, and the remainder had diagnoses such as mental retardation with psychosis (now, intellectual disability, with psychosis), childhood disorders, and brain disease in conjunction with an addiction (Torrey, 1997). Was it possible to effectively treat these issues outside of a hospital setting? For over 100 years,

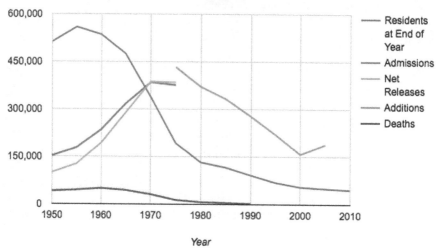

Fig. 1.5 Number of hospital residents, admissions, net releases, additions, and deaths, using CMHS data presented in a national report entitled, "Funding and Characteristics of State Mental Health Agencies, 2007" (SAMHSA, 2007) with year 2010 added from "Behavioral Health United States, 2012 (SAMHSA, 2012)

establishing effective treatments for these diagnoses eluded mental health professionals. Real change was finally happening, but was it positive change?

As these questions were being wrangled with, political pressure from various sources was pushing states to decrease the size of state mental hospitals. It was certainly easier to acquiesce to these pressures with the broader adoption of the phenothiazines; however, the combination of the Community Mental Health Centers Act of 1963 with the enactment of Medicaid and Medicare (via Title XVIII and XIX of the Social Security Act, signed into law by Lyndon B. Johnson) cemented the trend of treating mental illness outside of hospital settings (Torrey, 1997; SAMHSA, 2007). In particular, the Community Mental Health Centers Act was put in place to develop a network of community mental health centers at the local level, reversing the trend that Dorothea Dix promoted. Medicaid and Medicare helped to cover the cost of using these centers for patients. This shift may have led to positive results if, in fact, the nationwide mental health network could prove successful. This would mean that the system ensures that people with mental illness receive medication, rehabilitation services, and aftercare to ensure ongoing treatment compliance, yielding the best chances for personal success with treatment. Unfortunately, this great experiment is absent of success stories. In later decades, the narrative of mental health would become entangled in another failing policy shift of the twentieth century – American criminal justice reform, including its war on drugs.

1.1.5   The Media Coverage of Hospital Conditions and Homelessness and Social Awareness

As the Federal government pushed forward with policies favoring treatment of mental illness in local communities over state-run institutions, additional forces added to the momentum – or, at minimum, aided to continue to reduce the size and scope of state mental hospitals. The most potent of these forces is the effect of mass media coverage of the hospitals, which had become dilapidated and chaotic messes as their resources continued to dwindle in these years. For example, Life Magazine published Albert Q. Maisel's photo essay on the horrors of state-run mental hospitals, "Bedlam 1946: Most U.S. Mental Hospitals are a Shame and a Disgrace." The impact of visualizing the suffering in photographs was certainly palpable, with the captions reading "NEGLECT. In Cleveland Hospital's bare wards a patient lies unnoticed and unattended on stone floor," "RESTRAINT. This woman wears a camisole with sleeves tied behind her. Ulcers on leg are bandaged," "USELESS WORK. At Massillon Ohio State Hospital barefoot patients polish splintered wooden floor in 1890 building - a poor substitute for occupational therapy," and so on with explicit photographs depicting "NAKEDNESS... OVERCROWDING... FORCED LABOR... IDLENESS... [and] DESPAIR." The 13-page spread dedicated to the issue began to raise awareness on a growing problem, a problem that seemed intractable, until pharmaceutical and policy intervention. This copyrighted work – including its shocking visceral images – is available online at the time of this writing, easily searchable by the article's title.

This was certainly not the only instance of mass media's contribution to the conversation. One of the most iconic exposés of this era that brought these issues into the public spotlight was Geraldo Rivera's work on Willowbrook State School in Staten Island, New York, called "The Last Disgrace 1972."

> When Dr. Wilkins slid back the heavy door of B Ward, building No 6, the horrible smell of the place staggered me. It was so wretched that my first thought was that the air was poisonous and would kill me. I looked down to steady myself and I saw a freak: a grotesque caricature of a person, lying under the sink on an incredibly filthy floor in an incredibly filthy bathroom. It was wearing trousers, but they were pulled down around the ankles. It was shinny. It was twisted. It was lying in its own feces. And it wasn't alone. Sitting next to this thing was another freak. In a parody of human emotion they were holding hands. They were making a noise. It was a wailing sound that I still hear and that I will never forget. I said out loud, but to nobody in particular, "My God, they're children." Wilkens looked at me and said, "Welcome to Willowbrook." (Rivera, 2017).

There are some very notable contrasts and similarities of Rivera's words to Dix. First, the stark contrast each observer's characterization of the mentally ill is staggering: Dix refers to the vulnerable people she witnessed as idiots and lunatics, acceptable early medical labels for the mentally ill in that era, while Rivera uses the stigmatic word *freak*. Yet, the message was essentially the same. How was it possible for the government, at any level, to treat the vulnerable in such an inhumane way? In today's terms, the exposé would go viral. One cannot underestimate the impact of photojournalism and documentary-style exposes in their potential to elicit a grassroots and/or policy response. At minimum, the ongoing and visceral report- ing on the issue of mental illness reinforced the political sentiment of the era to increase resources for mental health services in communities while divesting in state-run institutions, and many would argue with convincing evidence that this set the stage to defund almost all state mental hospitals by the end of the twentieth century.

At this point in history, the issue becomes much more complex, and the follow- ing forces are at play: the mass media, professional medical organizations jockeying for authority, the pharmaceutical industry, policymakers and political figures, and a growing socially aware populace with broader access to political influence. Deinstitutionalization has triggered the process of reintroducing a sizeable popula- tion of individuals with severe mental illness to the public, whereas in the past, this group was kept vastly segregated and out of sight. Grob (1983) remarked that peo- ple with mental illness remained effectively invisible to the populace throughout his historical study. This was done largely without a scientific assurance that individu- als with mental illness could live successfully, with minimal symptoms, in the men- tal health networks created for their treatment. While the available treatment would, in fact, work well for some people, it would end up leaving many vulnerable, with- out access to care, and untreated. These individuals would soon become documented in a growing scientific literature on the failures of deinstitutionalization, namely for ending up in the swelling numbers of the homeless or criminally institutionalized in the nation's jails and prisons.

Yet, as deinstitutionalization would quietly criminalize untreated mental illness, American mass media would instead become focused on homelessness. Buck and Toro (2004) point to several reasons why this occurred in the 1980s. First, Ronald Reagan's administration led the initiative of making substantial cuts to social pro- grams in light of a recession. In response, Reagan's political opponents aligned with homelessness activists to begin a media campaign on the issue in sharp rebuke of the administration with hopes of political fallout. Second, many aging urban centers were redeveloping and becoming gentrified, leading to fewer affordable housing options. The combination proved to be excellent kindling for a crisis in a super- heated political environment, keeping this story circulating in the news for several years in the 1980s. The previous social ill of vagrancy, an often-stigmatized term with a lengthy negative connotation throughout American history, would become homelessness. Tramps and hobos would become the homeless.

In their 2002 study, Buck, Toro, and Ramos evaluated these trends in print cover- age from 1972 (well before media interest began on the issue) to 2001 (well after the issue attracted front covers) in four leading newspapers: *The New York Times, The Washington Post, The Los Angeles Times,* and *The Chicago Tribune.* These research- ers took 500 randomly selected articles and identified four distinct time periods, labeled preinterest (1972–1980), rise and peak (1981–1987), decline (1988–1993), and plateau (1994–2001). They argued that the rise and peak period seemed to be "the most revealing." It is during these years that the media departed from their previous view of the homeless and would, generally, cast a more sympathetic light on these individuals. But, while the media reported on mental health as a contributing factor and tied deinstitutionalization and related structural issues to the broader homelessness problem, Buck and Toro found that most of the coverage failed to talk about services or long-term programs designed to address homelessness, noting that few services or programs existed during that time. In the decline years, negative reporting returned in greater frequency, often bringing back stereotypes of skid row alcoholics and drug addicts, with the addition of the mentally ill and the dangerousness stigma. It is not that the media completely turned their backs to the plight of the homeless; instead, Buck, Toro, and Ramos argue that the American public grew to understand that homelessness is complex, and the media coverage of the time reflects that by its broad coverage of the issue.

Instead of a broad compassionate policy response as seen in previous eras, mental illness was on a collision course with criminal justice reform. For many with mental illness, deinstitutionalization increased the risk of substance use and abuse (called co-occurring disorders – more on this later) and illegal behaviors (some may be contributed directly to the illness). Many were left vulnerable and without a safety net as the community mental health networks never became comprehensive enough to effectively treat the population previously served by state-run mental hospitals. The war on drugs began with Richard Nixon's administration; but it was the Reagan administration and the 98th (1983–1985) and 99th (1985–1987) U.S. Congress that initiated the criminal justice reforms that would rapidly accelerate the growth of the rate Americans incarcerate their citizens. This trend would continue into the administrations of George H.W. Bush and Bill Clinton with the full support of Congress. With a fragmented mental health treatment network as the only option for many vulnerable people, their fate amounted to a different iteration of the incarceration faced by those in state-run mental hospitals. Except, this time, their experiences would be much worse as American jails, and prisons were hardly prepared to care for people with mental illness.

1.1.6   The Impact of the War on Crime and the Incarceration State

The primary drivers moving individuals with mental illness from the community and into jails and prisons are (1) substance abuse and (2) untreated or undertreated symptoms. Just as Kris and Carmichael may have predicted, untreated or undertreated symptoms would produce a return to the state hospital – except that these hospitals had shuttered, with remaining facilities having vastly reduced capacities and a bare bones operation that would only serve the most severe cases. Further, the struggles facing this vulnerable population do not occur in isolation; in other words, poverty, homelessness, substance use and abuse and self-medication, violence and victimization, and frayed social support, to name a few, can all influence each other and influence one's mental health to deteriorate or symptoms to appear – again, a theme that was foreshadowed by Kris and Carmichael's Thorazine® study.

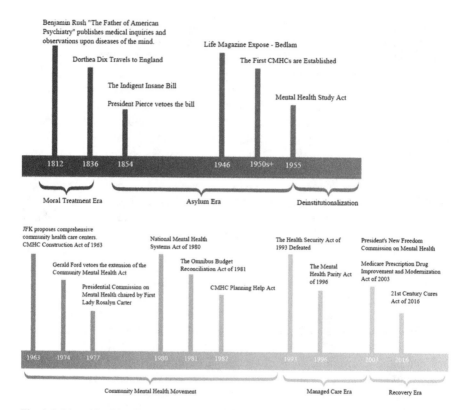

Fig. 1.6 Mental health policies over time

Figure 1.6 lists the policies, the timing of the policies, and their effects on mental health and criminal justice.

The "Tough on Crime" (or War on Crime) movement has led to dramatic changes. Foremost, jails and prison populations have increased exponentially. While *total* numbers are difficult to come by for this entire period, the Bureau of Justice Statistics (BJS) – an agency within the Department of Justice tasked with collecting data on the operation of justice systems among all levels of government – maintains a dataset called the National Prisoner Statistics Program that has followed the State and Federal prison population since 1925 (Bureau of Justice Statistics, 1982). While it excludes data on local (jail) inmates, the dataset clearly shows stability of the prison population around 100 per 100,000 persons in the United States until the mid-1970s (Fig. 1.5). By all accounts, this figure trended aggressively upward through the 1980s, 1990s, and into the new millennium – exceeding 500 per 100,000 persons. Yet, to truly understand the impact of deinstitutionalization apart from the "Tough on Crime" movement, one would also need to observe changes in all segments of the *justice-involved population*. Justice-involved is a broad term that refers to individuals in State and Federal prisons, in community corrections (e.g., State and Federal probation and parole), and in local jails either awaiting trial or serving

Incarceration rate of inmates incarcerated under state and
federal jurisdiction per 100,000 population, 1925-2020

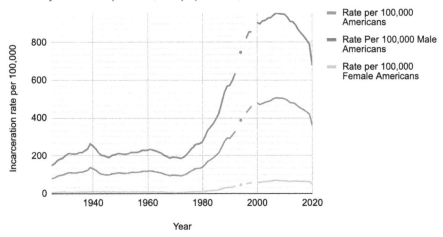

Fig. 1.7 Data from the National Prisoner Statistics Program, Bureau of Justice Statistics

time. Unfortunately, since consistent and reliable data on all segments of the justice-involved population only began to be collected in the late 1970s, it is truly difficult to follow the impact of deinstitutionalization on justice involvement.

Available data from the Bureau of Justice Statistics (see Fig. 1.7) certainly suggest the use of the criminal justice system as a broad intervention tool for substance use and abuse and "criminality." Starkly, the reach of the criminal justice system peaked in 2008 at 2405 per 100,000 adult Americans involved in the system in some way, up from 800 per 100,000 in 1980 (Bureau of Justice Statistics, 2016). Put another way, that amounts to just over two per every hundred adults in the United States were in prison or jail, or on probation or parole, in 2008. Many of these individuals were swept up into the system for nonviolent drug offenses as a direct result of the "Tough on Crime" movement, which focused so much of its efforts on drug policy. As Jonathan Rothwell (2015) points out, while 1 in 5 state prisoners are incarcerated for drug offenses on average, there were three million admissions (just above 30% of all admissions) to both state and Federal prisons for this type of offense from 1993 to 2011, far more than any other type (e.g., violent crimes, property crimes, and all other crimes). Quite simply, drug crimes continue to be the main driver of imprisonment, even in current times.

Yet, many questions still remain – how many of those adults are mentally ill? What was the true impact of deinstitutionalization? If deinstitutionalization trends began in 1955, how can one effectively explain why prison populations did not trend upward until the mid-1970s? The capacity to answer how many justice-involved persons have mental illness is growing, and the true impact of deinstitutionalization mostly relies on anecdotal conjecture as consistent and reliable data identifying justice-involved individuals with mental illness only has recently become routine.

After all, a scenario may exist that the proportion of mentally-ill, justice-involved persons has stayed consistent, with just the total population ballooning; yet, all available evidence does not bear this out.

Many observers, such as Lamb and Weinberger (2005), have argued that mental illness has effectively become criminalized over this period post deinstitutionalization. The exact numbers remain elusive to this date; however, there are a few ways to estimate the number of individuals with mental illness in the *current* justice-involved population. One way, Lamb and Weinberger suggest, is to take the estimation of the percentage of individuals in jails and prisons who could be diagnosed with serious debilitating mental illness (e.g., major depression, schizophrenia, bipolar disorders, and various other psychotic disorders) as published in current scientific literature, which at the time, ranged from 16% to 24%. Using a conservative approach, Lamb and Weinberger use the 16% for the year 2000 and estimated 113 per 100,000 individuals in jails and prisons to be severely mentally ill. "Severely mentally ill individuals who formerly would have been psychiatrically hospitalized when there were a sufficient number of psychiatric inpatient beds are now entering the criminal justice system for a variety of reasons (Fig. 1.8). Those most commonly cited are: (1) deinstitutionalization in the terms of limited availability of psychiatric hospital beds; (2) the lack of access to adequate treatment for mentally ill persons in the community; (3) the interactions between severely mentally ill persons and law enforcement personnel; and (4) more formal and rigid criteria for civil commitment."

Taking a more liberal approach, two BJS statisticians – James and Glaze (2006) – analyzed personal interviews with prisoners and local jail inmates in two surveys performed just a few years prior in a special report. In their analysis, James and Glaze were able to decipher individuals with mental health problems by one of two ways to gain better insight into this population: (1) recent history (within the last 12 months) of a clinical diagnosis and/or treatment by a mental health professional, and (2) exhibiting symptoms of a mental health disorder as determined by targeted questions on the two surveys. The results were staggering; 705,600 (56%) state prisoners, 78,800 (45%) federal prisoners, and 479,900 (64%) local jail inmates met criteria for having a mental health problem, amounting to just over *half* of the total population. These figures differ considerably from the first comprehensive accounting of mentally ill subpopulation by the BJS performed only a few years prior in 1999. At that time, BJS statistician Paula Ditton had access to survey questions asking participants directly if they suffer from a mental illness or if they had stayed overnight in a mental hospital. This line of questioning resulted in estimates of 283,800 individuals with mental illness in jails and prisons, with 16% of state inmates, 7% of federal inmates, and 16% of local jail inmates self-reporting mental illness in this manner. The differences between these two undertakings are essentially underscoring the potential undiagnosed mental health problems endemic to this justice-involved population. More on this in later chapters.

The updated report also included a more comprehensive description of mentally-ill, justice-involved individuals, giving supporting evidence to the anecdotal descriptions of this population in the literature at the time: state prisoners and jail inmates

Total Adult Correctional Population, By Rate, 1980-2019

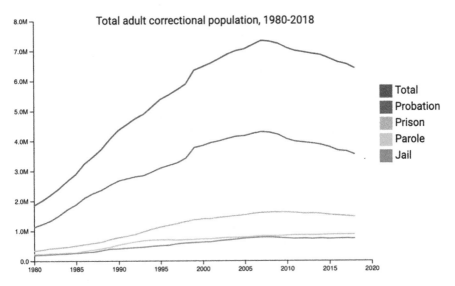

Fig. 1.8 Data from the Bureau of Justice Statistics, key statistic: total correctional population

with mental health problems are more likely to report being incarcerated three or more times relative to those who do not report mental health problems; female inmates reported mental health problems more than male inmates; about three quarters of the individuals reporting mental health problems also met criteria for substance use disorder or abuse; nearly two-thirds of these individuals used drugs in the month prior to their arrest; state prisoners with a mental health problem were twice as likely to be homeless and twice as likely to be injured in a fight since admission relative to individuals who did not (James & Glaze, 2006). There is little doubt that a sizeable portion of the people who need mental health services have, at minimum, a higher likelihood of contact with the criminal justice system since deinstitutionalization.

1.2   Current Policy

While the prognosis may appear grim, policy efforts to address the fallout from the "Tough on Crime" movement are ongoing. Further, a functional network of community-based mental health services is possible; in fact, these networks are already in place for those who have access through private health insurance. Much of the innovation for the vulnerable populations discussed above – the homeless, individuals with mental illness, and/or those with addiction – stems from the Second Chance Act of 2007 and Justice Reinvestment Initiative legislation. Briefly, the Second Chance Act was a bipartisan law easily passed under the George W. Bush administration that earmarked funding to invest in programs to reduce recidivism while ensuring public safety. Through 2018, over $695.2 million has been invested in promising programs via discretionary grants, marking a formal start to the "Reentry" movement. A primary caveat to receive these funds at the local or state level is to initiate programs or services that are *evidence-based*. Two Second Chance Act programs are specifically relevant here – Targeting Adults with Co-occurring Substance Abuse and Mental Health Disorders and the Statewide Adult Recidivism Reduction Strategic Planning Program. The first of the two has further refined our knowledge of what works to help individuals with mental illness return to the community and reduce their chances of being reincarcerated, while the latter has enabled states to develop the policy initiatives to help drive this sort of change for state prisoners and local jail inmates alike.

The Justice Reinvestment Initiatives are currently a collaborative project with states and localities and the Pew Charitable Trusts, with funds authorized by Congress in 2010 via the Bureau of Justice Administration. These initiatives require broad participation by stakeholders in each location to participate in a comprehensive analysis of their criminal justice system in order to define which evidence-based strategies could be put in place to reduce recidivism and cost while maintaining public safety. Generally, these initiatives tend not put direct focus on mental health issues; however, many initiatives have better defined the problems facing justice-involved individuals with mental illness and have generated plans to mitigate these problems (Table 1.1).

The key to both of these strategies is to promulgate evidence-based practices and services that are proven to reduce recidivism, while further vetting promising practices and services that may lead to beneficial results. For justice-involved individuals with mental illness, this means provision of adequate care in *all* settings – jails, prisons, and upon return to the community. This means that a comprehensive review of these settings are beginning to take shape or have been completed since 2002.

Table 1.1 Participants served by Second Chance Act programs, 2009–2015

SCA programming	Number served
Co-occurring	9048
Family-based	8375
Mentoring	25,573
Technology careers	6632
Reentry demonstration	61,105
Reentry court	2595
Overall	*113,328*

Courtesy of the Bureau of Justice Assistance

Progress is beginning to take shape across the United States, and never has American justice and mental health policy been closer to the ideal of providing mental health services in the *least restrictive* manner (Atkinson & Garner, 2002; World Health Organization, 1996) – that is, fewer locked doors, less incarceration or commitment, fewer shackles, chains, and restraints, and so on.

It also should be noted that both strategies placed substantial focus on overall cost reduction of criminal justice as overall expenditures were getting out of hand, particularly during times of recession. This emphasis on "smart" cost savings has enabled broad support for policies that are affecting change since the beginning of the century. While change has been slow to come, its momentum continues to expand the array of services available to the very same vulnerable population cast aside since the days of Dorothea Dix. One recent example was the passage of the twenty-first Century Cures Act – a bipartisan effort signed into law by Barack Obama at the end of his last term. Within the legislation, the 114th Congress embedded previous iterations of the Helping Families in Mental Health Crisis Act as Division B of the Cures Act. This section is dedicated to completely revisioning mental health services in the United States. Key provisions of the Act include: the creation of an Assistant Secretary for Mental Health and Substance Abuse and an Assistant Secretary of Planning and Evaluation within the Substance Abuse and Mental Health Services Administration, creating a biennial report to tabulate progress, and developing a strategic plan – all to bolster leadership and accountability of mental health services; encouraging the development of evidence-based programs and services and other innovation via grants, prioritize development of services based on need, and disseminating this information – to ensure these efforts keep up with the best and current science on mental health and substance abuse; supporting state innovation via block grants; and promoting access to mental health services via grants for homeless populations, jail populations, integration of primary and mental health care, revisioning suicide prevention, and much more.

Throughout the Cures Act, there are several mentions of expanding the use of inpatient beds in a strategic fashion. One priority is to use technology to better understand the availability of inpatient resources, their utilization, and their fit in a broader continuum of care by region and across the country. Thus, this reimagination of mental health care is a key, and bold, effort since deinstitutional-ization policies to address this persistent need of a vulnerable class of citizens. Notably, it expands Medicaid to cover a broader array of mental health services to stymie the use of jails and prisons as the new asylum for individuals with mental illness. Yet, these institutions will remain an important component of the "new" system of care it envisions.

One tangible accomplishment of the Cures Act pertaining to mental health – the expansion of Assisted Outpatient Treatment (AOT) programs – provides evidence of progress. AOT programs target individuals with mental illness at risk of relapse or harm to self and/or others *without* inpatient commitment. This is accomplished via court order, and a court officer (e.g., judge) supervises each client's dynamic outpatient treatment services. This powerful program has documented success in reducing suicidality, homelessness, substance use, physical harm, hospitalization, and arrest and incarceration. More in this novel program later in this text.

1.3 Key Problems Today

The four following problem areas need to be introduced early in this text: stigma, trauma, co-occurring disorders, and cost of services. Together, they represent per-sistent barriers to successfully addressing mental health care in the United States. In fact, "stigma" is directly addressed 4 times in the Cures Act; "trauma" 27 times; "co-occurring" 37 times; and "cost" 98 times. Recall that cost is the glue that makes the effort to re-envision mental health care possible; thus, any innovation will only prove to be viable if it can prove cost savings. Always keep this in mind when con-sidering the advances of science in future years.

1.3.1 Trauma

Trauma is often related to a significant untoward and problematic event in a person's life (SAMHSA, 2014, 2017a, b). It is more common than one may expect, and is not bound by age, gender, race, ethnicity, socioeconomic status, or other difference between people. While many people can persevere through traumatic events with-out experiencing lasting negative outcomes, a broadening array of research is revealing the importance of early treatment intervention. Individuals with a support system and those who have never or rarely experience trauma are typically more resilient, but not always. Unfortunately, this trauma can linger and become a larger problem, perhaps in the form of mental illness and/or substance abuse – especially when the trauma is persistent and/or occurs with increased frequency. Furthermore, it is important to note that the negative effects of trauma are magnified when they occur during childhood. Thus, children and teenagers are at most risk for develop-ing lasting conditions such as substance abuse disorder (including smoking cigarettes and drinking alcohol) and mental health problems (including depression, anxiety, and posttraumatic stress disorder), or engage in risky behaviors such as self-injury and risk taking.

Trauma may be the result of harm, violence, and victimization from a variety of experiences. In fact, SAMHSA offers toolkits (2014) that offer an excellent summary across the broad domains of experiencing trauma, and helpful resources that can help both laypersons and professionals link up with evidence-based treatments to address these sources of trauma. Broadly, these domains include: sexual abuse or assault; physical abuse or assault; emotional abuse or psychological maltreatment; neglect (e.g., failure of a caretaker to provide care, food, shelter, and other basic necessities); serious accident, illness, or medical procedure; victim of or witness to domestic violence; victim of or witness to community violence (e.g., gang violence, racial conflict, police–citizen confrontations, and riots); historical trauma (e.g., traumatic experiences tied to a group or culture, for example, American slavery, Jim Crow, and post-Jim Crow); school violence and bullying; natural or manmade disasters; forced displacement; war, terrorism, or political violence; military trauma (e.g., for military members and their families as a result of deployment and/or military service); victim of or witness to personal or interpersonal violence; traumatic grief or separation; and system-induced trauma and retraumatization. While this list may not be exhaustive, it does offer a structure to begin to investigate the sources of trauma.

Further, a great deal of recent research has been focused on early life trauma, called adverse childhood experiences (ACEs). This research has clearly shown that these events pose a significant risk factor for the development of mental health disorders in later life (in particular, substance use disorders) and can have an impact on future prevention efforts (SAMHSA, 2017a, b). This research was kickstarted by a collaborative effort between of the Centers for Disease Control and Prevention and Kaiser Permanente; in 1998, these entities published their research on ACEs in 17,337 participants studied across two waves in the *American Journal of Preventive Medicine* outlining. Their findings were remarkable: (1) ACEs are common – 28% of participants reported some form of physical abuse and 21% reported some form of sexual abuse; (2) ACEs tend to occur in clusters, or in multiples – that is, 40% of participants reported a history of two or more ACEs and 12.5% experienced four or more; (3) ACEs predict health problems with strong, positive statistical relationship – or, in other words, the more ACEs one experiences strongly predicts the risk of a variety of health problems in later life, including substance use and co-occurring disorders (see Fig. 1.9; read the next section for a definition of co-occurring disorders).

The reason why trauma is considered a key problem here is that the effects of trauma can be tricky to diagnose and treat, and without addressing this root cause of mental health and/or drug abuse problems, symptoms and negative outcomes can persist and can confound prevention efforts. For example, if an underage drinking prevention program with a proven track record of success is adopted in a high-risk community, it may not have the same level of success *or any success* if the programming does not address adverse experiences. Or, alternatively, if this program has the

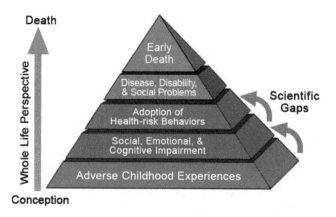

Fig. 1.9 Relationship among adverse childhood experiences and potential later life outcomes. (Courtesy of the U.S. Centers for Disease Control & Prevention. Use of this image does not imply endorsement by CDC, ATSDR, HHS or the U.S. Government of the authors, Springer, or this book. Original image available on CDC's website at no charge)

ability to recognize the signs of ACEs, it may link with other programming that can address coping skills, dysfunction in the home, the effects of divorce, and so on.

1.3.2 Co-occurring Disorders

Co-occurring disorders, once known as dual diagnosis, exist when a person has both mental health and substance use disorders at the same time. According to the National Survey on Drug Use and Health in 2014, more than 7.9 million Americans had co-occurring disorders. With this large number, adding on issues related the criminal justice system can only further complicate recovery for individuals.

One of the major hurdles with co-occurring disorders is establishing high quality and appropriate treatment. Treatment for this type of disorder lends itself to the "chicken or the egg" adage – does the mental health diagnosis occur before the substance use disorder or does substance misuse/abuse occur before other mental illness? The answer to this question can radically shape an appropriate treatment protocol in one direction or another very different direction. Even further, clinicians need to ask, do the mental health concerns fuel the struggles with substance use, or does the substance use struggle fuel the mental health concerns? From the clinician's perspective, the signs and symptoms of both mental health and substance use disorder can be difficult to separate, which leads to further difficulty in treating the disorders adequately. Clinicians may require longer periods of time to document and diagnose these issues, perhaps delaying the delivery of the best treatment to address these compounding symptoms. Yet, the system of care for mental health services in many locations may not allow for optimal care and treatment; Many treatment programs may only treat one disorder while not addressing the other which often does not help in the overall wellness and health of the individual. For example, a person may suffer from bipolar disorder and cocaine use disorder. With bipolar disorder, the individual can experience both depressive episodes and manic episodes. Cocaine is a stimulant, so in this scenario, it could be difficult to differentiate between symptoms from the manic episode from bipolar disorder versus the "highs" of the cocaine use disorder. Additionally, the idea of "self-medicating" can be often brought up in the clinical discussion regarding co-occurring disorders. For example, a person suffering from depression may use alcohol to "self-medicate" and mask negative feelings when experiencing tough times. In this way, alcohol will also fuel the depression and symptoms. Therefore, in both of these examples, treatment professionals may have difficulties with treatment plans. Often, to fully realize the true nature of the mental illness side, the person must fully detox from the substance(s).

Additionally, and further complicating matters for mental health professionals, the level of severity of co-occurring disorder can vary wildly across and within individuals. For example, both of the following may fit the "co-occurring" definition: (1) a person experiencing mild anxiety who misuses alcohol to help with sleep by engaging in frequent binge drinking, (2) a person diagnosed with schizophrenia may abuse opiates to avoid or shut out the hallucinations they may be experiencing. The intensity and frequency of the issues depicted here can vary in one's life depending on stressors, life circumstances, and so on. Since either the mental illness or the substance use disorder can develop first, it often can be difficult to determine which is fueling the other. Substances can pose a problem by also worsening or, at times, creating problems with a person's mood and throwing off one's brain chemistry leading to behavior issues. Therefore, most treatment options for co-occurring disorders involve an integrated approach.

According to information provided by the National Alliance on Mental Illness, "about a third of all people experiencing mental illnesses and about half of people living with severe mental illnesses also experience substance abuse" (NAMI, 2017). That is a significant number of people impacted by these illnesses, and these figures are important to keep in mind from a treatment perspective. In particular, helping the person and their loved ones understand how both mental illness and substance abuse interact and impact their daily life is important for transformative change. Further, "in the substance abuse community, about a third of all alcohol abusers and more than half of all drug abusers report experiencing a mental illness" (NAMI, 2017). It is also important to note that men are more likely to develop co-occurring disorders than women. Also, those of a lower socioeconomic status, people with more medical illnesses, and military veterans are more likely to be at risk of co-occurring disorders.

SAMHSA literature points out that "the consequences of undiagnosed, untreated, or undertreated co-occurring disorders can lead to a higher likelihood of experiencing homelessness, incarceration, medical illnesses, suicide, or even early death" (SAMHSA, 2017a; b). In the criminal justice system, many people have co-occurring disorders and using integrated treatment is essential to success. Further, appropriate screening to identify co-occurring disorders is important to ensure inmates are receiving the proper care within the system. Addressing both mental health and substance use both during and after incarceration can also reduce the likelihood of recidivism.

1.3.3 Dollars and ~~Cents~~ Sense

One of the biggest obstacles, and one major common theme throughout this book, is funding Recall that the most recent landmark mental health law, the Cures Act, mentioned cost more than any other concept; thus, this is not only a theme for this book, it is the top driving force for American policy decision-making. At the more localized level, budgets for jails and state prisons are being cut substantially, primarily due to the overuse of incarceration as a solution for social problems (largely, drug problems). Incarceration is a very expensive solution to maintain at current levels; the addition of any financial strains, such as from the fiscal pressures of recession, has resulted in cutting services to bare minimums in many circumstances. Further, expenses related to the justice and mental health services are more vulnerable (if not *the most* vulnerable) to cuts as lawmakers tend to be more protective over services that directly affect their constituents – such as schools, roads, parks, and local community services. Divestment in justice and mental health services lead to not only increases in need, but decreases in jobs and quality options. If funding for treatment is cut, then jobs and options for treatment providers are also diminished, making for a bleak outlook. Burnout and frustration in the workforce will also heighten; think – if our criminal justice and behavioral health systems were overwhelmed before budget cuts (as they have tended to be historically), how are they professionals in the aftermath of divestment?

One struggle with lack of mental health treatment options is the waste of the little resources involved primarily due to the inefficiency of the system; many critiques of the system do not account for this. Professionals often know of "frequent fliers," or individuals who are well-known for returning to facilities with recurrent symptomatology because their care is often incomplete. Their treatment is likened to a person with an open wound who is treated with a band-aid and an over-the-counter pain reliever instead of full ambulatory care (think stitches, antibiotics, and follow-up to ensure that an infection has not occurred). In other words, providing effective treatment for an individual suffering from mental illness costs a finite amount of resources, which depends on the type of treatment (inpatient, outpatient, etc.), medication, doctor visits, follow-ups, counseling services, and so on. Consider then, like any other illness, prolonging treatment by lack of options, resources, long wait times, or access to medication can often worsen the condition and time to achieve a healthy outcome – and cost volumes more in the long run. Further, the traumatizing experience of incarceration because one's symptoms cause legal problems can create additional negative mental health outcomes, and may complicate treatment in the long run. And, cost even more money.

Incarcerating a person in need of treatment puts the financial burden onto the criminal justice system, thus creating a different problem. In this case, the criminal justice system now bears the burden of housing and treating a person with mental illness. Currently, the system is overcrowded and underfunded. Adding more people to the situation only furthers the burden while also complicating matters with their illness. Utah, like many other states, has seen an increase of deaths in jails, specifically to suicide. In one county alone, Weber County, there have been 31 deaths in the jail since 2000, and 14 of those were to suicide.

1.4 Rethinking Mental Health

Removing the stigma associated with mental illness and treating it as any other concern is one of the major needs of our society. However, more central to fundamental change are the interconnected linkages that need to be built throughout a comprehensive system of care. This system must be able to communicate effectively across its entire footprint, including those tangibly involved or providing services but are not formally connected with the system.

What if mental illness was treated the way that cancer or diabetes is treated? If it was even viewed in a similar light, the outcomes could drastically be different. For example, with cancer, primary care physicians commonly are knowledgeable about how to refer patients out to specialists – at times, high profile specialists at the Moffitt Center or MD Anderson – and ensure that patients follow-up to be seamlessly handed off to their specialists for treatment. This treatment can involve imaging, labs, consultants with specialists, and so on. Each of these appointments can also be made seamlessly, often with reminders that occur automatically. What if we put this practice into commonplace mental health care?

1.4.1 A Continuum of Care

The continuum of care is a difficult but essential element of the process to ensure the health of an individual. The continuum of care refers to all of the steps and actions involved in the overall care cycle for a person – including all the key players at and between each point of contact and between the "system" and patient. For example, an individual exhibiting symptoms of depression may make an appointment with their primary care doctor. During their visit, the primary care doctor may refer the person to a psychiatrist. Upon seeing a psychiatrist, the individual may be prescribed an antidepressant medication and/or referred to a therapist to begin talk therapy. In an ideal situation, the psychiatrist and therapist would discuss that patient/client's treatment on a regular basis to ensure the wellness of the person continues throughout the span of their care.

In the criminal justice realm, there are many more professionals involved, which can often lead to many more options for problems or issues "falling through the cracks." The care and obstacles depend on many variables: is this person incarcerated in a jail or prison? If prison, is it state or federal? Has this person been treated before for mental illness or is their onset within jail/prison? (Fig. 1.10)

The term continuum of care, also known as organized delivery systems, has certainly become a "buzz" word in the health care delivery industry. As it progressed to include first responders, law enforcement, courts, and jails, the continuum of care is a complex concept that focuses on a simple outcome – that no patient or client falls through the cracks of a complex care system. In other words, as a patent enters the health care system, this person will be properly triaged and evaluated, referred to the best source(s) to handle the next steps in his or her care, and if further care is needed, follow-ups occur, further referrals are given, treatment is delivered, and this continues until the issue bringing this person into the system is resolved. Additional aftercare is delivered to ensure that success continues. With first responders, correctional officers, officers of the court, and more professionals being pulled into a broader continuum of care for many individuals, this has set the American mental health care system on a new paradigm to reevaluate previous conceptualizations of continuums of care across the nation – this includes the criminal justice system as a starting point or referral point into health care delivery systems.

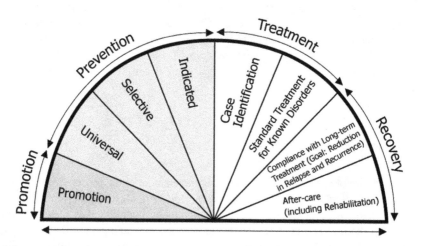

Fig. 1.10 The continuum of care protractor. Note that diagnosis occurs between prevention and treatment. Institute of Medicine. 1994. Reducing Risks for Mental Disorders: Frontiers for Preventive Intervention Research. https://doi.org/10.17226/2139. (Reproduced with permission from the National Academy of Sciences, Courtesy of the National Academies Press, Washington, D.C.)

1.5 Conclusion

With problems of awareness, in prevention, and with stigma, people will continue to suffer in their mental illness – particularly the vulnerable. Unfortunately, this can magnify the risk of contact by law enforcement and lead to the involvement in the criminal justice system. Further complicating the problem, mental health resources are scarce in most segments of the criminal justice system – whether it being federal or state prison, in local jails, or within community corrections. These institutions lack funding for programming and staff to fully attend to the needs of mental health inmates. Substance abuse often can further complicate mental health symptoms, creating an endless cycle of negative experiences for a vulnerable population.

This population was first brought into the public consciousness by Dorothea Dix. She brought compassion to a suffering class of people and sought to bring about the moral treatment of individuals with mental illness. While her efforts shifted people with mental illness from jails and prisons to state hospitals, most of these institutions ended up devolving into prisons themselves – with often "patient" treatment being worse than inmate life. This system continued until the abuses of the new system were brought to light by a new and powerful media. At the same time, psychiatric medicine (or psychopharmacology) experienced its most important breakthrough in the development of antipsychotic drugs. This enabled symptoms to be treated in what would be known as the least restrictive setting – often this means treatment in the community setting. From this moment through today, the ideal goal for the majority of special interests and advocacy groups alike was to enhance American communities to build the capacity to address mental health by setting up full systems of care. Thus, a trend set in to divest from state mental hospitals with hopes of setting up a comprehensive network of community mental health treatment services. After many decades of development, many gaps continued to exist to effectively treat many of those in need. At first, the most vulnerable have ended up homeless and, at times, in jail; and then, after the significant criminal justice policy shifts in the 1980s, an exponential increase of individuals with mental illness has occurred in jails and prisons. This has caused a notable strain on the criminal justice system, further complicating the overall system of care.

One solution is to develop a comprehensive continuum of care that involved both the public behavioral health and criminal justice systems. Professionals working to seek this change use data and evaluation methods to examine points in the system can be the most successful in intervening in mental health episodes or crises. This can be an encounter with a law enforcement officer, upon intake into a jail, at the emergency room, at a community clinic, and even can begin with a call to 911, crisis hotlines, or resource lines. This solution does not try to eliminate the criminal justice system as earlier advocates have pioneered; it includes it as one segment of many intervention points. In a perfect world, it would be the point of the last resort. In many circumstances, justice intervention can be a very salient one, however. As researchers and professionals acknowledge this, it can lead to stronger partnerships and better outcomes for the vulnerable.

Finances and investment will continue to be an impendent toward progress, especially in dire fiscal times. Both behavioral health and criminal justice services take higher priorities for lawmakers when they consider budget cuts. It is important to note that this trend is no longer absolute. With the twenty-first Century Cures Act, legislators have signaled an impetus for change. It dedicates resources, gives direction, and provides a template for progress. This progress may be incomplete without comprehensive criminal justice reform; however, *progress will still occur without it*, albeit at a slower pace and in fewer places across the country.

Discussion Questions

1. Reflecting on this chapter discussion of Dorothea Dix, how do you think she would be involved in mental health advocacy and/or reform in our current times?
2. Who makes decisions on criminal justice and mental health policy at the local level? State? Federal?
3. How can local areas change policy to better help funding for mental health, specifically within criminal justice?
4. How does a community ensure that they keep up with the needs of the people in said community?
5. This chapter presents the work of Buck, Toro, and Ramos, who present the evolving media coverage on homelessness across a thirty-year time period that ends in 2003 and the impact that such coverage has on society. How would you best summarize the media coverage on homelessness since 2003, particularly in light of the growing dominance of social media? How might this coverage impact our current perception of mental illness?

References

Atkinson, J. M., & Garner, H. C. (2002). Least restrictive alternative – Advance statements and the new mental health legislation. *Psychological Bulletin, 26*, 246–247.

Buck, P., & Toro, P. (2004). Images of homelessness in the media. In D. Levinson (Ed.), *Encyclopedia of homelessness, volume 1*. Sage.

Buck, P. O., Toro, P. A., & Ramos, M. A. (2004). Media and professional interest in homelessness over 30 years (1974–2003). *Analyses of Social Issues and Public Policy, 4*(1), 151–171. (2002).

Bureau of Justice Statistics. (2017a). National Prisoner Statistics Program. URL: http://www.bjs. gov. Last accessed: 2017, June 1.

Bureau of Justice Statistics. (2017b). Key statistic: Total correctional population. URL: https:// www.bjs.gov/index.cfm?ty=kfdetail&iid=487. Last accessed: 2017, June 1.

Carter, K. C., & Carter, B. R. (1994). *Childbed fever: A scientific biography of Ignaz Semmelweis*. Greenwood Press.

Grob, G. N. (1983). *Mental illness and American Society, 1875–1940*. Princeton University Press. https://doi.org/10.2307/j.ctvct00bz

Haller, J. S. (1981). *American medicine in transition, 1840–1910* (Vol. 185). University of Illinois Press.

Hatzenbuehler, M. L., & Link, B. G. (2014). Introduction to the special issue on structural stigma and health. *Social Science & Medicine*.

Healy, D. (2009). *The creation of psychopharmacology*. Harvard University Press.

James, D. J., & Glaze, L. E. (2006). *Mental health problems of prison and jail inmates*. Bureau of Justice Statistics.

Kris, E. B., & Carmichael, D. M. (1957). Follow-up study on patients treated with thorazine. *The American Journal of Psychiatry, 114*(5), 449–452.

Lamb, H. R., & Weinberger, L. E. (2005). The shift of psychiatric inpatient care from hospitals to jails and prisons. *Journal-American Academy of Psychiatry and the Law, 33*(4), 529.

Link, B. G., Cullen, F. T., Struening, E., Shrout, P. E., & Dohrenwend, B. P. (1989). A modified labeling theory approach to mental disorders: An empirical assessment. *American Sociological Review, 54*, 400–423.

Link, B. G., Phelan, J. C., Bresnahan, M., Stueve, A., & Pescosolido, B. A. (1999). Public conceptions of mental illness: Labels, causes, dangerousness, and social distance. *American Journal of Public Health, 89*(9), 1328–1333.

Maskel, A. Q. (1946, May 6). Bedlam 1946: Most U.S. mental hospitals are a shame and a disgrace. *Time Magazine.*

Muckenhoupt, M. (2004). *Dorothea dix: Advocate for mental health care.* Oxford University Press.

Packard, F. R. (1901). *History of medicine in the United States.* Lippincott.

Pescosolido, B. A., Monahan, J., Link, B. G., Stueve, A., & Kikuzawa, S. (1999). The public's view of the competence, dangerousness, and need for legal coercion among persons with mental health problems. *American Journal of Public Health, 89*, 1339–1345.

Rivera, G. (2017). Geraldo Rivera. URL: http://geraldo.com/folio/willowbrook. Last accessed: 2017, June 1.

Rothwell, J. (2015). *Drug offenders in American prisons: The critical distinction between stock and flow.* Brookings Institute. URL: https://www.brookings.edu/blog/social-mobility-memos/2015/11/25/drug-offenders-in-american-prisons-the-critical-distinction-between-stock-and-flow/ Last accessed: 2017, June 1.

Substance Abuse and Mental Health Services Administration. (2007). *Funding and characteristics of state mental health agencies, 2007.*

Substance Abuse and Mental Health Services Administration. (2010). *Behavioral health, United States, 2012.*

Substance Abuse and Mental Health Services Administration. (2014). *TIP 57: Trauma-informed care in behavioral health services.*

Substance Abuse and Mental Health Services Administration. (2017a). Prevention of substance abuse and mental illness. URL: https://www.samhsa.gov/prevention. Last accessed: 2017, October 21.

Substance Abuse and Mental Health Services Administration. (2017b). Types of trauma and violence. URL: https://www.samhsa.gov/trauma-violence/types. Last accessed: 2017, June 1.

Torrey, E. F. (1997). *Out of the shadows: Confronting America's mental illness crisis.* Wiley.

Trent Jr., J. W. (2017). Moral treatment. Disability History Museum. URL: http://www.disability-museum.org/dhm/edu/essay.html?id=19. Last accessed 2017, June 1.

United States National Library of Medicine. (2017). Digital collections. URL: https://collections.nlm.nih.gov/. Last accessed 2017, October 1.

World Health Organization. (1996). Mental health care law: Ten basic principles. URL: http://www.who.int/mental_health/media/en/75.pdf. Last accessed: 2017, October 31.

Chapter 2
Stigma

> *By definition, of course, we believe the person with a stigma is not quite human. On this assumption we exercise varieties of discrimination, through which we effectively, if often unthinkingly, reduce his life chances. Erving Goffman, 1963.*

Stigma, as we have come to define it today, was officially launched as a sociological concept by Erving Goffman over 60 years ago. In his book, *Stigma: Notes on the management of spoiled identity*, Goffman describes how people tend to make characterizations on others' social identities based on attributes. When others possess an attribute "of a less desirable kind – in the extreme, a person who is quite thoroughly bad, or dangerous, or weak," people tend to reduce such individuals as tainted persons. This type of person is someone who could be "justifiably" discredited or is discreditable. Goffman defines this sort of attribute to be a stigma. Yet, it goes deeper. Goffman describes how, in some situations, an attribute that could be stigmatizing may be interpreted in differing ways, depending on context. Stigma, then, is better described as when attributes and stereotypes collide. This stigma could fit within three broad domains: (1) physical deformities, (2) "blemishes of individual character," which could range from proclivities toward deviance, mental illness, criminal behavior and incarceration, alcoholism and drug use, and so on, and (3) inherited attributes from familial lineage to include race, national identity, and religion. Modern approaches to stigma continue to focus on the concept of devalued identities as the direct or indirect result of the interactions Goffman describes.

2.1 Defining Stigma

Graham Davey (2013), writing for *Psychology Today*, has a great description of mental health stigma and both the outward discussion as well as internal: "Mental health stigma can be divided into two distinct types: *social stigma* (or public stigma) is characterized by prejudicial attitudes and discriminating behaviour directed towards individuals with mental health problems as a result of the psychiatric label they have been given. In contrast, *perceived stigma* or *self-stigma* is the internalizing by the mental health sufferer of their perceptions of discrimination, and

J. Hector, D. Khey, *Criminal Justice and Mental Health*,
https://doi.org/10.1007/978-3-031-15338-9_2

perceived stigma can significantly affect feelings of shame and lead to poorer treatment outcomes" (Davey, 2013; emphasis as in original; citing Link et al., 1989; Perlick et al., 2001). The stigma associated with mental illness can be a barrier for many to seek treatment in the first place; in other words, people's resistance and reluctance to be labeled mentally ill – officially or unofficially – often makes them think twice about reaching out for help, even to those they trust. Also, friends and family members often struggle with overcoming stigma and stereotypes to remain supportive to those suffering from mental illness. Increasingly concerning, as with many illnesses, lack of treatment leads to worsening of symptoms and severity. Typically, better outcomes are tied to addressing an illness as early as it can be detected – mental health included. This is the basis of why the concept of stigma is so important, and it is vital to understand why it endures.

Beyond public- and self-stigma, a third related type or classification of stigma includes *structural* stigma. Hatzenbuehler and Link define structural stigma as "societal-level conditions, cultural norms, and institutional practices that constrain the opportunities, resources, and well-being for stigmatized populations" (2014: 2). Structural stigma can include well-entrenched attitudes among correctional officers regarding mental illness, for example. Not only could these cultural attitudes inhibit referrals to mental health services, but they can also repress individual correctional officers working in this cultural environment from seeking help themselves when they experience symptoms of depression, anxiety, and so on (Ricciardelli et al., 2021).

The typical stereotype of mental illness is a "crazy" person who commits acts of violence and could be a harm to themselves or others (Angermeyer and Matschinger, 1996; Nunnally, 1961; Pescosolido and Boyer, 1999; Penn et al., 1999). In reality, most individuals with mental illness are not violent. One widely cited study by Link and his colleagues (Link et al., 1999) details the power of this misconception through an experiment with five vignettes placed on a massive social science survey in 1996 (the General Social Survey). The vignettes were written about people with mental illness in a nonclinical way to gauge people's reaction about (1) alcohol dependence; (2) major depression; (3) schizophrenia; (4) drug dependence; and (5) a "troubled person." Importantly, the "troubled person" vignette represented a person experiencing a rough time in their life, but did not meet any criteria for mental illness, giving the researchers a basis for comparison. For example,

> John is a [ETHNICITY] man with an [EDUCATIONAL LEVEL] education. Up until a year ago, life was pretty okay for John. But then, things started to change. He thought that people around him were making disapproving comments and talking behind his back. John was convinced that people were spying on him and that they could hear what he was thinking. John lost his drive to participate in his usual work and family activities and retreated to his home, eventually spending most of his day in his room. John was hearing voices even though no one else was around. These voices told him what to do and what to think. He has been living this way for six months – the vignette for schizophrenia.

The results from 1444 survey participants detail the depth of the issue of stigma and the stereotype of the dangerousness of mental illness. When directly asked, "In your opinion, how likely is it that [NAME] would do something violent toward other

people – very likely; somewhat likely; somewhat unlikely; very unlikely," the average responses indicated that people viewed cocaine dependence as the most dangerous (87% of respondents either chose very or somewhat likely), followed by alcohol
dependence (71%), and schizophrenia (61%). This reaction is in the face of volumes
of empirical evidence consistently finding that only a minority of individuals with
mental illness become violent. Perhaps even more telling, when Link and his colleagues asked whether the people surveyed would be willing to live next to this
person, spend an evening with them, work closely with them, and react to them
marrying a relative, most respondents sought to distance themselves from the person in the vignette. The results were in line with perceived dangerousness – the vast
majority of people surveyed would distance themselves from cocaine dependence
(90%), alcohol dependence (70%), and schizophrenia (63%). Even the individual
depicted as having major depressive disorder would be isolated by many respondents (47%).

Importantly, the researchers also felt as though the respondents felt hesitant to
use the term "mental illness" when asked about the people in the vignettes.
Specifically, when respondents were asked if they believed the person detailed in
the vignette was experiencing a mental illness, most, but not all, responded affirma-
tively. This was especially the case with major depressive disorder (69% of respondents thought the person had a mental illness), alcohol dependence (49%), cocaine
dependence (44%), and a troubled person (22%). Yet, when confronted with the
specific condition of the people depicted in the vignettes, the vast majority of
respondents were convinced that the individuals had alcohol dependence (98%),
cocaine dependence (97%), major depression disorder (95%), and schizophrenia
(85%). The differences in responses here show the weight of the words "mental
illness."

Over the course of the next decade, the General Social Survey probed the
American public about stigma. By 2016, the majority of adults (80%) agreed that
treatment is effective, with adults living in states with lower mental health expenditures trending to agree to a lesser extent (National Academy of Sciences, 2016). In
fact, people living in states with less expenditures also tended to report seeking
mental health services to a lesser extent. Yet, the data seemed to point out something
perplexing: "by 1996, public knowledge had increased such that respondents dif-
ferentiated between 'problems of daily living' and standard psychiatric disorders.
Stigma levels for the former decreased between 1996 and 2006 but stigma related to
psychiatric disorders remained high" (National Academy of Sciences, 2016: 4).
Further, the General Social Survey findings are able to tell us how American adults
general attitudes about psychiatric illness and substance use disorder, yet we still do
not really know how these attitudes impact actual behaviors toward individuals perceived to have or who indeed have mental and substance use disorders. This presents us with a conundrum – awareness of public stigma seems to be increasing
among the populous, yet public stigma persists to a considerable degree.

Stigma, social distancing, and labels are incredibly powerful interrelated and
complex concepts. Not only do these concepts shape the experience of mental illness, but the science in this area also details the interconnectedness of deviance

(including drug use/abuse), crime and criminality, vulnerability and victimization, homelessness, and mental illness with stigma as a central component. Thus, it is important to fully explore stigma and its role in the lives of people with mental illness.

2.1.1 Double and Multiple Stigma – Layered Stigma

For sure, stigma can be a difficult obstacle to overcome. Within the criminal justice system, the label of "criminal" can be harsh, misunderstood, and almost impossible to wipe clean. In the mental health realm, stigma can be just as harsh and limit or prevent an individual from seeking treatment. Now, imagine the stigma of incarceration *and* mental illness together. Having both labels and negativity piled on can be the catalyst to harmful and tragic outcomes. For example, the statistics for suicide in both populations are high in isolation, but the compounded stigma of both being a "criminal" and "crazy" often placing these individuals at greater risk of self-harm and/or suicide.

Double stigma, or layered stigma, is defined as the presence of two stigmatized qualities present in one person. This can be a criminal history and mental health concerns. Some researchers have attributed a double stigma to be present among transgendered individuals who have mental health concerns, others have argued a double stigma among Muslim Americans who have mental health concerns, and so on. Beyond double stigma, multiple stigmas are simply the presence of additional stigmatized qualities in one person. Each stigmatized status arguably confounds and magnifies each other, leading to poorer and poorer outcomes and lessens the likelihood of healthy, "normal" lives.

While this simplistic terminology does not appear in many mainstream sources, its underlying assertions are clear. This will be addressed more fully in a subsequent chapter, but it is important to note here that stigma and labels can often be likened to a snowball effect – in other words, stigma and labels and build off of each other to knife off potential opportunities the legitimate and pro-social world, pushing those with stigma away from society and leaving them vulnerable to victimization, self-medication, homelessness, and much more.

2.1.2 A Review of Recent Stigma Research

A study by Sickel et al. (2014) provided a deep review of the consequences of mental health stigma. This unearthed recent trends in stigma research with focus across several domains – mental health stigma and the resulting barriers to seeking care, the negative impact on self-esteem and self-efficacy, discrimination in employment and housing opportunities, conflicts and strain in interpersonal relationships, increased physical health comorbidities, and reduced treatment adherence and coping. As a result, "research suggests that greater sophistication is needed when looking to examining [mental health stigma] and its consequences" (208). Specifically, Sickel, Seacat, and Nabors describe an indirect relationship between the perception of stigma and the outcomes described above. A similar systemic review of the literature by Sharac et al. (2010) revealed consistent findings across 27 studies regarding the impact of mental health stigma on employment and income. These findings are being confirmed using sophisticated analytical techniques, such as structural equation modeling (Sickel et al., 2019). Essentially, this statistical approach is able to confirm that self-reported mental health stigma impacts attitudes about seeking help for mental and physical health concerns.

This general theme – that stigma continues to persist in society, yielding harmful outcomes among individuals with mental and substance use disorders – is at the core of the most comprehensive assessment on the topic of stigma to date. This study, undertaken by the National Research Council and Institute of Medicine, published by the National Academies of Sciences (2016), digs deeper into the unsettled science about "what works to change negative behavioral health social norms" (19). Specifically, the committee who worked on this report focused their effort on three key areas: "(1) the change in behavioral health norms needed to support individuals with mental and substance use disorders to seek treatment and other supportive services; (2) discrimination, negative attitudes, and stereotyping faced by individuals with mental health and/or substance use disorders; and (3) public knowledge about behavioral health, including how to seek help for people with such disorders" (20). The report goes into great detail into the current knowledge of stigma of mental and substance use disorders, reviews the science of communication and why our words matter in shaping norms, thoroughly identifies and examines the approaches in reducing stigma, examines prior research strategies regarding stigma and explores ways to fill gaps in our knowledge on the topic, and wraps up with six recommendations.

Given the emphasis placed on the need to explore effective strategies to change negative behavioral health norms, this text will selectively highlight broad strategies in place discussed in the report. The types of underlying strategies vary and include (1) educational strategies, which present factual information to correct for misinformation and stereotypes, (2) mental health literacy campaigns, a type of educational strategy that focuses on improving knowledge, attitudes, and help-seeking behaviors of strategic target populations, (3) contact campaigns, putting people in *direct* touch with people with mental and substance use disorders (either face-to-face or via video-conference), (4) peer services, or linking up individuals with mental and substance use disorders (or their family members) with others with lived experiences with these human conditions (or, family members with lived *vicarious* experiences, and (5) protest and advocacy campaigns, led by grassroot efforts to bring attention to issues that surround mental and substance use disorders, and legislative and policy change.

The report goes on to describe three large-scale efforts to meaningfully address stigma and the negative behavioral norms that may result – Opening Minds (Canada), Time to Change (England), and beyondblue (Australia). Many others, particularly some in the United States, made honorable mentions (the Eliminations of Barriers Initiative and the What a Difference a Friend Makes campaign, for example), yet the report focuses on Opening Minds, Time to Change, and beyondblue due to their comprehensive approaches with ongoing and robust evaluation research designs. Each of these efforts utilized an array of strategies described above in their campaigns with a focus on *changing* behaviors. In addition, they build in ways to determine whether behavioral changes were ongoing as a direct or indirect cause of exposure to the campaigns included in these efforts. For example, the researchers evaluating Time to Change in England measured both reported and intended changes in behavior using an eight-item scale designed to measure this concept – the aptly named Reported and Intended Behavior Scale (RIBS). Upon evaluation, the social marketing campaign featuring public service announcements was the most impactful in changing behavior. After 300 million media impressions (see: bring change to mind, 2022), researchers found those surveyed reported consistent improvement in one important item on the RIBS – "In the future, I would be willing to live with someone with a mental health problem" (National Academies of Sciences, 2016: 84). Other such findings were unearthed with beyondblue, a cornerstone of which is Mental Health First Aid. This powerful curriculum was social marketing campaigns, sponsored events, community education programs, and normalizing an official day – RUOK Day – to ask check in on fellow Australians simply by asking, "Are you okay?" This commemorative day continues through present-day – last year, it was held on September ninth, 2021. National self-report surveys have indicated decreases in social distancing since launch of beyondblue, yet the perception of mental illness as dangerous and unpredictable persists. Last, while not to downplay the positive developments found through comprehensive study of the Opening Minds campaign in Canada, the most crucial findings presented were twofold: the large-scale media campaigns were ineffective in changing attitudes and grassroot networks and local champions were perceived as crucial to success. In addition, the stakeholders behind Opening Minds realized the need to develop a curriculum for emerging journalists to help shape the media coverage of mental and substance use disorder as a critical element to ensure broad success in changing attitudes – and subsequently, behaviors.

A broad review of the National Academy of Sciences study recommendations is summarized as follows:

- A comprehensive approach to tackling stigma is not new for many countries around the globe. Stakeholders have made substantial gains in addressing stigma among persons with HIV/AIDS, for example. The lessons learned from these efforts are invaluable.
- "The experiences of the U.S. campaigns related to HIV/AIDS and of anti-stigma campaigns in Australia, Canada, and England demonstrate the need for a coordinated and sustained effort *over 2 or more decades* to reduce the stigma associated with mental and substance use disorders" (115–116; emphasis added).

- As a result, "Recommendation 1: The U.S. Department of Health and Human Services should take the lead responsibility among federal partners and key stakeholders in the design, implementation, and evaluation of a multi-pronged, evidence-based national strategy to reduce stigma and to support people with mental and substance use disorders" (116).
- To affect change in a lasting way, any broad effort needs to include a coordinated effort among a diverse array of stakeholders with an outsized focus on consensus building.
- "Recommendation 2: The U.S. Department of Health and Human Services should evaluate its own service programs and collaborate with other stakeholders, particularly the criminal justice system and government and state agencies, for the purpose of identifying and eliminating policies, practices, and procedures that directly or indirectly discriminate against people with mental and substance use disorders," thus addressing structural stigma that currently is embedded in our institutions (118).
- A strategic plan (to be maintained by the Substance Abuse and Mental Health Services Administration) should be created to structure iterative change and effective monitoring.
- "Recommendation 3: The Substance Abuse and Mental Health Services Administration should conduct formative and evaluative research as part of a strategically planned effort to reduce stigma" (119).
- Effective social media campaigns are designed in a way that first develops well-defined goals for each target population/audience. Messages should be customized to each audience and directly align with the goal(s) defined.
- "Recommendation 4: To design stigma-reduction messaging and communication programs, the Substance Abuse and Mental Health Services Administration should investigate and use evidence from formative and evaluative research on effective communication *across multiple platforms* (120, emphasis added).
- The potential expansion of contact-based programs should be carefully studied before developing such campaigns with careful considerations of the risks and benefits of disclosure of lived experiences of those who would be involved.
- "Recommendation 5: To decrease public and self-stigma and promote affirming and inclusive attitudes and behaviors targeted to specific groups, the Substance Abuse and Mental Health Services Administration should work with federal partners to design, evaluate, and disseminate effective, evidence-based, contact-based programming" (121).
- Peer support specialists do not have an accepted set of standards.
- "Recommendation 6: The Substance Abuse and Mental Health Services Administration should work with partners to design, support, and assess the effectiveness of evidence-based peer programs to support people with mental and substance use disorders along their path to recovery and to encourage participation in treatment" (121).

2.2   Champions for the Cause

In a later chapter, this text will discuss grassroot and nonprofit organizations to combat stigma, raise awareness, and increase access to mental health care in depth. Some organizations have been founded by celebrities and athletes – or other influencers with a broad public reach – as a means to decrease stigma and inform the public about mental health and self-care. Given the findings of the National Academies of Sciences report, this chapter will focus on the message and challenge each reader to determine whether each campaign has achieved the elusive goal of changing behaviors and reducing harmful stigmas of all type, public, self-, and structural. As the authors of the report have noted, public awareness seems sustained and ubiquitous throughout the country and in many nations around the globe. However, behavioral change has been intractable.

Recently, celebrities, and especially athletes, have been using their own platforms (news media, social media, books, podcasts, etc.) to share their own experiences dealing with mental health. This type of a novel contact-based approach is interesting in that many such efforts occur organically. One model example is the story of Simone Biles, the multimedal winning Olympic gymnast. At the 2020 Tokyo Olympic summer games, Simone Biles withdrew herself from competition for some events due to her own mental health. That raw moment and the moments that led up to that decision – one that had the opportunity to be exposed to many of the estimated 3.05 billion unique viewers of the Games (International Olympic Committee, 2022) – no doubt received broad, mostly supportive media coverage. A study by the Pew Research Center (Shaw, 2021) revealed that Ms. Biles was the most-mentioned Team USA athlete (e.g., across all sports and events – 598 athletes in total) on Twitter during the Games. Specifically, Biles had received more than 2.1 million mentions on the social media platform. The Pew report analyzed these impressions and found substantial patterns of the use of such words and phrases as "love and support," "courage," and "brave." Yet, other patterns of language used in Biles impressions did include "quitter," "mental health," and "abuse." Publicly, Biles was vocal on social media about feeling the weight of the world placed on her shoulders, which came to a head during competition finals. On July 28th, 2021, U.S. Gymnastics tweeted: "After further medical evaluation, Simone Biles has withdrawn from the final individual all-around competition. We wholeheartedly support Simone's decision and applaud her bravery in prioritizing her well-being. Her courage shows, yet again, why she is a role model for so many."

In an effort to create change, Simone partnered with the mental health app Cerebral and subsequently became their Chief Impact Officer in October 2021. "Cerebral mission is to improve access to high-quality mental health care to everyone who needs it. Mental health issues to do not discriminate" (Cerebral, 2021a). The app creators thought Simone's experience and ability to speak publicly about her struggles at the Olympics would make her a great partner for their platform. The main focal point of the campaign is to normalize help-seeking by noting that "even the strongest of us need support." Cerebral has developed into a low-access-barrier telehealth platform, funded by a monthly subscription fee for clients to receive access to care for anxiety, depression, insomnia, postpartum depression, and menopausal depression (fees currently range from $85 to 325/month, without insurance and do not cover the cost of prescription medication). Further, the platform offers treatment options for ADHD, bipolar disorder, PTSD, and alcohol dependence in states they have licensure to do so. At the time of this writing, they offer prescription management in all US States and offer medication and therapy or standalone therapy plans in 32 states. Cerebral has served over 100,000 unique members since its launch in January 2020. In terms of impact, the for-profit company claims to reduce the average cost of psychiatric care (by as much as three-fold) while rapidly speeding up the time to first be seen by a clinician (80% of clients are offered to be seen in minutes compared to month-long wait times with traditional psychiatry; Cerebral, 2021b). Further, in their deal with Biles, the company has committed to set aside an allocation to provide services in underserved communities and be support aspiring athlete wellness efforts at the World Championship Centre and WCC Academy.

Even the highest paid female athlete in the world – Naomi Osaka – recently spoke on her own mental health (Forbes, 2021; Blinder, 2021). She advocated for a break from her sport (tennis) by withdrawing from the French Open competition in the Summer of 2021. She spoke openly about her own difficulties with the media and the impact on her mental health, a similar refrain shared by Biles in the moments that led up to her withdrawal from the Olympic Games the year before. The broad message Osaka exuded to the public was to say that taking a break when needed was important for self-care. Her message on Instagram, with well over two million followers at the time, read:

> Hey everyone, this isn't a situation I ever imagined or intended when I posted a few days ago. I think now the best thing for the tournament, the other players and my well-being is that I withdraw so that everyone can get back to focusing on the tennis going on in Paris. I never wanted to be a distraction and I accept that my timing was not ideal and my message could have been clearer. More importantly I would never trivialize mental health or use the term lightly. The truth is that I have suffered long bouts of depression since the US Open in 2018 and I have had a really hard time coping with that. Anyone that knows me knows I'm introverted, and anyone that has seen me at the tournaments will notice that I'm often wearing headphones as that helps dull my social anxiety. Though the tennis press has always been kind to me (and I wanna apologize especially to all the cool journalists who I may have hurt), I am not a natural public speaker and get huge waves of anxiety before I speak to the world's media. I get really nervous and find it stressful to always try to engage and give you the best answers I can. So here in Paris I was already feeling vulnerable and anxious so I thought it was better to exercise self-care and skip the press conferences. I announced it preemptively because I do feel like the rules are quite outdated in parts and I wanted to highlight that. I wrote privately to the tournament apologizing and saying that I would be more than happy to speak with them after the tournament as the Slams are intense. I'm gonna take some time away from the court now but when the time is right I really want to work with the Tour to discuss ways we can make things better for the players, press and fans. Anyways hope you are all doing well and staying safe, love you guys I'll see you when I see you (Osaka, 2021).

A New York Times article points out that at about the same time as Osaka's public announcements and withdrawal from the French Open, several other athletes publicly shed light on their personal struggles through self-disclosure – Michael Phelps spoke on his bouts of depression and anxiety, Aly Raisman (U.S. gymnast) spoke on her experience with PTSD, and Brandon Marshall (NFL wide receiver and six-time Pro Bowl player) spoke openly about his borderline personality disorder (Blinder, 2021). Of particular note, Michael Phelps (28-time medal winning Olympic swimmer, the most of any single Olympian to date) became vocal about mental health causes after retiring from the sport. In a feature on the South China Morning Post (2021), its Style Magazine, the article discusses his philanthropy and advocacy even before retirement – just that his efforts began to focus on mental health postretirement (2021). For example, he repurposed a one-million-dollar bonus from Speedo after the 2008 Olympic Games to start the Michael Phelps Foundation. That Foundation is now at the center of various mental health campaigns, at times featuring Phelps himself, such as "It's okay not to be okay." It was in 2018 when he began to openly discuss his experiences with ADHD and depression, launching a new career of sorts as a mental health advocate. He *defines* himself as a mental health advocate (Park, 2020). Similar to Biles, Phelps partnered with an online therapy company, Talkspace, to appear in ads for the company by sharing his story. On the Talkspace website (2022), Michael shares his own story by describing just how much anxiety and depression had impacted his life by saying "I hadn't left my room for 5 days. I questioned whether I wanted to be alive anymore. I realized I am the strongest person I know, but I felt like the weakest." This statement coming from a man who has won multiple Olympic medals says a lot about just how powerful his negative thoughts and feelings were at the time. Yet another, multimedal winning Olympian speaking out about their struggles can shed light on what many others face as well. During live TV coverage of the Olympic games, Michael Phelps spoke on Simone's bravery in speaking out as well as advocating for all who are in need to help with mental health to seek treatment.

Simone, Naomi and Michael are three Olympians, but also three humans who know the *impact* of mental health. Many more celebrities and athletes have begun to speak on mental health and including their own experiences and stories of those of family and friends. Even further, many in the public arena have begun to create change with stigma as well as access to treatment and care for mental health by creating their own charitable organizations. Some of those will be discussed in a later chapter. In addition to many Olympic athletes choosing to speak out about their own mental health, there have been many players within the National Football League (NFL) to discuss mental health – coming to a head when the NFL featured mental health issues on live broadcasts during week 8 of the 2021 season. These efforts were truly ongoing, with the league agreeing with the NFL Players Association on the need to create a Comprehensive Mental Health and Wellness Committee in May 2019 (Clemmons, 2021). On the NFL's website (2022) they state, "in collaboration with the NFLPA, the NFL is committed to helping build a positive culture around mental health by providing players and the NFL family with comprehensive mental health and wellness resources and equipping them with the tools to succeed, on and off of the field, over the course of their lives." This includes mandating that all teams have a behavioral health clinician on staff. The NFL's website also includes a video featuring a number of current players in the league promoting the destigmatization of mental health.

While all of these athlete efforts began in recent years, it is a step in the right direction to have individuals in the spotlight speaking on a cause – champions for the cause. And while the National Academies of Sciences report speaks on local champions, *layered* efforts can be predicted to yield best outcomes. Certainly, these efforts bring awareness to a broader audience. They are each making an effort to show the importance of recognizing mental health and seeking help. Each conversation is one more to lessen the stigma – but, will they impact behaviors? Our top researchers seem to think that these efforts will take sustained effort across decades. Yet, the momentum to begin could never have been better given these highly-visible stories.

2.3 Pop Culture and Real Life

The topic of stigma is prevalent in many aspects of pop culture. Movies, television shows, and entertainment, writ large, all have some level of impact of the perception of mental illness. In the past, these stereotypes and perceptions tended to be mostly negative. Luckily, more recently a positive outlook with positive change has begun to emerge with mental health stigma in pop culture – much in line with the watershed moments of athlete self-disclosures. More *visible* and direct efforts are being made to depict people and characters in a more accurate sense – in ways that normalize mental health struggles. Additionally, showing both people and characters seeking help has, arguably, become more commonplace and typical. However, many remnants negative connotations, innuendo, and stigma persist.

Consider the characters portrayed in movies and TV even for children. One study from Lawson and Fouts (2004) examined mental illness in animated Disney films. The researchers examined 34 films made by The Walt Disney Company like Beauty and the Beast, Dumbo and The *Lion King*. The results showed that 85% of the films studied "contained references to characters with mental illness." Furthermore, "21% of all principal characters were referred to as mentally ill (for instance, Maurice of Beauty and the Beast, Jafar of Aladdin, and Mrs Jumbo of Dumbo)." While mentioning mental illness itself is not inherently negative, the use of stigma-inducing language can be. For example, in these films, the average number of mental illness references per film was 4.6, with the 3 most prevalent words being (in descending order) "crazy," "mad" or "madness," and "nut" or "nutty." While this research only addresses Disney films, it is safe to say that language can be powerful when discussing stigma. Exposure to language for children begins the cycle of stigma of mental illness before many children have even begun to understand mental health.

2.3.1 Media Scrutiny – A Case Study

Another pop culture example of stigma that then bleeds into real world is that of the character Jar Jar Binks from Star Wars. Jar Jar is described as "a clumsy, well-meaning Gungan outcast on Naboo, Jar Jar Binks struggled to prove his worth throughout his life. Putting his awkward past behind him, Jar Jar left the swamps of Naboo to enter the even murkier waters of Coruscant politics, becoming a representative for his people in the galactic capital. There, his best intentions and eagerness to serve were exploited by scheming Senators and others in positions of power" (Star Wars, 2022). Even without being a fan of the Star Wars franchise, one can see the hints of language that could lead to concern with his mental health. Describing the character of Jar Jar as "clumsy" with an "awkward past" that would then later be exploited tells the reader there may be some potential for stereotypes that interplay with attributes to yield stigma. Many did speculate on what mental health disorders could relate to Jar Jar, including some researchers. Hall and Friedman (2015) noted that they theorized Jar Jar Binks had Attention Deficit Hyperactivity Disorder (ADHD).

While some viewers and fans of the franchise found the character of Jar Jar Binks endearing, many did not. In fact, Jar Jar was such a disliked characters to the extent that the fan backlash led to concerns for the actor who him. Ahmed Best, the actor who portrayed Jar Jar, discussed his thoughts of suicide after his experience from fan backlash for the character several years after his experience. He even shared in an interview that he had received death threats after playing Jar Jar (BBC, 2018). He played the character when he was 25 years old, and in 2018, stated that it was still affecting his career. While the backlash against Best, largely had to nothing to do with Jar Jar's behavior or depiction of mental illness, it is ironic the impact this had on the actor in his own life.

For someone who is not accustomed to being in the limelight, particularly when cast in a negative light, media and social media attention can result in damage to one's identity – in the very same stigmatizing process that Goffman describes in his work back in the early 1960s. While society has come a long way from the twentieth century in terms of awareness, we often find many instances where stigma persists, leading to negative outcomes. With the power of social media to direct ire and stigmatizing language at everyday people around the world to a degree unimaginable in Goffman's era, we must realize that efforts to combat stigma are critical to societal health.

2.4 Conclusion

The use of language is extremely important when speaking about stigma. In fact, at workshops held by the Committee on the Science of Changing Behavioral Health Norms, many experts with international reputations on behavioral health mentioned the importance of language when addressing stigma, particularly for mass media (National Academies of Sciences, 2016). With profit focused on fresh content, impressions, and clicks and less on engagement and scientific accuracy, reducing stigma-laden language may be seen as counterintuitive as any salacious language is easy pickings for click-bait. Even simply using a term, like "mental illness," can evoke a certain reaction. The assumption often goes directly to severe examples of disorders despite stereotypes being dispelled, even by influencers with massive followings. Many people across the world continue to correlate mental illness with violent tendencies both overtly and passively. This includes people living in countries with successful antistigma efforts.

Readers should evaluate all aspects of television shows, movies, and social media to detect stigmatizing content. Consider common phrases describing mental illness in our discourse in everyday life and better understand their origins and use. At the moment, the science is able to show that societies across the world have robust levels of awareness, even before the wave of positive social media sourced by athletes (primarily) and pop culture icons (such as Alyssa Milano and Selena Gomez). At the time of this writing, we are beginning to engage the mechanics of change that may exist beyond our acknowledgement that a global "mental health crisis" confronts us.

Discussion Questions
1. What are the things in everyday life (language, media, etc.) that influence stigma for mental health, substance use, or justice-involved individuals?
2. How is stigma prevalent in different communities? Consider what an individual considers to be their community. Think about different points of view.
3. How do you think celebrities and/or athletes as champions for the cause impact the message? Positive or Negative? Why?
4. How is mental health viewed in relation to other medical conditions? How does that impact treatment?
5. The chapter emphasizes that the public is often aware of stigma and stigmatization, however what, if any actions, are being made to lessen stigma?
6. How did the COVID-19 pandemic impact the stigma of mental illness?
7. How are certain types of mental health conditions like depression or anxiety seen differently than others like schizophrenia or substance use?

References

Angermeyer, M. C., & Matschinger, H. (1996). The effect of violent attacks by schizophrenic persons on the attitude of the public towards the mentally ill. *Social Science Medicine, 43*, 1721–1728.

BBC News. (2018). Star Wars: Jar Jar Binks actor Ahmed best considered suicide. URL: https://www.bbc.com/news/entertainment-arts-44708983. Last accessed: 2022, February 6.

Blinder, A. (2021). With her candor, Osaka adds to conversation about mental health. *The New York Times*. URL: https://www.nytimes.com/2021/06/01/sports/tennis/mental-health-osaka.html. Last accessed: 2022, February 6.

Bring Change to Mind. (2022). Schizo. URL: https://bringchange2mind.org/learn/psas/schizo/. Last accessed: 2022, February 5.

Cerebral. (2021a). Introducing Simone Biles, Cerebral's new Chief Impact Officer. URL: https://cerebral.com/blog/simone-biles-cerebral-chief-impact-officer. Last accessed: 2022, February 6.

Cerebral. (2021b). Final press kit. URL: https://prismic-io.s3.amazonaws.com/cerebral/d6954c9e-a3f2-417b-b738-8cc11791de0a_FINAL+Press+Kit+(updated+10_21_21).pdf. Last accessed: 2022, February 6.

Clemmons, A. K. (2021). Pushed by players, the NFL works to embrace mental health. *The New York Times*. URL: https://www.nytimes.com/2021/11/26/sports/football/nfl-mental-health.html. Last accessed. 2022, February 6.

Davey, G. C. L. (2013). Mental health & stigma. *Psychology Today*. URL: https://www.psychologytoday.com/blog/why-we-worry/201308/mental-health-stigma. Last accessed: 2022, February 5.

Forbes. (2021). The highest paid female athletes of 2021. URL: https://www.forbes.com/pictures/61ddfb9e53295bec9dd3caeb/1-naomi-osaka/?sh=4a7438692d0c. Last accessed: 2022, February 6.

Goffman, E. (2009). *Stigma: Notes on the management of spoiled identity*. Simon and Schuster.

Hall, R. C., & Friedman, S. H. (2015). Psychopathology in a galaxy far, far away: The use of Star Wars' dark side in teaching. *Academic Psychiatry, 39*(6), 726–732.

International Olympic Committee. (2022). IOC launches new long-term study of Olympians to protect athletes' physical and mental health. URL: https://olympics.com/ioc/news/ioc-launches-new-long-term-study-of-olympians-toprotect-athletes-physical-and-mental-health

Lawson, A., & Fouts, G. (2004). Mental illness in Disney animated films. *The Canadian Journal of Psychiatry, 49*(5), 310–314.

Link, B. G., Cullen, F. T., Struening, E., Shrout, P. E., & Dohrenwend, B. P. (1989). A modified labeling theory approach to mental disorders: An empirical assessment. *American Sociological Review, 54*, 400–423.

Link, B. G., Phelan, J. C., Bresnahan, M., Stueve, A., & Pescosolido, B. A. (1999). Public conceptions of mental illness: Labels, causes, dangerousness, and social distance. *American Journal of Public Health, 89*(9), 1328–1333.

National Academies of Sciences, Engineering, and Medicine. (2016). *Ending discrimination against people with mental and substance use disorders: The evidence for stigma change*. The National Academies Press.

National Football League. (2022). Player health and wellness: Mental health. URL: https://www.nfl.com/playerhealthandsafety/health-and-wellness/mental-health/. Last accessed: 2022, February 6.

Nunnally, J. (1961). *Popular conceptions of mental health*. New York, NY.

Osaka, N. (2021) Instagram post. URL: https://www.instagram.com/naomiosaka/?utm_source=ig_embed&ig_rid=a03dcf3f-09bb-41d0-a51d-78ad7f15c062. Last accessed: 2022, February 6.

Penn, D. L., Kommana, S., Mansfield, M., & Link, B. G. (1999). Dispelling the stigma of schizophrenia: II. The impact of information on dangerousness. *Schizophrenia Bulletin, 25*(3), 437–446.

Perlick, D. A., Rosenheck, R. A., Clarkin, J. F., Sirey, J. A., Salahi, J., Struening, E. L., & Link, B. G. (2001). Stigma as a barrier to recovery: Adverse effects of perceived stigma on social adaptation of persons diagnosed with bipolar affective disorder. *Psychiatric Services, 52*(12), 1627–1632.

Pescosolido, B. A., & Boyer, C. A. (1999). How do people come to use mental health services? Current knowledge and changing perspectives. In A. V. Horwitz & T. L. Scheid (Eds.), *A handbook for the study of mental health: Social contexts, theories, and systems* (pp. 392–411). Cambridge University Press.

Park, A. (2020). Michael Phelps opens up about retirement and mental health awareness: 'I struggle through problems just like everybody else.' URL: https://time.com/collection/davos-2020-mental-health/5402066/michael-phelps-mental-health-activism/. Last accessed: 2022, February 6.

Ricciardelli, R. R., Haynes, S. H., Burdette, A., Keena, L., McCreary, D. R., Carleton, R. N., et al. (2021). Mental health, stigma, gender, and seeking treatment: Interpretations and experiences of prison employees. *Applied Psychology in Criminal Justice, 16*(1), 107–127.

Sharac, J., Mccrone, P., Clement, S., & Thornicroft, G. (2010). The economic impact of mental health stigma and discrimination: A systematic review. *Epidemiology and Psychiatric Sciences, 19*(3), 223–232.

Shaw, S. (2021). *Simone Biles by far the most-mentioned team USA athlete on Twitter during Tokyo Olympics*. Pew Research Center. URL: https://www.pewresearch.org/fact-tank/2021/09/16/simone-biles-by-far-the-most-mentioned-team-usa-athlete-on-twitter-during-tokyo-olympics/. Last accessed: 2022, February 6.

Sickel, A. E., Seacat, J. D., & Nabors, N. A. (2014). Mental health stigma update: A review of consequences. *Advances in Mental Health, 12*(3), 202–215.

Sickel, A. E., Seacat, J. D., & Nabors, N. A. (2019). Mental health stigma: Impact on mental health treatment attitudes and physical health. *Journal of Health Psychology, 24*(5), 586–599.

South China Morning Post. (2021). Michael Phelps today. URL: https://www.scmp.com/magazines/style/celebrity/article/3143482/michael-phelps-today-olympic-legend-shares-mental-health. Last accessed: 2022, February 6.

Star Wars. (2022). Jar Jar Binks. URL: https://www.starwars.com/databank/jar-jar-binks. Last accessed: 2022, February 6.

Talkspace. (2022). Michael X Talkspace: Michael's mental health story. URL: https://www.talkspace.com/michael. Last accessed: 2022, February 6.

Chapter 3
Size and Scope of Justice-Involved Mental Illness

> *Research on mental health epidemiology shows that mental health disorders are common throughout the United States, affecting tens of millions of people each year, and that, overall, only about half of those affected receive treatment – National Institute of Mental Health, 2017.*

Before starting a discussion on just how many justice-involved individuals have a diagnosable mental illness, what those diagnoses tend to be, their severity of symptoms, and their rates of relapse, it will be helpful to keep a few caveats in mind. First, diagnosing mental illness can prove difficult as it impinges on the full cooperation of the patient. This cooperation may be influenced by stigma, varying levels of acceptance of mental health care by gender, race, and culture, and, likely, the "us versus them" relationship of medical staff to inmate, probation and parole officer to client, drug court case manager to client, and so on. Second, there is evidence of moderate amounts of malingering in the justice-involved population; in other words, justice-involved individuals are known to feign illness, including mental illness, if doing so will provide a benefit, such as getting out of assigned work duties, obtaining higher quality meals, to get out of their jail or prison cell, to be able to be in an air conditioned facility, or just to feel the reward of gaining a privilege or advantage, no matter how trivial it is to an average person. Last, there is considerable variation in applying mental health screening tools in professional circles, and further, there can be dynamic differences in how mental health professionals apply diagnoses over time, by place or region, or other given factors (that will be discussed later). Long story short, there is a substantial amount of gray area when trying to estimate the *prevalence* of mental illness among the justice-involved population. This chapter will discuss the most current prevalence estimates – or the overall rate of mental illness among each segment of the justice-involved population.

J. Hector, D. Khey, *Criminal Justice and Mental Health*,
https://doi.org/10.1007/978-3-031-15338-9_3

3.1   What We Know – It's Complicated

To begin, and most importantly, there has been no comprehensive record-keeping of mental illness for justice-involved individuals. Further, the epidemiological tracking systems on mental health for all Americans is addressed by the Centers for Disease Control; yet, the organization only recently began its first deep assessment in 2011 by piecing together data from several of its monitoring programs (Centers for Disease Control, 2021a). Ideally, one centralized source would build the capacity to collect data on the extent of mental illness in the United States as well as within the subpopulation of justice-involved individuals; but instead, existing data on the topic come from a series of special governmental reports, state reports, and sporadic independent research endeavors. This persistent problem was, in fact, acknowledged by the twenty-first Century Cures Act. For example:

- Sect. 14015, entitled "Improving Department of Justice Data Collection on Mental Illness Involved in Crime," requires the U.S. Attorney General to gather and report data on homicides (including homicides of police officers), serious injuries, assaults, serious injury or death by law enforcement officers "with respect to the involvement of mental illness in such incidences, if any,"
- Sect. 14016, entitled "Reports on the Number of Mentally Ill Offenders in Prison," includes a mandate to the Comptroller General to estimate the cost of imprisoning individuals with "serious mental illness by the Federal Government or State or unit of local government."

While these efforts of expanding our tracking systems are ongoing and are beginning to be fleshed out, it is important to understand our most current tools. As a helpful resource, William Reeves (2013) of the Centers for Disease Control offers a comprehensive summary of the American mental health surveillance systems. Reeves begins by defining seven key public health functions of these systems, which underscores the importance of this section. First, the public health surveillance systems are put into place to inform interventions with the benefit of data to help shape decision-making. In other words, the systems are set up in a way that allows for trends to be monitored, providing an easy mechanism to discover, identify, and describe changes – or potential signs of problems – and act on them. Second, these systems provide a way to estimate the impact of health conditions, including mental illness. Third, surveillance provides an ability to experts to follow the progression of health conditions and how our responses and treatments shape outcomes. This "natural history" offers a learning tool to help professionals refine future responses and treatments. Fourth, they aid in providing a big picture description of how conditions are distributed in society and how often they occur. Fifth, and related to the second function above, these systems provide structure for hypothesis creation and seeds research ideas. Sixth, they further allow for the evaluation of prevention efforts and control measures. Last, they help professionals plan programs strategically.

As Reeves describes it, surveillance is accomplished through a diverse multilayered approach deployed in unison to give us "a complete mosaic" of the health issues being explored. Specifically, three broad types of surveillance systems exist that collect data on mental illness: population surveys, health care surveys, and vital statistics. Each provides a slice of information that assist in the *triangulation* of data. According to George Rutherford and his colleagues, "public health triangulation is a process for reviewing, synthesizing, and interpreting secondary data from multiple sources that bear on the same question to make public health decisions" (Rutherford et al., 2010). In fact, triangulation goes deeper than this; in other words, surveillance systems use different research methodologies and/or sampling strategies to access information in unique ways. The key triangulation is to look for convergence and divergence in the data for further exploration.

3.1.1 Population Surveys

Population surveys examine health issues of *all* citizens (or a subpopulation) through the use of representative samples of the American public at the national, regional, state, and local levels. This survey technique relies heavily on self-reported information to determine the occurrence of mental illness in the wider population. While there is not any one population survey that solely deals with mental health, the U.S. Department of Health and Human Services embeds an array of mental health surveillance into a suite of ongoing programs. For example, the National Survey of Drug Use and Health (NSDUH – administered by SAMHSA) has been tracking mental health since 1994; this survey tool is an annual, nationally-representative, self-report survey of Americans aged 12+ designed to capture a broad array of data on substance use and abuse as well as general and mental health. It has become a leading tool for surveillance and has led to an array of special governmental reports and independent research on overall mental health trends in the United States. As such, it can easily be considered the flagship mental health population survey tool at this time. Specifically, it was equipped with the ability to track two key mental illness measures in 2008, both at the state and national level: (1) severe mental illness and (2) any mental illness (SAMHSA, 2013). The drive for this upgrade to the NSDUH in 2008 was, in fact, made over 15 years earlier when Congress passed the Alcohol, Drug Abuse, and Mental Health Administration Reorganization Act, thus showing how slowly innovation can occur after policy shifts.

The NSDUH currently utilizes sets of questions, called scales, to determine whether a survey respondent has severe mental illness or any mental illness. Such scales include psychological distress and functional impairment, which largely makes up the clinical interview section of the survey – the Structured Clinical Interview (SCID-I/NP; includes mood, anxiety, eating, impulse control, substance use, and adjustment disorders as well as a screen for psychotic symptoms). In addition, the NSDUH includes questions on thoughts of suicide and depression within the last year and these questions help shape the estimations of both severe mental illness and any mental illness in the population. Using the most up-to-date methods available, the survey estimated that 4.6% of American adults have a serious mental illness (19.1% have any mental illness) in 2018 (SAMHSA, 2019). Importantly, this prevalence is not impacted by diagnoses – that is, this information is gathered in a way that does not require a diagnosis if the scales deployed in the NSDUH have been vetted properly and are sufficiently reliable. Ongoing research is being done to ensure that these estimations are reflective of the American reality of mental illness (see Figs. 3.1, 3.2, and 3.3). In fact, these most recent estimations were recently recalibrated in the 2011 edition of the NSDUH in a collaboration project between SAMHSA and the National Institute on Mental Health (NIMH). These recalibration efforts will continue to be ongoing as our understanding of mental illness evolves. For example, in October 2015, the American Psychiatric Association released its newest Structured Clinical Interview (First, Williams, Karg, & Spitzer 2016). As such, it is important to remember that there will be a lag of ability to receive the latest intelligence of mental health prevalence on the American population using population surveys. It is also important to remember that the diagnostic criteria for many mental illnesses do not change substantially over the years. In other words, there will be relatively negligible amounts of error in the population data collected. It still is important to note the shortcomings of each data type, especially when trying to account for changes in mental health conditions over time.

Additionally, it is also important to note that the NSDUH reaches respondents who have a physical address. While this can include some "non-institutional group quarters" such as shelters, boarding houses, university dorms, migrant worker

Fig. 3.1 Latest prevalence of mental health illnesses in American adults by gender, age, and race/ethnicity, reported in 2020, by SAMHSA. (Last column in Race/Ethnicity is 2 or more races/ethnicities reported). (See also: https://www.nimh.nih.gov/health/statistics/mental-illness)

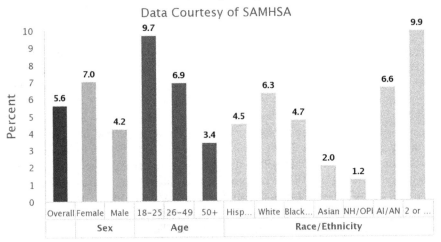

Fig. 3.2 Latest prevalence of *serious* mental health and serious mental health illnesses in American adults by gender, age, and race/ethnicity, reported in 2020, by SAMHSA. (Last column in Race/Ethnicity is 2 or more races/ethnicities reported). (See also: https://www.nimh.nih.gov/health/statistics/mental-illness)

Fig. 3.3 Prevalence of mental health and serious mental health illnesses from 2008 to 2018 in American adults by age, reported in 2019, by SAMHSA. In this 2019 report, SAMHSA notes that there are statistically significant increases in prevalence rates of any mental illness and severe mental illness in 2018 relative to 2016 for all age groups except for "50 or Older." Of particular note, the "18–25" age group has seen steep, statistically significant increases in both any mental illness and severe mental illness in recent years

camps, and halfway and quarter houses, NSDUH *does not* reach many homeless or transient Americans who do not consistently seek shelter. Most importantly for the current discussion, NSDUH further excludes individuals in jails and prisons, nursing homes, state mental health hospitals, and individuals in long-term care facilities. In other words, it excludes a wide swath of the vulnerable populations we are interested in studying. These vulnerable populations must be accounted for in some other way; but we also should consider the prevalence of mental illness will always be underestimated when reviewing the findings of the NSDUH results each year.

To expand and refine mental health surveillance further into states, and more importantly, down to the county level, the Centers for Disease Control and Prevention have relied on the Behavioral Risk Factor Surveillance System (BRFSS). This effort began in 1984 to annually interview a representative sample of Americans in all states to record and track information on health-related risk behaviors, chronic health conditions, and the use of local preventative services. It has since become one of the largest routine health surveys in the world with over 400,000 participants each year. In regard to mental health, the BRFSS has historically used some core questions to ascertain number of mentally unhealthy days and has since 2007 included optional modules (with states given the option to opt-in) for anxiety and depression as well as mental health and stigma. For the states that opt-in to examine mental health issues, the BRFSS can provide basic information about the prevalence of mental health issues at the local level. It can also assist mental health professionals in realizing the capacity of services in the local area or estimate the numbers of underserved individuals needing mental health care. This will become important for justice-involved populations as states and communities begin seeking alternatives to jails and prison and need the data to inform change. In 2007, the BRFSS mental health module was robustly delivered in half of the United States: Alaska, Arkansas, California, Connecticut, District of Columbia, Georgia, Hawaii, Illinois, Indiana, Iowa, Kentucky, Louisiana, Minnesota, Mississippi, Missouri, Montana, Nevada, New Hampshire, New Mexico, Puerto Rico, Rhode Island, South Carolina, Vermont, Virginia, and Wyoming. Overall, 36 states had originally opted into the mental health and stigma module, with only 16 states opting-in to receive follow-up data in 2009, 13 in 2012, and 10 in 2013 (SAMHSA, 2017). Thus, while this BRFSS module offers some additional coverage, the NSDUH continues to be the dominant population survey tool for mental health surveillance.

Reeves (2013) further points out that additional in-depth population surveys occur sporadically, typically at near-10-year intervals. Examples of these include the National Comorbidity Surveys and the National Epidemiologic Survey on Alcohol and Related Conditions. This also includes three special editions of surveys performed by the Bureau of Justice Statistics to expand this surveillance into the justice-involved population: (1) the 1996/2002 Survey of Inmates in Local Jails, (2) the 1997/2004 Survey of Inmates in State and Federal Correctional Facilities, and (3) the 2011–2012 National Inmate Survey. The last substantial special edition (the 1997/2004 update) mimics the methodology of the NSDUH by utilizing a modified clinical interview (for the DSM-IV). The findings for incarceration populations, not surprisingly, are *very different* from the general public. About 56% of state prisoners, 45% of Federal prisoners, and 64% of local jail inmates indicated any mental health problem, with many symptoms being severe in nature (James & Glaze, 2006). This update also disentangled substance dependence (or abuse) from mental health problems. When doing so, the results show just how enmeshed these problems are (Table 3.1):

Table 3.1 Prevalence of mental health problems among prison and jail inmates (James & Glaze, 2006); note the levels of individuals with mental health problems

Selected characteristics	Percent of inmates in —			
	State prison		Local jail	
	With mental problem	Without	With mental problem	Without
Criminal record				
Current of past violent offense	61%	56%	44%	36%
3 or more prior incarcerations	25	19	26	20
Substance dependence or abuse	74%	56%	76%	53%
Drug use in month before arrest	63%	49%	62%	42%
Family background				
Homelessness in year before arrest	13%	6%	17%	9%
Past physical or sexual abuse	27	10	24	8
Parents abused alcohol or drugs	39	25	37	19
Charged with violating facility rules[a]	58%	43%	19%	9%
Physical or verbal assault	24	14	8	2
Injured in a fight since admission	20%	10%	9%	3%

[a]Includes items not shown

The special report (James & Glaze, 2006) entitled, "Mental Health Problems of Prison and Jail Inmates," provides a summary of the findings from the special editions of the Survey of Inmates in Local Jails (2002) Survey of Inmates in State and Federal Correctional Facilities (2004). The modified clinical interview in these surveys reliably estimated 23% of state prisoners and 30% of jail inmates had symptoms of major depression, and 15% of state prisoners and 24% of jail inmates had symptoms of a psychotic disorder. Notably, while a substantial portion of prisoners and inmates had a recent history of mental illness (24% of state prisoners; 21% of jail inmates; 14% of Federal prisoners), many more exhibited symptoms of mental illness (49% of state prisoners; 60% of jail inmates; 40% of Federal prisoners). More troubling, very few receive services to address these issues (33% of state prisoners who exhibited mental health problems; 17% of jail inmates who exhibited mental health problems; 24% of Federal inmates who exhibited mental health problems). Much more detail will be provided in subsequent chapters on the nature of these findings:

- Roughly one in four of state prisoners and jail inmates with a mental health problem served three more prior incarceration periods relative to state prisoners and jail inmates without mental health issues.
- Female inmates exhibited higher rates of mental health problems relative to male inmates (73% of female state prisoners compared to 55% male; 75% of female jail inmates compared to 63% male).

• State prison inmates who exhibited a mental health problem were about twice as likely to experience homelessness relative to those without a mental health issue.

In the most recent report updated to reflect 2011–2012 data, Bronzon and Berzofsky (2017) reveal that 14% of prisoners (in both state and Federal facilities) and 26% of inmates in U.S. jails report experiences meeting or exceeding the threshold for serious psychological distress in the past 30 days before being surveyed – findings that seem in line with previous surveillance efforts. In addition, they find that 36.9% of prisoners and 44.3% of inmates in U.S. jails report a history of a mental health problem. While the underlying assessment of mental illness is completely different than other special editions (e.g., the Kessler 6 nonspecific psychological distress, scale capable of reliably screening adults for *severe* mental illness, versus the more sensitive modified clinical interview), the critical features of this report helps us understand some of the nuances of incarcerated individuals with mental health concerns (Table 3.2).

Bronson and Berzofsky dig deeper into the National Inmate Survey to reveal nuances in the data that provide deeper context. For example, respondents who graduate from college are more likely to have a history of mental health problems relative to those with a high school degree; respondents who are married are less likely to experience severe psychological distress than those who are not married; and Federal prisoners experiencing severe psychological distress did not differ in

Table 3.2 Prevalence of mental health indicators among prisoners and jail inmates, by type of indicator, 2011–2012

Mental health indicator	Prisoners*	Jail inmates
No indication of a mental health problem[a]	49.9%	36.0%**
Current indicator of a mental health problem[b]		
Serious psychological distress[c]	14.5%	26.4%**
History of a mental health problem		
Ever told by mental health professional they had mental disorder	36.9%	44.3%**
Major depressive disorder	24.2	30.6**
Bipolar disorder	17.5	24.9**
Schizophrenia/other psychotic disorder	8.7	11.7**
Post-traumatic stress disorder	12.5	15.9**
Anxiety disorder[d]	11.7	18.4**
Personality disorder[e]	13.0	13.5

Source: Bureau of Justice Statistics, National Inmate Survey, 2011–2012
Note: See appendix Table 4 for standard errors
*Comparison group
**Difference with the comparison group is significant at the 95% confidence level
[a]Includes persons with a score of 7 or less on the K6 scale and who had never been told by a mental health professional they had a mental disorder
[b]Current at time of the interview
[c]Includes persons with a score of 13 or more on the K6 scale. See *Methodology*
[d]Includes panic disorder and obsessive compulsive disorder, and excludes post-traumatic stress disorder
[e]Includes antisocial and borderline personality disorder

their sentence lengths. Interestingly, the amount of time served at a respondent's current facility did not correlate with any increases in severe psychological distress. In fact, for jail inmates, time served at one's current facility correlated with reductions in severe psychological distress. Perhaps the most revealing discovery of this most recent special edition was a breakdown of mental health treatment for those respondents indicating a history of mental health problem (see Table 3.3 below). It is interesting to note that the vast majority of respondents *who revealed they were diagnosed with a mental health disorder by a psychiatrist* or those who experienced

Table 3.3 Mental health treatment received by Federal prisoners and jail inmates who indicate a mental health problem, by type of indicator, time period, and treatment type as reported by Bronson and Berzofsky

Mental health treatment received by prisoners and jail inmates with an indicator of a mental health problem, by type of indicator, time period, and treatment type, 2011–2012

Time period and treatment type	Serious psychological distress[a]		History of a mental health problem[b]	
	Prisoners[*]	Jail inmates	Prisoners[*]	Jail inmates
Ever received mental health treatment during lifetime	74.2%	72.7%	88.1%	90.3%[**]
Ever overnight hospital stay[c]	41.8	43.1	44.8	51.3[**]
Ever taken prescription medication	62.8	61.3	76.4	80.4[**]
Ever had counseling/therapy from trained professional[d]	60.9	54.9[**]	74.6	73.9
Mental health treatment since admission	54.3%	35.0%[**]	63.0%	44.5%[**]
Prescription medication	45.8	30.0[**]	52.6	38.3[**]
Counseling/therapy from trained professional[d]	42.2	17.8[**]	48.9	23.5[**]
Prescription medication and counseling/therapy	33.9	12.9[**]	38.7	17.5[**]
Currently treated for a mental health problem[e]	35.6%	29.7%[**]	37.0%	37.8%
Prescription medication	29.1	25.7	29.9	33.0
Counseling/therapy from trained professional[d]	25.8	12.6[**]	26.7	16.4[**]
Prescription medication and counseling/therapy	19.5	8.7[**]	19.7	11.8[**]

Source: Bureau of Justice Statistics, National Inmate Survey, 2011–2012
Note: See appendix table 11 for standard errors
[*]Comparison group
[**]Difference with the comparison group is significant at the 95% confidence level
[a]Includes inmates with a score of 13 or more on the K6 scale. See Methodology
[b]Includes inmates who reported they had ever been told by a mental health professional they had a mental disorder
[c]Includes inmates who stayed overnight or longer in any type of hospital or other facility to receive treatment or counseling for any problems with their emotions, nerves, or mental health
[d]Includes a psychiatrist, psychologist, social worker, or nurse
[e]As of the time of the interview

serious psychological distress in the last 30 days reported some history of treatment during their lifetime. Yet, it is also critical to note that the current treatment rates among this population remain low.

These issues are central to this text and will be explored into great depth. Data such as these are critical in providing context to some of the broader concerns among this vulnerable population. For example, Bronson and Berzofsky reveal that Federal prisoners and jail inmates with serious psychological distress and who report a history of a mental health problem are statistically more likely to be written up or charged with a verbal or physical assault against correctional staff or against another inmate. Thus, under- or untreated mental illness has direct and indirect consequences beyond sentencing that continues to shape the lives of these individuals – perhaps by leading to further isolation, longer stays in jails or prisons, or other harmful outcomes. At this point, consider the value of this type of research and surveillance tool in understanding mental illness, particularly within vulnerable populations.

3.1.2   Health Care Surveys

Health care surveys are only recently gaining more significance in the surveillance of mental illness. The reason for this is that the data come directly from healthcare and insurance providers; historically, mental health professionals use the Diagnostic and Statistical Manual of Mental Disorders, or DSM, to diagnose a patient whereas hospitals, medical providers, and insurance companies use the International Statistical Classification of Diseases and Related Health Problems as managed by the World Health Organization, or ICD. The latest edition of the DSM – the DSM-V – has only recently been aligned with the ICD, which is now in its tenth revision (ICD-10). While mental health is yet to be effectively tracked in this manner, it is only a matter of time before the professions adjust to report on more indicators than it has been able to reliably track in the past. To date, suicide is one of the few reliable indicators being tracked by this system of surveillance (Reeves, 2013).

One prime example of a health care survey is the National Ambulatory Medical Care Survey, again led by the CDC. This survey, conducted annually since 1973, randomly selects physicians providing direct patient care to participate. It has since been expanded to cover community health centers in 2006. Specifically, the survey tool asks physicians to provide information on roughly 30 patient visits in a randomly-selected one-week timeframe (see Table 3.4). Mental health-related questions have been asked in a few different ways since the 2001, including asking physicians about whether they screen their patients for mental health concerns, such as depression or anxiety. The most recent data available are revealing – only 8.5% of primary care office visits in 2016 included a screening for depression (Healthy People 2030, 2022). Other examples of health care surveys include the National Hospital Discharge Survey and the National Nursing Home Survey.

Table 3.4 Primary diagnosis at office visits, classified by major disease category in 2013 (NAMCS; Center for Disease Control and Prevention, 2021b)

1.	Supplementary classification (follow-up care, including routine care).	18.2%
2.	Diseases of the musculoskeletal and connective tissue	10.1%
3.	Diseases of the circulatory system	9.0%
4.	Symptoms, signs, and ill-defined conditions	8.4%
5.	Diseases of the nervous system and sense organs	8.1%
6.	Diseases of the respiratory system	8.1%
7.	Mental disorders	6.7%

To date, there has not been any survey to medical providers in jails or prisons that replicates these surveillance techniques. Even if most of these providers wanted to engage in a surveillance program, lack of resources proves to be a significant roadblock in doing so. For example, medical records may not be kept electronically, or if they were, the systems in which the information is kept may be out of date and incompatible with modern surveillance systems. It is for these reasons that reports of this nature are limited to states with well-resourced criminal justice systems.

3.1.3 Vital Statistics

Vital statistics generally include births, deaths (and fetal deaths), marriages, and divorces. For the current discussion, deaths are the important component of public health surveillance. Suicide is the leading mental health indicator that can easily be tracked by current surveillance methods. As of 2019, suicide is the second to accidents as the leading cause of death for Americans aged 10 to 34 and the tenth leading cause of death in all Americans (CDC, 2021c). Another notable indicator that can be included among vital statistics is substance use disorder. For example, medical examiners or coroners can determine that substance abuse contributed to a decedent's cause of death, such as in a case of a long-term cocaine abuser who died from a heart condition. It could very well be determined that this user's heart was damaged by chronic cocaine use, which is very possible with the stimulant family of drugs. Yet, it is important to note here that death investigation systems are quite vary across the United States. It is true that the vast majority of deaths (99% according to the CDC) are recorded, not every jurisdiction has equal access to a comprehensive death investigation system. As such, many deaths may not be classified correctly or completely. In the same example of a long-term cocaine abuser, it may be that his death is simply recorded as cause of death: myocardial infarction (immediate cause); manner of death: natural without any mention to cocaine dependence as a mechanism of death. Thus, the heart attack would not be noted as a direct consequence of the long-term cocaine use on a death certificate and in vital records.

Suicide has been the leading cause of death for jail inmates for quite some time (deaths in custody was first tracked by the Bureau of Justice Statistics in 2000, so certainly since then; Noonan, 2015). About one-third of jail inmate deaths are attributed to suicide (or 46 suicides per 100,000 inmates), with deaths from heart disease close behind. Compare this to 5.5% of prison inmate deaths attributed to suicide (or 15 suicides per 100,000 prisoners), and the vulnerable population becomes clear – much more about this will be discussed in later chapters.

3.1.4 Putting It All Together – A Summary of Mental Health in America Today

The National Alliance of Mental Illness, a leading advocacy organization for mental health, keeps an array of easy-to-follow briefs on the most up to date compilation of mental health statistics available to aid in spreading its message. For example, in their most recent *Mental Health Facts in America* infographic, the following facts are the most salient:

- 43.8 million American adults experience mental illness in any recent year; that is 1 in 5 adults in the United States.
- A subset of these Americans – ten million, or close to 1 in every 25 adults – lives with a serious mental illness.
- Half of all chronic mental illness begins to occur by age 14, with the average delay between the onset of symptoms and initial intervention being 8 to 10 years.
- Depression is the leading cause of disability worldwide.
- Serious mental illness is estimated to cost the United States $193.2 billion in earning losses each year.
- 90% of those who commit suicide have an underlying mental illness; suicide is the tenth leading cause of death in the United States.
- The majority of adult American living with mental illness – 60% – did not receive mental health services in the previous year; half of youths (aged 8–15) with mental illness did not receive services in the previous year.
- Black and Hispanic Americans are half as likely to seek and use mental health services compared to their white American counterparts; Asian Americans utilize mental health services even less, about one-third the rate of their white American counterparts.

This information largely draws from the National Institute of Mental Health resources and is updated frequently to promulgate the latest intelligence on mental health in the most user-friendly way.

3.2   What We Don't Know

With only six targeted population surveys on justice-involved individuals, the three most recent being much more comprehensive than the previous ones, we still may not know the "true" size and scope of justice-involved mental illness. Also disconcerting, the latest available data date to 2011–2012 – over a decade ago – and much has changed since then. In particular, a steady stream of Federal investment in evidence-based practices and programming has shown the potential to ameliorate the issues being discussed here; on the other hand, a perfect storm was also brewing for massive cutbacks in criminal justice and mental health within the same time frame: (1) the level of mass incarceration crested at a peak of 506 inmates and prisoners per 100,000 citizens in 2007–2008; and (2) this coincides perfectly with a substantial economic recession, the so-called "Great Recession," beginning December 2007. Consider these findings from a recent SAMHSA (2016) review of behavioral health spending and use: the broad trend in mental health spending from 1986 to 2014 indicated a deeper divestment in inpatient and residential treatment coinciding with an increase in the use of and expenditures in outpatient treatment; during the same timeframe, Medicare, Medicaid, and private insurance use increased while out-of-pocket expenditures decreased; conversely, decreases in Medicaid (26–25%) and local spending (16–14%) occurred from 2008 to 2014. If one were to dig deeper into these expenditures, they would find a mix bag of successes and failures – with the successes masking the failures when observing this summary data.

For example, the National Alliance on Mental Illness (2015) published its results of an annual survey on state legislation on, and investment in, mental health. In this study, NAMI cites a loss of $4.35 billion in state cuts to mental health care systems since the recession. From the initial results of this survey published in 2013, many states have begun to reinvest in these systems upon recovery, yet some states have been unable to reform while others have been in decline. Perhaps more troubling, the results in 2015 show slowed growth and progress relative to previous years for states that were able to make headway. Alaska, North Carolina, and Wyoming are cited by NAMI to be in states of steady decline, with signs of problems occurring in Kentucky, Arkansas, Iowa, Kansas, Ohio, and the District of Columbia. While not mentioned directly in the narrative of the study's findings, Louisiana also has been struggling to reform; in fact, its state constitution will only allow for cuts to higher education and health care during nonbudget legislative sessions (e.g., every other year). While other states may not be so restrictive, mental health and criminal justice are often higher on the chopping block for cuts than other essential services.

Thus, information about the level of need that exists for mental illness and substance use disorder treatment, or both, is ill defined. What is clear is that the number individuals in jails and prisons who require treatment far exceeds the number who receive it – the latest justice-involved population surveys verified this. Specifically, "over 1 in 3 State prisoners and 1 in 6 jail inmates who had a mental health problem received treatment since admission" (James & Glaze, 2006). In other words, *66% of prisoners and 83% of jail inmates do not get the mental health treatment that they need according to the most up-to-date and comprehensive investigation into the justice-involved mental health population.* Remember, these bleak figures were obtained before mental health systems were further stressed by the recession. Ongoing treatment lapses are further documented in a subsequent report, reflecting the lack of momentum to resolve under- and untreated mental illness in this population.

Not knowing much more beyond this is a barrier to progress. Recall that Reeves (2013) describes seven key functions of public health surveillance systems: (1) to inform interventions with the benefit of data, providing an easy mechanism to discover, identify, and describe changes – including signs of problems – and act on them, (2) to estimate the impact of health conditions, (3) to provide a natural history of health conditions and how our responses and treatments shape outcomes, (4) to provide a big picture description of how conditions are distributed in society and how often they occur, (5) to structure hypothesis creation and seeds research ideas, (6) to enable thorough evaluation of prevention efforts and control measures, and, perhaps most importantly, (7) to help professionals engage in strategic planning. Without further investment into mental health surveillance, these functions become much more difficult to achieve. One truth in all of this is that, historically, the United States has prioritized mental illness behind other matters.

3.3   What We Know We Don't Know – Hidden Mental Illness

It is entirely possible – in fact, it is very probable – that not all illnesses are addressed while an individual is incarcerated. Further, these illnesses may not be addressed in time to help the patient, fully addressed in the best way possible, or diagnosed in a way to offer the best treatment. On that last point, proper diagnosis may require several visits and observations by a mental health professional, all of which may benefit greatly by comprehensive medical records for the current provider to understand prior assessments, treatments, and so on. Often, for many reasons, a person's medical history may be disjointed and/or lack current information. Consider visiting a doctor as an adult and being asked for a complete medical history from childhood. Even for a person with little to no medical history, it may be difficult to recount all that is needed for a current report. Now, imagine this scenario again from someone who has felt stigmatized many times for a mental health concern and criminal history. The mental illness alone may have prompted denial or a reluctance to report symptoms. Add in a criminal history, this yields all the more reason for a person to fear stigma. Further, the chain of information is broken after incarceration and return to society. Often, this continues to repeat again and again resulting in stagnation for the individual in the process of recovery and health.

Broadly speaking, inmates may not disclose their illness for fear of discrimination, negative treatment, or just plain lack of knowledge. Often, individuals feel shame surrounding their mental health. Mental health concerns are often seen as a sign of weakness – a label that is perhaps one of the most problematic for inmates – which only further perpetuates the stigma. Masking the signs and symptoms of depression or anxiety, or any other psychological disorder can be a major setback for a person as these issues will go untreated, potentially leading to significant problems, decompensation, and higher risks of bad outcomes (e.g., suicide, drug overdose, violent confrontations, and so on). Seeking help as soon as symptoms arise is important to the health of the person affected, yet this has not historically been the case for jail inmates or prisoners thanks largely to the effects of stigma. Additionally, knowing one's own triggers is essential for future prevention and proactive efforts to remain healthy.

Taking that ideal a step further, mental illness in a male prison there is less likelihood of disclosure of mental illness and seeking of treatment. According to the World Health Organization (2022), there are differences in both prevalence of mental health and substance abuse as well as reporting by gender. This gap is supported by a stream of literature; for example, Kartalova-O'Doherty and Tedstone Doherty, (2010) published their analysis of the HRB National Psychological Wellbeing and Distress Survey in 2010. The data in this telephone survey revealed significant gender differences between males and females that influence seeing general practitioners for mental health concerns. In particular, an array of sociodemographic and psychological factors (such as feelings of limited physical activity and social activity, educational level, employment status, marital status, self-reported physical health, self-reported quality of life, and whether these men live in a rural or urban setting) influenced male visits to general practitioners while females were only influenced by social factors (e.g., feeling like mental health limits social activities) and access to healthcare (e.g., price), thus leading to broader differences among the genders in seeking mental health help from practitioners. The main point here is that we generally know less about individuals who do not seek help or are not willing to seek help and that the rate of untreated mental illness is likely higher in some groups relative to others, gender being a prime example.

Another issue surrounding the idea of prisons or jails as it relates to mental health, is time. The intake process is limited and only a small amount is spent addressing the immediate needs of the incoming inmate as well as acclimating them to the policies and procedures of the prison. Also, keep in mind the mindset of the individual being brought into the facility. Obviously, none of this is ideal for the typical psychosocial interview. In a hospital setting, a trained mental health professional would complete a psychosocial interview upon intake with a patient. This interview would include questions regarding background and history on both physical and mental health in order to gain a baseline for the individual. This allows the treatment staff to have somewhat of a comparison for behavior. Additionally, this information is kept in the patient's medical record for future use if needed. If the same patient returns for treatment, the staff would then be able to review past notes and information to best treat the person. Jails and prisons, however, do not have similar processes in place (oftentimes), leading to an utter lack of knowledge about the people within these facilities. Thus, mental health diagnoses often remain undiagnosed, yielding to a lack of ability to adequately describe the issues within justice-involved populations. Other than the few major surveys of jail and prison inmates, which offer limited glimpses into the "true" picture of mental health within these facilities, there is a major disadvantage in the lack of ability to track issues over time, track the emergence of new problems, understand the impact of policies on mental health, and so on.

3.3.1 Marginalized Groups and Cultural Differences

Marginalized groups struggle within the criminal justice system as they do in regular society. Persons of different races, religions, sexual orientation, et cetera often experience difficulties in seeking help, maintaining treatment regimes, or even being considered for treatment services (for example, in the case of justice-involved transgender individuals). These groups often experience higher rates of victimization, isolation, stigmatization, and so on, and often are less likely to report mental health concerns and seek treatment. Without knowing the full picture and extent of these issues with relevant data, it is difficult to intervene in the lives of these vulnerable individuals. This certainly can add to their trouble receiving help. Without factual information to support the need, most facilities cannot justify providing further programming – particularly when trying to justify costs. And unfortunately, with little to no information and data being collected on these vulnerable subpopulations (let alone, on individuals with mental illness, generally), it is difficult to assess the extent of the problem(s) in the first place. Part of the lack of information lies in the lack of understanding of different marginalized groups or cultures even outside of the criminal justice system. Even further, without research and information, it is also difficult to determine any further disparities that may exist; most research suggests this to be the case.

For example, recent stories of violence against transgender persons has emerged as a widely-publicized issue in late 2016 and early 2017. With recent national attention on issues of this population, advocates are helping to aid in equality for transgender persons in criminal justice settings as well by tapping into this surge of attention. The National Center for Transgender Equality (NCTE) – a leader in this movement – advocates for protections and accountability through the development of advocacy tools focused on gender nonconforming people's interactions with the criminal justice system, law enforcement officers, and the broader public (2021). Within the literature found on their website, the NCTE makes reference to the daily humiliation, increased risk of physical and sexual abuse, and fear of harm if individuals use legal solutions to report these problems. In particular, the Prison Rape Elimination Act (PREA) was designed specifically to include dedicated provisions to help protect incarcerated transgender individuals against sexual assault. However, prisoners (and staff) often lack respect for the PREA process, with many left thinking that it could be considered "a joke" or just a window dressing on the realities of prison life (Khey, unpublished research).

Mental health professionals are trained on cultural competencies to work with different cultural groups, particularly with an understanding of the issues described above to encourage sensitivity to the deficiencies primarily caused by the social realities of vulnerable populations. The dilemma, as mentioned many times within in this book, often rests with a lack of professional staffing to accommodate all inmates within a jail or prison. This means, that despite adequate training for mental health professionals, there being one person for an entire jail or prison means that there may not be the means to assess all inmates to ensure proper care and adherence to cultural etiquette. At that point, administrators tend to focus their efforts on meeting and maintaining what is currently understood as the constitutionally-acceptable level of mental health services. Much more on this concept will be explored in subsequent chapters; however, it is important to understand that typical levels of mental health services throughout American corrections tend to only allow for crisis care and exigent problems as they may present themselves. Vulnerabilities can often be magnified in criminal justice settings, including those inherent in cultural differences.

To be sure, there are many various cultural barriers that may exist within society that also are relevant within the criminal justice system. For example, language barriers can be difficult to overcome in everyday life, let alone the difficulties that language barriers can present when entering a jail upon arrest. A language barrier can particularly exacerbate the issue of obtaining proper and accurate information (of special note: health information). Also, it is further important to recognize that certain cultures are far less likely to adhere to American cultural norms. Some people of Asian descent tend not to make eye contact, which to some may be perceived negatively or disrespectful – or, more notably in this instance – may be a sign of deception for some trained law enforcement and corrections personnel. In addition, in some Asian cultures, as well as in others such as Orthodox Hasidim, it is wholly inappropriate to have any interaction between females and males who are not married. With this in mind, consider the harsh environment of a jail or prison; if a male inmate were to be approached by a female corrections officer and who subsequently avoids eye contact and does not respond, there could be potential trouble (e.g., insubordination). The inmate would be doing this as a sign of respect to his culture, but for the officer and other staff, this would be viewed as disrespect and could lead to possible infractions inside the jail/prison. Furthermore, different races, religions, and other cultural subgroups may have other barriers and specific behaviors. Consider differences among Islamic inmates, women of color, American Indians, and so forth.

On a final note, it is often important to consider one's perceived social status when discussing mental health outcomes. In other words, it may not be enough only to consider membership in a vulnerable subpopulation or class (e.g., transgender male prisoner) in isolation. Importantly, mental health problems may be attenuated by one's own perception of being marginalized. In research published by Friestad (2010), male Norwegian prisoners were surveyed to understand how perceived social status in prison affected potential inequalities in health (and mental health). As expected, prisoners who perceived that they were marginalized exhibited increased odds of experiencing mental health problems. More work needs to be done in this area to better understand the impacts of vulnerable individuals, particularly at the point when these individuals are set to reenter society.

3.4   Conclusion

Many professionals suspect that most mental illnesses are underreported. In fact, this chapter remains brief as the American epidemiological understanding of mental illness continues to take a back seat to other, less-, or nonstigmatized problems. This is truly the result of the lack of investment in mental health research relative to other American priorities. There appears to be a shift in this trend, however. The twenty-first Century Cures Act was recently enacted into law; it sharply responds to this problem through policy, by earmarking funds, and by shifting governmental agencies in a way that will enable progress in this area. While it is not exactly clear when these changes will start producing results, changes have already started to occur to ensure transformation in America's struggle with mental health.

One key issue that is not always discussed or even thought of in regard to the lack of mental health treatment options, is the waste of the resources earmarked for this purpose. This waste can take many forms. Consider then, like any other illnesses, the effect of prolonging/delaying treatment in that this can often result in an increase the cost/investment necessary to achieve a healthy outcome. Further, the traumatic experiences of incarceration, one of America's primary responses to mental health diagnosis, often serves to only push vulnerable people toward further or compounding negative outcomes. Therefore, if treating the person in the community early in the disease process could be given a certain dollar amount, it most certainly would be monumentally less than the amount necessary when the cost of incarceration is factored in for those individuals that fall in the cracks of this safety net. Incarcerating a person in need of treatment has placed a large financial burden onto the criminal justice system, thus creating a different problem. To date, this problem has been largely ignored; yet, progress is slowly occurring in the form of broad partnerships and fresh ideas to address this problem.

Discussion Questions

1. What information regarding mental health within the criminal justice system is provided for other countries?
2. Why are data crucial in the discussion surrounding mental health/criminal justice system?
3. How can we improve collection of data and appropriate use to improve the issues within these areas?
4. How transparent are states about addressing mental health within their criminal justice systems? Should they be more or less transparent?

References

21st Century Cures Act. Public Law 144–255. 2016.

Bronzon, J., & Berzofsky, M. (2017). *Indicators of mental health problems reported by prisoners and jail inmates, 2011–12*. Bureau of Justice Statistics. URL: https://bjs.ojp.gov/content/pub/pdf/imhprpji1112.pdf. Last accessed: 2022, January 24.

Center for Disease Control and Prevention. (2021a). CDC report: Mental health surveillance among U.S. adults. URL: https://www.cdc.gov/mmwr/preview/mmwrhtml/su6003a1.htm. Last accessed: 2021, January 24.

Center for Disease Control and Prevention. (2021b). Ambulatory health care data. URL: https://www.cdc.gov/nchs/ahcd/index.htm. Last accessed: 2021, January 24.

Center for Disease Control and Prevention. (2021c). Facts about suicide. URL: https://www.cdc.gov/suicide/facts/index.html. Last accessed: 2021, January 24.

First, M. B., Williams, J. B., Karg, R. S., & Spitzer, R. L. (2016). *User's guide for the SCID-5-CV Structured Clinical Interview for DSM-5® disorders: Clinical version.* American Psychiatric Publishing, Inc..

Friestad, C. (2010). Socio-economic status and health in a marginalized group: the role of subjective social status among prison inmates. *European Journal of Public Health, 20*(6), 653–658.

James, D. J., & Glaze, L. E. (2006). *Mental health problems of prison and jail inmates.* Bureau of Justice Statistics. URL: https://www.bjs.gov/content/pub/pdf/mhppji.pdf. Last accessed: 2021, January 24.

Kartalova-O'Doherty, Y., & Tedstone Doherty, D. (2010). Recovering from recurrent mental health problems: Giving up and fighting to get better. *International Journal of Mental Health Nursing, 19*(1), 3–15.

National Alliance on Mental Illness. (2015). State mental health legislation 2015: Trends, themes, & effective practices. URL: https://www.nami.org/About-NAMI/Publications-Reports/Public-Policy-Reports/State-Mental-Health-Legislation-2015/NAMI-StateMentalHealthLegislation2015.pdf. Last accessed: 2021, January 24.

National Center for Transgender Equality. (2021). Issues: Police, jails, & prisons. URL: http://www.transequality.org/issues/police-jails-prisons. Last accessed: 2021, January 24.

Noonan, M. (2015). *Mortality in local jails and state prisons, 2000–2013 – Statistical tables.* Bureau of Justice Statistics. URL: https://www.bjs.gov/content/pub/pdf/mljsp0013st.pdf. Last accessed: 2021, January 24.

Reeves, W. (2013). Mental health surveillance. In M. D. Gellman & J. R. Turner (Eds.), *Encyclopedia of behavioral medicine.* Springer.

Rutherford, G. W., McFarland, W., Spindler, H., White, K., Patel, S. V., Aberle-Grasse, J., ... & Stoneburner, R. L. (2010). Public health triangulation: approach and application to synthesizing data to understand national and local HIV epidemics. BMC public health, 10(1), 1–10.

Substance Abuse and Mental Health Services Administration. (2013). Revised estimates of mental health from the National Survey on Drug Use and Health. URL: https://www.samhsa.gov/data/sites/default/files/NSDUH148/NSDUH148/sr148-mental-illness-estimates.htm.   Last accessed: 2021, January 24.

Substance Abuse and Mental Health Services Administration. (2016). Behavioral health spending & use accounts: 1986–2014. URL: https://store.samhsa.gov/sites/default/files/d7/priv/sma16-4975.pdf. Last accessed: 2021, January 24.

Substance Abuse and Mental Health Services Administration. (2017). State-level comparisons of mental health issues from the National Survey on Drug Use and Health (NSDUH) and the Behavioral Risk Factor Surveillance System (BRFSS). URL: https://www.samhsa.gov/data/sites/default/files/NSDUH-N12-NSDUHBRFSS-2015.pdf. Last accessed: 2022, January 24.

Substance Abuse and Mental Health Services Administration. (2019). Key substance use and mental health indicators in the United States: Results from the 2018 National Survey on Drug Use and Health (HHS Publication No. PEP19–5068, NSDUH Series H-54). URL: https://www.samhsa.gov/data/sites/default/files/cbhsq-reports/NSDUHNationalFindingsReport2018/NSDUHNationalFindingsReport2018.pdf. Last accessed: 2022, January 24.

Substance Abuse and Mental Health Services Administration. (2022). Reports and detailed tables from the 2020 National Survey on Drug Use and health. URL: https://www.samhsa.gov/data/report/2020-nsduh-detailed-t2ables. Last accessed: 2022, January 24.

World Health Organization. (2022). Gender disparities and mental health. URL: https://www.who.int/mental_health/media/en/242.pdf. Last accessed: 2022, January 24.

Chapter 4
The Frontline: EMS, Law Enforcement, and Probation and Parole

Mental health continues to be a topic people would rather ignore, especially management.

Survey Respondent, National Association of Emergency Medical Technicians, 2017

First responders – which typically include emergency medical services (EMS), "line" (or patrol) law enforcement officers, and firemen – are workers who are dispatched to crime scenes, accidents, and emergencies. Aside from bystanders and witnesses, they are often the first to encounter people in crisis and even more likely to be the first to engage with these individuals. These professionals routinely encounter the turmoil, panic, and pain in its rawest form, and thus are often dealing with difficult and serious situations – perhaps even daily. In regard to confronting mental illness, the primary concern lies in the lack of relevant training for the vast majority of these professions. For example, EMS personnel commonly have *some* level of training to enhance their ability to work with individuals experiencing mental health crises and/or who have a mental illness (diagnosed or undiagnosed); on the other hand, law enforcement officers commonly have *little to no required training* in mental health-related topics. This training deficiency is beginning to be addressed as some departments are moving to require officers, or a subset of law enforcement agencies' patrol units, to be trained to serve on Crisis Intervention Teams (CIT), but this is not yet universal. Therefore, it is imperative to carefully consider the unintended consequences of having citizens routinely encountering professionals who are not properly trained to work with individuals experiencing mental health crises when emergency services are dispatched. While many urban and suburban areas have created a mobile crisis unit that provides immediate services in the event of a mental health crisis, these units are often underfunded or work in isolation. Ideally, these mobile crisis units work together with local law enforcement when emergency services are called. This chapter discusses the current picture of first responders' work with individuals with mental illness and citizens experiencing mental health crises. It further identifies probation and parole officers as part of the first responder definition as these professionals confront the very same issues as do their colleagues in patrol law enforcement and EMS.

© The Author(s), under exclusive license to Springer Nature Switzerland AG 2022
J. Hector, D. Khey, *Criminal Justice and Mental Health*,
https://doi.org/10.1007/978-3-031-15338-9_4

4.1   Know the Role

Dealing with people who are ill day in and day out can be difficult for almost anyone. Much like any other illness (in particular, chronic illness), those with mental illness also may seek treatment repeatedly with varying levels of success (and failure and/or setbacks). Also, many illnesses can progressively worsen over time particularly with lack of treatment, including undertreatment. Seeing the same person over and over as a first responder or treatment provider – often colloquially called frequent fliers – can take its toll. Imagine if you perceive that whatever you do on your job, that very little of it seems to be helping or that you feel like you are simply "doing the motions" without anything to show for it.

"Helping professionals" often get into the business directly due to a passion or desire to want to help people. For example, on a top police news and blogging site – PoliceOne.com – a post entitled "7 reasons I'm still a police officer" explained that the unnamed author cherished "protecting those who cannot protect themselves," and "getting help to someone who needs it" as his or her main reasons for continuing to serve while the recent political climate seems to have given rise to a downturn in confidence in American law enforcement officers (Police One, 2019). With a broken continuum of care and a consistent lack of systematic resources, protecting vulnerable citizens and proving help to those who need it can be a very difficult and often frustrating task. Factor in the bureaucracy of local, state, and federal government and you can begin to envision a series of roadblocks that can often demotivate American first responders, leading to further unintentional consequences. For example, these barriers commonly lead to burnout, and this burnout leads to mental health concerns for these helping professionals and first responders.

Unfortunately, these concerns have become self-evident in the number of suicides within these professions. In a study by the Centers of Disease Control and Prevention, "protective service" professionals including law enforcement and firefighters were found to have the sixth-highest suicide rate and well over double the national average suicide rate of that year (30.5 per 100,000 versus 12.6 per 100,000 average for American Adults, both in 2012; McIntosh et al., 2016). Even more stark, female protective service professionals experienced the highest suicide rate relative to other adult females in any other occupation (14.1 per 100,000). Of note, this is not an American issue – it is an issue endemic to the profession itself. In a study of suicide among protective service professionals in Australia, the suicide rate followed a similar pattern (Milner et al., 2017). The suicide rate for male and female protective service professionals was double that of male and female counterparts in any other profession, with the highest risk of suicide among those employed by the defense force, prisons, and ambulance agencies (more on this in the Self Care chapter).

It is far from clear what level of impact deinstitutionalization has had on the mental health of these professionals themselves; however, it is clear that deinstitutionalization has starkly increased the interaction of helper professions with individuals with mental illness and/or individuals at high risk to experience mental health crises. On its website, the National Alliance on Mental Illness strongly suggests that "law enforcement agencies have increasingly become the de facto first responders to people experiencing mental health crisis" while citing indirect evidence to support this claim. From the evidence presented in the last chapter, this bold claim appears to have a lot of truth to it in the absence of direct study; either way, it is certain that these interactions are common, frequent, and have an impact on both responders and respondees in ways we are yet to completely understand.

Probation and parole officers also struggle with these very issues, yet have been largely forgotten in the growing research in this area. Further, probation and parole officers often must contend with increased caseloads and decreased resources due to the nature of recent justice reforms and policies set in place to decrease prison overcrowding/populations. As revealed in the previous chapter, the vast majority of individuals in need of services are not receiving them in jail or prison settings. At this point, the vast majority of treatment resources continue to remain in the communities probationers and parolees return to; however, connecting these individuals with services often remain challenging. Research is direly needed in this area as probation and parole officers often have caseloads that include individuals with varying degrees of mental illness and co-occurring disorders who may require routine care.

For supervisees with serious mental illness, community corrections agencies have often adapted a special agent role or "unit" to address "extreme" cases, and thus focuses training resources on agents with the most challenging caseload (Lurigio, 2001). Yet, the job also demands that *all* agents confront individuals when they are having mental health crises. Relative to patrol police officers, it appears that many in community corrections has broader experiences with individuals with mental illness and/or at risk of experiencing mental health crises. A litany of research questions arises from these interactions and are yet to be explored.

For example, probation and parole officers aid in the success of individuals in lieu of incarceration or postincarceration. The transition of leaving jail, prison, or court-ordered treatment can be the most difficult period for person; in fact, a wide array of literature focuses on this transitional period as a particular moment of high risk of problems (most likely, relapse, recidivism, rearrest, and/or reincarceration; Begun et al., 2016; Lolita Jacob & Poletick, 2008; Stewart & George-Paschal, 2017). Consider that the mission of community corrections agencies often highlights and prioritizes the assurance of accountability among their supervisees to promote successful outside of jail and prison facilities and to ensure public safety. One must rhetorically consider, then, the level of accountability to be placed on individuals with mental illness and co-occurring disorders. Perhaps the following question should be carefully considered: how should probation and parole officers respond to supervisees who are in violation with their conditions of supervision or release directly due to mental illness and/or substance abuse?

The frontline of first responders are people who truly get to be pillars of support in times of crisis. They often help those in need when the worst has happened, quickly becoming the worst moments in people's lives and memories. The level of empathy and concern for others is truly a remarkable feat that often gets overlooked when assessing the problems of tending to individuals with mental illnesses.

4.1.1 EMS and Trained Firefighters

Emergency Medical Services (EMS) refers to the medically-trained professionals (and their agencies) who are dispatched to incidents of medical emergencies to provide acute out-of-hospital care, triage, and transportation services to medical facilities for further assessment and treatment. They include (1) paramedics – highest level of training and licensure of their class, paramedics are skilled in ambulatory medicine delivery, heart monitoring, intubation, establishing an airway when it is occluded, and other advanced life support procedures (e.g., defibrillation); (2) emergency medical technicians (EMT) of varying levels of training and expertise including EMT-Intermediate (one step lower in training relative to paramedics – to be phased out in upcoming years), Advanced-EMT (limited range of ambulatory medicine delivery, yet fully trained in advanced airway procedures and set to replace the EMT-I level of certification), and EMT-Basic (limited range of emergency care procedures, yet include the most important such as defibrillation, procedures in case of potential spinal injury, and oxygen therapy); and (3) ambulance personnel (who are, at times, cross-trained in a certification listed above). As mentioned earlier, EMS personnel work closely with law enforcement and fire departments when responding to various types of emergencies. In fact, in most major metropolitan areas, when EMS is run as a public venture, it often falls under fire services in organizational charts. Further, EMS has been increasingly privatized as noted in a recent New York Times expose entitled, "When you dial 911 and Wall Street answers" (Ivory et al., 2016), leading to new challenges yet to be adequately researched and assessed.

As with most medical-related occupations, EMS personnel do receive some training as it relates to mental health, albeit minimal at this time. Most critically, it should be noted that EMS personnel and firefighters have consistently and historically retained a medical orientation to care coming from a *nonlaw enforcement* perspective. In other words, as first responders to incidents featuring mental illness and/or mental health crises, law enforcement professionals have been criticized for their paramilitary orientation and approach which often is contraindicated for these types of incidents. So, while the level of training may not be substantially different in the certification and licensure process (and recertification process) for law enforcement and EMS personnel, the orientation should theoretically produce significantly different results on the street.

In Florida, training often consists of lectures relating to excited delirium (e.g., symptoms of bizarre and aggressive behavior, psychomotor excitement (high rate of breathing and feelings of "on edge"), paranoia, panic, and potential violence), combative patients, and the use of restraint and drugs such as ketamine. In all actuality, these topics are covered within broader lectures on interfacing with patents, often lasting a few hours (at best; Strate, 2017). In New Orleans, similar coverage was confirmed with a local training manager and community liaison (Belcher, 2017). As such, the majority of the EMS and firefighter workforce remain critically undertrained in mental health across the nation. Further, there is a dearth of literature on the impact of privatization of these services on the quality of care given to individuals with mental health concerns. This is a critical issue as privatization has become more prevalent since the economic downturn and recession in the United States in 2008. Anecdotally, it appears that there is a great potential for more problematic interactions between private sector EMS personnel and firefighters; the New York Times expose detailed worsening response times, failing and faulty equipment, and poor service that has led to the death of at least two patients (Ivory, Protess, and Bennett, 2016).

4.1.2   Law Enforcement

The vast majority of "line" law enforcement personnel across the country attend standardized training, called Peace Officer Standards and Training (POST). The POST standards are created and maintained by state-level commissions and vary across states. As such, the level of mental health training police cadets receive varies and it remains difficult to decipher which areas provide robust training versus scant or minimal training. For example, in California, cadets attending POST-certified police academies across the state will receive at least one module that addresses the following: (1) an introduction to the laws put into place that protect people with mental illness and disabilities, (2) training in recognizing the behaviors that can be a red flag or serve as indicators of mental illness or disability, (3) training in de-escalation skills, (4) training in responses that are appropriate to differing situations that include indirect referrals for the individual and direct referrals to community partners, and (5) educate cadets in mental health and disability stigma to ensure reduction in stigma (California Commission on Peace Officer Standards and Training, 2022). This content was developed in partnership with the National Alliance on Mental Illness, local mental health professionals, and POST subject matter experts to ensure best results; and while the hours of training dedicated to this module may vary, most this Regular Basic Course receive a minimum of 664 hours of training (yet most academies average over 850 hours of overall training, signifying that most academies go above and beyond the minimum to ensure adequate training of new cadets). As a comparison, Louisiana has 25 unique training academies (not including satellite academies run by the same agency) with varying curriculum. At the time of this writing, the Louisiana Peace Officer Standards and Training Council *does not require any specific* mental health training nor does any specific academy list dedicated mental health curriculum on their websites *as a part of the basic training process* (Louisiana Commission on Law Enforcement, 2022). Yet, the minimum training requirements for all Louisiana peace officers – detailed in Louisiana Revised Statute 40:2404.2 – was recently updated to require the state's Training Council to include "curriculum for de-escalation, bias policing recognition, sudden in-custody death, and crisis intervention training, which shall include training for law enforcement interaction with persons with mental illness and persons with developmental disabilities, for peace officers that consists of classroom or internet instruction, or both." Thus, training in Louisiana has come online for adoption across the state, yet standards requiring a specific minimum array of training are not detailed by statute. This may result in differential training practices across the state, at least in the short-term.

Since 2017, California leads the United States in the development of this type of embedded training in POST academies. This is directly due to state legislation that was signed into law in October of 2015. California Senate Bill 11 created a statutory mandate directing the Commission on Peace Standards and Training to include "adequate instruction in the handling of persons with developmental disabilities or mental illness, or both....[and] to establish and keep updated a continuing education classroom training course relating to law enforcement interaction with developmentally disabled and mentally ill persons" (California Legislative Information, 2015). As time passes, it will be interesting to see if other states follow suit, take an alternative approach to ensuring better training practices (such as in Louisiana), or remain stagnant. As training systems adopt change, many peace officers may continue to receive training that mirrors the status quo for EMS personal explained above. This status quo tends to focus on "containment and transportation" (Strate, 2017). Such training can include tactics of restraint, which again, can be contraindicated in some situations. One popular alternative may include general de-escalation skills in the form of "Verbal Judo" or something quite similar. Verbal Judo is training program developed by George Thompson (whose doctorate was in English and was further trained in rhetoric) that focuses on the power of persuasion and verbal communication to redirect behavior. It remains empirically unclear whether these tactics show statistical improvement in outcomes when encountering individuals with mental illness and/or citizens who are experiencing a mental health crisis. Yet, Verbal Judo remains incredibly popular as a training option for developing crisis intervention skills in the United States and abroad.

A recent study by Fiske, Songer, and Schriver (2021) provides more context on the current state of mental health training among peace officers. In their review of peer review literature, Fiske and her colleagues discovered that researchers began surveying police agencies about mental health and crisis training in the late 1990s and early 2000s. This earlier research found that the departments surveyed reported a median of 6.5 hours spent on mental health training at police academies and a median of 1 hour of training during in-service training (e.g., after graduating from the academy and while on the job). In addition, one-third of responding agencies to this earlier research effort reported having no training at all after their officers complete the academy. This research also details that the mental health and crisis training that was available typically focused on substance use, mental disabilities, and containment and transportation to manage unruly citizens (Hails & Borum, 2003). Fisk and her colleagues set out to determine the amount of training and content offered by training academies in the late 2010s. To do so, they compiled a list of 224 law enforcement academies and 489 police departments across the United States with email contact information available to training officers or heads of agencies. They received responses from 31 academies from 30 states and 128 departments in 38 states.

While these survey efforts are not necessarily representative of American training academies or police agencies nationwide, the findings from the Fisk and colleagues' study are promising. They detail that training on a *variety* of mental health topics has increased substantially since the early 2000s. Specifically, Fisk, Songer, and Schriver report that their respondents had a median of 20 hours of training during academy training and a median of 4 hours after graduation. By the late 2010s, these agencies and departments reporting topical coverage including mental illness de-escalation, suicide de-escalation, suicide prevention, psychosis, intellectual disabilities, neurocognitive problems, autism, substance abuse, and mental health resources. These results are encouraging, but one must be cautious of extrapolating these results broadly. Given that the sampling techniques used during this study does not provide for representativeness among academies and departments in the United States due potential selection bias, we should not interpret this to believe that mental health training is now commonplace for *all* peace officers. It is, however, promising to compare these results to those reported in the early 2000s as their sampling strategies are very similar. There seems little doubt that, overall, specific mental health training for peace officers is increasing both in time spent and by topical area.

While broad training for all would be ideal, the most concentrated and promising investment in affecting change among law enforcement, EMS, and trained firefighters has been in building Crisis Intervention Team (CIT) programs and its related training. This in-service training has become robust, evidence-based, and is thought to be the leading solution to the current state of affairs of underserving vulnerable mental health populations and individuals with disabilities. CIT is explained further below.

4.1.3 Probation and Parole

Probation and parole officers face a different challenge working with individuals after their criminal convictions and postincarceration. The agent's role involves supervising individuals who have been arrested of a crime and are sentenced to a probationary period or individuals who are being released from incarceration. Typically, supervision involves case management, frequent random drug tests, and regular visits and/or check-ins. Policies can differ across states as well as with the Federal approach; however, the basic approach and routine are essentially very similar.

In urban areas with adequate resources, special units within community corrections have been created to address the mental health caseload that these agencies may have. For example, in New York City, the New York City Probation offers a Forensic Mental Health Unit to "help their clients adjust to probation supervision while also addressing…mental health needs…., [including] working individually with clients and tracking their progress, sometimes through periods of hospitalizations and homelessness" (2017). This is a relatively new unit, with mandates that began their formation in 2008 after a formal review of gaps in services performed by New York City. It is difficult to determine the effectiveness of this type of program; yet, it does appear that it and others like it deploy evidence-based practices and services designed to show improvements in outcomes for this target population. Much more research on the effectiveness of these programs is slated to emerge in upcoming years.

One recent study, by Wolff and her colleagues show that there is great promise in deploying specialized mental health caseloads (Wolff et al., 2014). This study used a mixed-methods approach to first ensure that trained special agents in New Jersey were staying true to their training and evidence-based approaches while also following up to observe any potential differences in outcomes among probationers with mental illness who are supervised on a specialized caseload versus those who are not. Their findings show that the special caseloads were deployed with rigor and probationers who received these special services had statistically improved criminal justice and mental health outcomes (e.g., fewer violations of probation resulting in arrest and jail days, improved mental health symptoms, better quality of life, et cetera) relative to those who were not placed on a special caseload (although they did qualify). This study is robust, yet the researchers urge future researchers to examine special caseloads with a random-control treatment design to be able to understand whether other potential confounding factors are interfering with these results.

Probation and parole officers will be as important as first responders in managing mental health in American communities in the upcoming years. In fact, there will likely be more burden directly placed on their shoulders to be on the frontlines of this response. Initial findings from studies of specialized caseloads are promising. Beyond the Wolff study, Skeem, Manchak, and Montoya find that probationers with mental illness paired with a probation officer with a specialized caseload substantially reduced rearrest rates *almost by half*, with enduring reductions that lasted 5 years when compared to a matched probationer assigned to a typical probation officer with a "standard" caseload. Thus, probation officers can play a key role to reducing mass incarceration among people with mental illness.

4.2   Common Interactions

The vast majority of interactions between first responders and individuals with mental illness and/or experiencing mental health crises are often perceived as negative. Yet, "[a]pproximately one-third of individuals with severe mental illness have their first contact with mental health treatment through a law enforcement encounter" (Treatment Advocacy Center, 2019). Textbooks, advocacy groups, and research often uses a lens of the perspective of individuals with mental illness, which is compelling and offers great insight into the plight of this target population. This text does make light of this perspective, often heavily, to ensure adequate assurance of busting myths that plague this topic, to improve understanding in the area, and to help make sense of the broken nature of our mental health care systems. Yet, exploring these interactions from this perspective alone will only be able to depict a smaller part of the broader problem. To gain better understanding into and compassion for the issues explored in this text, it will be important to understand both sides of the interaction.

4.2.1 Frequent Flyers: An Example of Typical and Common Interactions (and Frustrations)

In Austin, Texas, Travis County Emergency Medical Services grew curious about the number repeated calls to 911, often from the same patients time and time again (Plohetski, 2008), a common occurrence experienced by EMS professionals across the country (Belcher, 2017; Strate, 2017). One such example described a man calling emergency dispatchers three times in 1 day, resulting in three separate trips to local hospitals. Further research into this case uncovered that over the course of 2 years, paramedics were called to this man's home 290 times (an average nearing three times a week). As a result of such cases, Travis County began to track repeated-call data in order to better serve the community and identify a better solution for such patients with extraordinary need. Of note, this study found:

- "Ten patients made up more than 1% of the system's 130,000 contacts with patients in 2 years. Their most common complaints were stomach or chest pain, injuries or respiratory problems. Paramedics also responded to calls when the patients exhibited behavioral problems.
- Nearly all of the patients went to a hospital emergency room each time, sometimes crowding into already overflowing facilities.
- The patient who was seen 290 times in the two-year period was evaluated by paramedics twice on 36 days and nine times in a separate seven-day period."

This new tracking system and database has allowed for Travis County EMS to take a better look at their processes and where their time and resources were being spent (and wasted). For example and at that time (in 2008), Travis County was spending $300 on labor, gasoline, and medical equipment costs for the average call and was putting in more than an hour of time commitment. The cumulative drain repeated and unsuccessful calls for service has on the system had become a critical issue with regard to the *quality* of services for the entire service area. Adding to the emerging crisis, cutbacks were occurring contemporaneously to Austin's mental health centers and hospitals, resulting in increased activity in emergency rooms (and, by default, emergency medical services) in addition to the lack of resources and reduced quality care available in the area at the time.

Common problems arise in situations where these inefficiencies in the system promulgate. In other words, frequent fliers in the system can cause a ripple effect. For example, patients may end up in emergency room beds to too long, possibly even days or weeks without medical history or medication information. The emergency room, particularly at hospitals serving the vulnerable and underserved populations, can also have less capacity to provide thorough treatment or assistance for patients experiencing mental illness. In Travis County's case, local stakeholders were compelled to search for alternatives after this critical introspection into its mental health care system's inefficiencies in order to overcome these obstacles and have even attempted to resolve things directly with patients in need. They have since explored better triage plans and policies for mental health patients by EMS, adding a nurse to emergency services dispatch to assess patients over the phone who appear to have mental health concerns, and developing a community health paramedic position. In one instance, Travis County EMS actually met with a patient and her caregiver directly to discuss ways to help and avoid frequent calls/hospital trips. The effort was successful temporarily until the patient was arrested and upon her release, the cycle of frequent calls began again. Yet, the willingness to explore out-of-the-box options are now on the table for many jurisdictions dealing with the very same issues.

"Frequent flyers" is common jargon among first responders (Belcher, 2017). Interventions with particular focus on the emergency room have been created, tested, and show promise (Michelen et al., 2006). For example, a relatively recent study of in New York City showed that an emergency department diversion program featuring health priority specialists and community health workers successfully reduced the return rate to the hospital. It appears that many areas are exploring broader community partnerships to engage on fixing this problem rather than having an approach spearheaded from a sole source (such as EMS like in Travis County or by a hospital, such as in this case in Manhattan).

4.3   Common Problems

The Treatment Advocacy Center is a nonprofit working to safeguard for the "effective treatment of severe mental illness" by removing barriers to services and care; this nonprofit also clearly documents the common problems facing American mental health services today (Treatment Advocacy Center, 2017a, b, c). Relevant to this discussion, the Center recently released a study discussing the interactions between law enforcement and individuals with mental illness. The study laid out some alarming statistics initially to drive its focus; for example, "people with untreated mental illness are 16 times more likely to be killed during a police encounter than other civilians approached or stopped by law enforcement" (Fuller et al., 2015). This particular study, entitled "Overlooked in the undercounted: The role of mental illness in fatal law enforcement encounters," explores additional data angles and alternative sources for estimates when data are unavailable to continue its point. Using publicly available data, Fuller, Lamb, Biasotti, and Snook uncover that while only a few individuals shy of 1 in 50 Americans are said to have untreated and severe mental illness, this segment of the population seems to be involved in *at least* a quarter of fatal shootings by law enforcement. In fact, their estimates put this statistic closer to half of these shootings involve this particular segment. When looking deeper, these researchers estimate that roughly one in 10 citizen-police encounters also involve this segment. While it may be tempting to also assert that these statistics are being sourced by an advocacy group who may be well-served by articulating these problems in the most negative light to get a reaction or to seed change, the report clearly recognizes its close partnership with the National Sheriffs' Association in evaluating these issues facing law enforcement.

Recall our discussion above about frequent flyers as well. Imagine having 10% of your workload (roughly) dedicated to citizens who have untreated severe mental illness, many of whom you (and/or your fellow coworkers) routinely encounter. Also imagine feeling powerless to do anything about it as your training offers you few options, certainly fewer options *that work*. The viewpoint of the Center is to develop a strategy to scale down confrontations between individuals with mental illness and law enforcement in order to diminish the number of fatal police shootings; it has worked closely with law enforcement over the years to begin promulgating solutions. Co-author and Executive Director John Snook makes his point clear – "By dismantling the mental illness treatment system, we have turned from a mental health crisis from a medical issue to a police issue. This is patently unfair, illogical, and is proving harmful to both the individual in desperate need of care and the officer who is forced to respond." To address these concerns, the report recommends: (1) a reinvestment and "restoration" of mental health care services, particularly for individuals with severe mental illness, (2) to establish a centralized (at the Federal level) tracking and reporting system of police use of deadly force, even if these incidents do not result in death, and (3) assure that any data collection has the capacity to identify the role when law enforcement utilizes use of deadly force. See Table 4.1 for a summary of the report.

While death is the most extreme result of problematic encounters between law enforcement and an individual with mental illness, this remains a very rare event and relatively uncommon. It could be said that these events are becoming increasingly common; however, it is the goal of this section to emphasize routine results from these often-problematic encounters. This is explored further below.

4.3.1 Police–Citizen with Mental Illness Encounters

Unfortunately, with the prevalence of mental health and dwindling treatment options, come the prevalence of conflicts, as made clear with the Treatment Advocacy Center report. These issues have since clearly spilled over into the public consciousness as partially evidenced by recent incidents in the news involving law enforcement and those suffering from mental illness – particularly when these encounters turned deadly. For example, there was the incident in July 2016 with social worker of an autistic man being shot by police in Miami that reverberated in news cycles around the country, with shares on social media with links to Internet sources rehashing the incident (Rabin, 2016). Perhaps the level of attention this story received sparked some conversations about the real issue: fear and

Table 4.1 Summary of undercounted: The role of mental illness in fatal law enforcement encounters (Treatment Advocacy Center, 2017c; Findings, Recommendations, and Since the Study elements are directly quoted from source below)

Overview: This study reviews law enforcement homicide reporting, examines the role of mental illness in the use of deadly force by American law enforcement, and recommends practical changes in policy to aid in reducing fatal police shootings
Findings:
The risk of being killed while being approached or stopped by law enforcement in the community is 16 times higher for individuals with untreated serious mental illness than for other civilians
By the most conservative estimates, at least 1 in 4 fatal law enforcement encounters involves an individual with serious mental illness. When data have been rigorously collected and analyzed, findings indicate as many as half of all law enforcement homicides ends the life of an individual with severe psychiatric disease
The arrest-related death program operated by the Bureau of Justice Statistics within the U.S. Department of Justice is the only federal database that attempts to systematically collect and publish mental health information about law enforcement homicides. The program was suspended in 2015 because the data available to the agency were not credible enough to report
Recommendations to policymakers:
Restore the mental illness treatment system sufficiently that individuals with serious mental illness are not left untreated to the point that their behavior results in law enforcement action
Accurately count and report the number of fatal police encounters in a reliable federal database
Accurately count and report all incidents involving use of all deadly force by law enforcement, not only those incidents that result in death
Systematically identify the role of mental illness in fatal law enforcement encounters
Since the study:
The 21st Century Cures Act, passed by Congress and signed by President Obama in December 2016, included a mandate for the U.S. attorney general to collect and report data on the role of serious mental illness in fatal law enforcement encounters
The Bureau of Justice Statistics overhauled its system for collecting law enforcement homicide data and, in December 2016, resumed reporting arrest-related death statistics. Using the new methodology approximately doubled the number of arrest-related deaths that were verified and reported by the Department of Justice. The role of mental illness in them has not yet been reported

misunderstanding as it relates to mental illness. Was this a case of fear and misunderstanding? With all of the officer-involved shootings and social unrest as of late, has the fear of violence led to more aggressive response by police? Would understanding autism have helped to ensure everyone's safety in this situation?

In this Miami incident, police were dispatched to a scene with the information that a man was on a city street threatening to commit suicide with a gun. This turns out to be not the case. After the chaos settled, police learned that a 23-year-old man with autism was holding a toy truck. When the officers reached the scene, they rightly identified the man who created the disturbance that prompted the call to 911; yet, this man was not responding to their orders. A caretaker from a nearby mental health facility attempted to intervene and explain the nonthreatening situation. Somehow the situation escalated to the point that the officers on the scene fired upon the autistic man and his caretaker, and both were injured. Bystander cell phone video was delivered quickly to the local media, which depicted the caretaker laying prone, hands clearly in the air, next to the man creating the disturbance who was sitting Indian-style with an object in his hand. The caretaker's attempts to intervene were obviously unsuccessful. This bystander-shot video is one of many recently shared on the Internet that have been a potent tool of critique of law enforcement tactics. These videos can also be a useful training tool and conversation starter on common problems that have been long simmering beneath the surface of public scrutiny.

Law enforcement officers hold difficult jobs for many reasons, as it is the nature of the position and the need for quick, split-second thinking that can have considerable consequences. Further complicating police use of force decisions described above are the instances colloquially called "death by cop" or "suicide by police." In this scenario, an individual provokes and intends to be shot and killed by a police officer. This is not only disturbing for the individual involved, but also by law enforcement. For example, in the suburban and rural areas just north of New Orleans – an hour's drive away from the city – two citizens recently confronted law enforcement with the intent of having officers end their lives by forced execution (within two days of each other; Rodrigue, 2017). In one case, officers attempted to engage in a traffic stop for a simple violation, the man in the car began to speed away and led officers on a high-speed chase. This resulted in a crash, with the man leaving the car with a machete and subsequently yelling at officers to "shoot me, just shoot me." In the second case, a woman in a rural area armed with a gun was engaging in similar behaviors when police were called to her house. In both cases, police were successful in de-escalating the situation and able to connect these "suspects" with mental health services in lieu of arrest. These starkly different outcomes from Miami story versus the one out of the New Orleans area are striking. The case where no deadly weapon was found to be in play turned out to be potentially fatal for two citizens while the cases where deadly weapons were clearly identified resulted in no one being harmed. Actually, the latter resulted in real help for the two individuals that needed it.

Maybe further investing in TRT (Tactical Response Teams) SWAT (or Special Weapons and Tactics team) training can help in these situations? According to the National Tactical Officers Association (NTOA, 2018), a Special Weapons and Tactics (SWAT) team whose members are trained to respond and resolve *all* of the following: "hostage rescue, barricaded gunman, sniper operations, high-risk warrant service and high-risk apprehension, high-risk security operations, terrorism response, special assignments and other incidents which exceed the capability and/or capacity or an agency's first responders and/or investigative units" (10). A TRT is a subtype of SWAT that, by definition, handles a single or combination of capacities above, yet not all of them. For SWAT (and, at times, for TRT), both law enforcement and emergency personnel train and work together to complete the missions of the specialized team. Also, as one would assume with the term "high risk," these missions can involve some potentially life-threatening or violent scenarios. For instance, take high-risk warrant service and apprehensions. Often these involve a person who is wanted for murder or a violent crime. The SWAT team would be engaged and briefed on the mission to serve the warrant and apprehend the wanted individual prior to going out in the field. Then, the team would travel to the location and attempt, and ideally successfully apprehend the individual. Obviously, much of this process involves potentially risky engagement. It is possible that the wanted individual is armed and willing to "put up a fight" if needed. Additionally, there may be a group of individuals armed with weapons at the location of interest. Also, if the individual does resist arrest in any way, the SWAT team may use force, including deadly force. All of these potential scenarios put both the law enforcement, medical personnel, wanted individual(s), and even bystanders/witnesses at risk of injury or death.

Yet, the often-aggressive tactics and appearance of SWAT is almost certainly contraindicated in most cases discussed here. A simple Internet search of SWAT and mental health uncovers some signs of trouble regarding the use of SWAT for individuals with mental illness. For example, an expose of the Chicago Police Department's use of SWAT for mental-health-related events revealed at least 38 clear cases that met these criteria, some with tragic outcomes (Lazare & Southorn, 2017). In fact, it appears that Chicago Police Department's use of SWAT in these situations is increasing. A Boston Globe reported recently featured a heartbreaking interview with a father in Hingham, Massachusetts who lost his son in a mental health-related SWAT raid. On July 8, 2017, Austin Reeves locked himself in his bedroom with his dog and a gun and told his family he needed some time alone. Leading up to this situation, Austin, age 26, was speaking with his ex-girlfriend on the phone. He was reeling from their recent breakup, and he was clearly distraught – to the point she hung up with Austin and quickly called the police to check on his welfare. As a result, the police had called the Reeves' house phone and got a hold of Russell Reeves, Austin's father. Learning about what was going on, Russell checked the guns in his house and found that they were all locked, as always. Austin arrived at the family house shortly thereafter and was met by his father explaining the situation and asking if he was okay. Austin grew upset when he learned the police had called the house, which he fled to his bedroom to be alone as a result. Russell, feeling out of options, called the police back asking for help. This escalated over a period 10 hours from the moment two uniformed police arrived at a full SWAT response and standoff with the police. How did a routine call about a family in distress turn into SWAT response? His father pleaded with police just to leave the family alone at that point, yet the police did not stand down. Eventually, the SWAT team infiltrated his bedroom and shot Austin, resulting in his death. To further intensify the pain of the Reeves family, the Hingham Police Department left a message on the family answering machine sometime after the standoff that was intended for the neighbors also impacted by this event: "Hello, this is a message from the Hingham Police Department. the Hingham Police Department would like to thank you for your cooperation this morning and notify you that the incident on Edgar Walker Court has been resolved. Thank you" (Russell, 2017).

Can some of the SWAT training can be applicable to or hinder decision-making when officers are serving on their regular duties? Many SWAT training materials cover crisis response, but it is unclear exactly how much mental health programming is delivered across the country. In fact, in the latest national SWAT standards guide, only two mentions to mental health/illness are made – suggesting that SWAT add a mental health liaison to serve as an advisor to SWAT when deploying a crisis negotiation team (as an "optimal" option) and that SWAT teams *should* train their personnel to determine the presence of mental illness among barricaded suspects (NTOA, 2018). Much more research is direly needed in this area to address these emerging and potentially more common interactions, particularly as these trends are perceived to be on an upward trend.

4.3.1.1 Baltimore, Maryland: A Model Story for Systemic Failure on the Frontline

The Baltimore Police Department (BPD) has been in the news a number of times, unfortunately most have been for extremely negative circumstances and events relating to mental illness (Young, 2016). According to the U.S. Department of Justice's (DOJ) Civil Rights Division report on the BPD:

- BPD's use of force against individuals with mental health disabilities or experiencing crisis violates the Americans with Disabilities Act.
- BPD's officers routinely use unreasonable force against individuals with mental health disabilities or those experiencing a crisis in violation of the Fourth Amendment. Additionally, by routinely using unreasonable force against individuals with mental health disabilities, BPD officers repeatedly fail to make reasonable modifications to void discrimination in violation of Title II of the American Disabilities Act of 1990.
- Since 2004, BPD has provided some specialized training to its new officers on how to interact with individuals with disabilities and those in crisis. But this training has not been provided to all officers (Department of Justice, 2016).

In many investigated situations, officers have assaulted vulnerable citizens, many of which have not committed a crime. Some of these assaults escalated into the use of unnecessary nonlethal force (e.g., deploying a Taser device) and lethal force resulting in at least one death. According to a recent Baltimore Sun article, "ACLU-Maryland reports that of the 109 people who died in police interactions from 2004-2014, 38 percent (41 people) were likely individuals with mental health and/or substance abuse issues" (Young, 2016). Again, these conflicting statistics underscore the need of monitoring such practices as indicated in the Treatment Advocacy Center report highlighted earlier in this chapter.

The BPD is only one department with clear and substantiated evidence of "engag[ing] in systemic disability-based discrimination" despite the many investigated across the nation done by DOJ. This is extremely disheartening for many reasons since these issues include both concerns with regards to individuals with disabilities as well as race concerns. The article discusses further that the police being the first responders to mental health calls is part of the overarching problem in not only Baltimore, but the criminal justice system as a whole. Community responses have begun to offer suggestions to overcome the struggles of those with mental illness in the area. Those responses begin with the idea of addressing this issue as a "healthcare matter" rather than a criminal justice/law enforcement issue. As stated over and over in this book and research surrounding this topic, the outlook by both the community and the DOJ is to gear toward more community care those with mental illness. The goal here is not only to reduce individuals re-entering the criminal justice system, but also to avoid entry to begin with in the first place. Baltimore is in dire need of a crisis response team to help with the increasing problem of caring for those with mental illness. This would not only take the burden from the police department, but also ensure those who need would receive proper care.

4.3.1.2   Not All Is Lost: Positive Law Enforcement Interactions

A little training can, in fact, go a long way. Consider an expose featured on Vox, entitled, "How America's criminal justice system became the country's mental health system," which details the story of Kevin Earley of Fairfax County, Virginia. At the time the article was published in 2016, Kevin was 37 and the interviews of himself and of his father shed light on the struggles he has had with his own mental health and how this has subsequently intersected with law enforcement. Both Kevin, and his father Pete, share multiple experience with police in Kevin's time of crisis with his mental illness. In one instance, Kevin explains his experience with a police officer during an encounter that resulted in his arrest and further paranoid, while in his last serious encounter is much more positive:

> One encounter began shortly after a psychotic episode that briefly landed him in an emergency room in 2002. Within 48 hours, Kevin wrapped tinfoil around his head, claiming that the CIA was reading his thoughts. He slipped out of the house and broke into a stranger's home to take a bubble bath, and eventually several officers and a police dog arrested him and took him into custody.

> [Yet, in] Kevin's last serious encounter with police in 2006, he was staying at a safe house, where people with mental health problems could relax for a night. There, he took off his clothes – thinking it made him invisible – and walked outside. A police officer, with training for mental health crises, approached Kevin. Kevin was scared, remembering the last time police approached him (and tased him). But this officer talked softly, reasoned with him, and, finally, convinced him to get into the car – no violence necessary. The cop didn't take Kevin to jail – he took him to a hospital. There, Kevin got a case manager. She fended off criminal charges, got Kevin into a "housing first" program for aid, and helped him sign up into a jobs program where he learned to become a peer-to-peer support specialist. (Lopez, 2016)

This last encounter with police in Fairfax county significantly changed Kevin's life situation. For the past 10 years, he has not had any negative police contact and has been under proper medication and care for his illness. Just a change in the approach taken by first responders can have lifelong positive outcomes. Kevin's story is a success story. He and his father believe that his final encounter resulted in transformative change as he was treated as a mental health patient and not a criminal. He was approached in a different manner by professionals who understood his illness and were focused on providing help in his time of need. While the systemic changes needed for agencies such as the Baltimore Police Department will take time, the good news is that there are plenty of documented stories of success to keep the faith that, in time, things can improve with dedicated positive momentum.

4.3.1.3 The Treatment Advocacy Center Issues Road Runners Report

In 2019, the Treatment Advocacy Center issued a new report in partnership with the National Sheriffs' Association and the New York State Association of Chiefs of Police detailing the results of a national survey of sheriffs' offices and police departments on the "outsized role law enforcement plays in psychiatric crisis response and transportation… [to provide] a glimpse into the burdens being shouldered by law enforcement, and the fiscal and society implications of that reality" (2). In essence, by focusing on crisis response and transportation, the report claims that we can better understand the full scope of crisis caused by failing to adequately address mental health concerns in our communities.

To fully research the topic, the study employs a survey and in-depth interviews with key leaders of select jurisdictions to aid in the development of case studies. The survey was electronic, sent out to the National Sheriffs' Association membership (over 3000+ Sheriffs' offices) and the state association of chiefs of police email listserv (to forward on the message to each state's chiefs of police). In response, 355 law enforcement agencies participated – a response rate indicative of Internet-based surveys. While the results should be interpreted with some caution, the key findings were compelling. In 2017: (1) a substantial portion of agency budgets were spent responding to and transporting individuals in a mental health crisis – an average of 10% of their budget overall across responding law enforcement agencies; (2) for agencies that were able to report actualized costs, the report found that a total of $17.7 million dollars was spent on transportation costs alone; (3) at times when law enforcement is able to transport individuals in a mental health crisis to a medical facility instead of a jail, these facilities tend to five times farther away, on average, yielding significant time, effort, and expense on transportation alone; (4) for agencies that were able to report actualized time and effort for transportation, these agencies reported 165,295 hours solely spent on this task, *or 21% of total staff time*; (5) the mean time officers had to wait at emergency departments after transport was 3 hours, versus a mean wait time of 37 minutes after transport to jail.

These findings help us understand the importance of developing tailored solutions that include law enforcement to some degree. The survey that drives the Road Runner study requested some feedback from agencies on a nonexhaustive list of emerging solutions, such as Crisis Intervention Team (CIT) training, coresponder teams that feature mental health professional and law enforcement partnerships to address these calls for service, mobile crisis or assertive community treatment teams to aid or displace law enforcement with these calls for service, and/or develop a centralized crisis receiving center to serve in any of the aforementioned designs to be able to accept individuals in lieu of jails or emergency departments, when warranted. The main point is – the system is spending so much time, effort, energy, and money into a broken system. This report reveals actual costs in a way that promotes some self-reflection. The system is spending substantial time and money, why not spend it on evidence-based solutions that can yield positive outcomes?

4.3.2   Interfacing with the Homeless or Near Homeless Population

One interrelated issue worth mention here is the lack of trust vulnerable populations have with police and emergency medical services, largely due to years of misunderstanding, miscues, and problematic encounters. This trust may be further eroding giving the unresolved issues described above, exacerbating the crisis on the street. In 2004, Kakrison, Hamel, and Hwang published a study focusing on the trust homeless people in Toronto have with local police and paramedics, and potential health-related outcomes. Perhaps their findings are not so surprising; among their sample of 160 homeless Canadians staying at a local shelter when surveyed, there was a wide margin of difference in willingness to call the police in times of emergency relative to emergency medical services (69% of the sample compared to 92%, in the same order as listed). This was surely related to the differences in the level of trust these homeless individuals had in these professionals (a median of 3 out of 5 for police versus a 5 out of 5 for emergency medical services personnel, with one representing the lowest trust and five representing the highest trust). Additional responses from this sample are quite compelling: about one in ten self-reported an assault by a police officer in the last year while none reported such an action by emergency medical services personnel.

What if there is no assurance on who would arrive on a scene of an emergency if emergency dispatch was called? What if, since 2004, these levels of trust have further eroded, especially in the United States that does not feature universal health care coverage as its neighbor to the north? Answers to such questions still allude us, as is common theme for this text.

4.4   Evidence-Based Solutions

Great strides have been made in the development of evidenced-based services and programs to address the ongoing mental health crisis in the United States. For law enforcement, the Bureau of Justice Assistance (2022) and its partners have produced the Police-Mental Health Collaboration Toolkit that can educate key stakeholders and community partners on the most progressive and research-informed practices available today. The dedicated website for the toolkit features an easy-to-follow, step-by-step guide to the ten essential elements of police and mental health collaborations that have proven to be successful in the jurisdictions that have implemented it: (1) collaborative planning and implementation, (2) program design, (3) specialized training, (4) call-taker and dispatcher protocol assessment and revision, (5) stabilization, observation, and disposition, (6) transportation and custodial transfer, (7) information exchange and confidentiality, (8) treatment, supports, and services, (9) organizational support, and (10) program evaluation and sustainability. The most recent toolkit, updated in 2020, features new content that expands this endeavor to include supports for people with mental illness and/or intellectual and developmental disabilities (I/DD). The updated content also features a self-assessment tool law enforcement agencies and their stakeholders can utilize to assess their local progress of instituting interventions.

Currently, the website includes the learning experiences and successes of the Arlington, Houston, Los Angeles, Madison (Wisconsin), Miami-Dade, Portland, Salt Lake City, Tucson, the University of Florida, and Wichita Police Departments as well as the Bexar County (TX), Harris County (TX), and Yavapai County (AZ) Sheriffs' Offices in customizing programming to meet their needs as well as their communities' needs. The common features of each are explored below.

4.4.1   *Crisis Intervention Teams:* **The** *Preferred Solution*

Crisis Intervention Team (CIT) programs "[are] community partnership[s] of law enforcement, mental health and addiction professionals, individuals who live with mental illness and/or addiction disorders, their families and other advocates" (Crisis Intervention Team International, 2022). First developed in Memphis, and sometimes known as the "Memphis Model," CIT programming offers police-based training from an inventive first-responder model. The *team* aspect of CIT primarily involves law enforcement and local mental health providers and other related service providers. The overarching goal of the partnership is to aid in working with a person in crisis and route these individuals to medical treatment in lieu of criminal justice processing that has become so common, creating a seamless flow for individuals with mental health concerns to receive services in the community. This often starts with dispatch flagging calls for service, relaying relevant information over to officers who receive dedicated CIT training, and linking up with professionals in the community who are plugged into the CIT partnership to address potential clients' needs. Each CIT is customized to the local community, and as such, are nimble to adapt to changes in the community. The model prioritizes and promotes the best welfare for people in crisis as well as concretely connecting them with the best option for success and recovery. Additionally, CIT provides for a safer interaction for law enforcement in the event of a crisis situation.

The National Alliance on Mental Illness and their local affiliates have been key in promulgating CIT training across the country. These trainings have become standardized, and feature 40 hours of training on the following topics:

- *Learning from mental health professionals and experienced officers in your community.* One of the reasons CIT is successful is that it connects officers with a team of clinicians and fellow officers who can advise, problem-solve and support them when a challenging situation occurs.
- *Personal interaction with people who have experienced and recovered from mental health crisis and with family members who have cared for loved ones with mental illness.* NAMI members present at the training, providing officers a first-hand opportunity to hear stories of recovery, ask questions and learn what helps (and harms) when a person is in a crisis.
- *Verbal de-escalation skills.* CIT teaches a new set of skills for ensuring officer safety – the words, approach and body language that convince a person to get help, or defuse a potentially violent encounter.
- *Scenario-based training on responding to crises.* With the help of volunteers or actors, officers practice their skills in common crisis situations, and get immediate feedback from instructors and classmates. (NAMI, 2022).

The standardized curriculum was developed through a partnership of the National Alliance on Mental Illness, the University of Memphis Crisis Intervention Team Center, CIT International, and the International Association of Chiefs of Police. Since implementation, research has shown the difference coordinated training can make: in Memphis, dispatch calls for "mental disturbances" fell substantially, by 80%; CIT-trained officers surveyed by researchers reveal that they feel they spend less time on such calls and feel more effective on meeting the needs of people with mental illness in their community; and CIT makes a clear difference in connecting citizens to the services that they need (e.g., counseling, medication, and other forms of treatment) relative to individuals being processed by the criminal justice system (Borum et al., 1998; Compton et al., 2011; Dupont & Cochran, 2002; NAMI, 2022; Tully & Smith, 2015).

With such enthusiasm and empirical support, many cities are moving toward positive and proactive measure to help educate local law enforcement and better help the citizens they serve. One way this is happening is to have officers trained in mental health practices. For example, New Orleans Police Department (NOPD), now trains officers regularly in CIT with the hopes to continue with more and more both new and veteran officers trained. This is a new concept and will hopefully prove to be effective for the city of New Orleans when dealing with individuals in crisis. On the downside, the state of Louisiana continues to have budget cuts that directly affect the amount of treatment, specifically inpatient hospitals, in order to treat those with mental illness properly.

Having law enforcement trained in handling individuals with mental illness and those in crisis is essential because they are often the first to arrive on the scene when emergency services are called. Also, keeping in mind that not all information is accurate when a phone call is made for emergency assistance. For example, a bystander may call 911 if a person is wandering through a public setting yelling at strangers. The bystander may have little to no information about the person or the situation but observes an individual in an irate situation. A police officer is then dispatched to the scene with no information regarding the mental status of the irate person. It is important that the officer approach the scene with caution for many reasons.

4.4.2 Mental Health First Aid

Originating in Australia, the Mental Health First Aid curriculum was developed in 2001 by a nurse with a background in health education, named Betty Kitchener, and a professor of mental health literacy, named Tony Jorm. It has become known to be a rigorous, yet "light" course that is delivered in eight hours. Mental Health First Aid has been likened to the mental health equivalent of CPR for nonclinicians when attending to a heart attack, with the goal of being able to appropriately and effectively intervene until "the real help arrives" – the trained professionals (Mental Health First Aid USA, 2022). The curriculum features ways to understand stigma, basic mental health knowledge, and related topics; however, the main focus of the course is to be competent in a five-step action plan in cases of a panic attack, suicidality, or an overdose situation. As such, it gives a practical and evidence-based approach to tending to these situations when they occur. Further, Mental Health First Aid appeared on SAMHSA's National Registry of Evidence-Based Programs and Practices as a promising strategy in improving knowledge, attitudes, and beliefs about mental illness as well as nonspecific mental health disorders and symptoms (SAMHSA, 2022). This registry has recently been relaunched as the Evidence-Based Practices Resource Center; while MHFA is not specifically listed on the resource center, it will likely be featured there someday soon given the robust evidence in the literature supporting the program's ability to increase mental health awareness among participants.

For first responders, Mental Health First Aid appends their knowledge, skillset, and tools to effectively attend to mental health crises. Anecdotally, this evidence-based practice is proving effective in these professions. For example, in a recent article from the Department of Homeland Security First Responder division (formerly under the website firstresponder.gov), a fire and rescue captain expressed his observations of the Mental Health First Aid Curriculum:

> Law enforcement is beginning to recognize that some of the situations they have found themselves in recently have been misjudgments of people with mental health issues…and if they had been able to recognize certain symptoms, they may not have taken the, you know, forcible action that they took….[If first responders] don't have a baseline training for these guys,… they can only draw on their own experience. And if they don't have any experience [dealing with mental illness], then they're going to come up with their own idea of whether it's right or wrong. We'd rather make a decision than not make a decision. (Department of Homeland Security, 2015)

The article expresses other first responder leadership's impression of the training in a positive light while explicitly suggesting others consider joint investment in both CIT and Mental Health First Aid. Notably, Mental Health First Aid is much cheaper and quicker to deploy, while also allowing for easily local sustainability through the form of "train-the-trainer" curriculum. That is, Mental Health First Aid offers standardized courses for individuals interested in becoming certified instructors. Thus, if a local jurisdiction wishes to make Mental Health First Aid available to a wide array of consumers, including first responders, they may simply invest in an initial round of training while also selecting a subset of trainees to receive instructor certification. These local instructors would then continue training until the local goal is met. This is the approach a regional National Alliance on Mental Health affiliate of Louisiana took in late 2015, continuing on through the current day. As of this writing, this NAMI office has trained several hundred trainees, including local judges, law enforcement, probation and parole, emergency medical services personnel, jail correctional officers and staff, and so on. While the impact of this initiative is unknown, the perception of the trainees has been positive (Richard, 2017).

4.4.3   Alternative Destination Pilot Project: North Carolina

North Carolina developed a novel approach to for emergency medical services working with patients with mental illness – called the Alternative Destination program. Rather than transporting the patients to the emergency room and waiting for a psychiatric evaluation, EMS enabled their personnel to transport them directly to a psychiatric facility. This was piloted initially in 2009, and has been expanded upon in recent years. The wait times in North Carolina emergency rooms were looming, medical professionals were overwhelmed, and resources were strapped. The Alternative Destination pilot project in Wake County, North Carolina set out to alleviate these problems in a smarter way.

The Alternative Destination protocol was strictly defined to focus resources on those who need it the most, yet who are not in exigent need of *emergency* medical services: (1) primarily, patients must not be experiencing a mental health crisis to a point that may require sedation or show an acute change in mental health status, (2) a patient's pulse is no more than 120 (signifying potential agitation or excited delirium, for example), (3) a patient cannot present with other acute medical symptomatology, (4) an extremely liberal blood alcohol content level must be met (up to 0.40, or anything less than five times the legal limit; note: if this condition is met with a high BAC while the other conditions presented here are met, this is an indicator of high alcohol tolerance), (5) each patient must be able to perform the activities of daily living (ADLs, or self-feeding, bathing, personal hygiene, dressing, using the bathroom and toilet hygiene, and walking and/or mobility), and (6) a patient must have a blood-glucose level of less than 300 mg/dL. If all of these qualifiers are met, EMS can redirect the patient to other medical facilities qualified to handle these patients with available space. To implement this protocol and its strict guidelines, "advanced practice paramedics" were trained using a 240-hour course, including topics such as available mental health resources within their own community as well as patient evaluation and assessment. By 2015, 20 trained advanced practice paramedics were active in Wake County, with over thirty others trained and ready to activate. Initial internal evaluations have been compelling: Miller (2015) reports that the pilot project has reduced emergency department transports by 20% from 2013 through 2015 by directing 764 patients to other facilities out of 3831 total mental health and/or substance abuse evaluations by advanced practice paramedics.

Over the length of a year, it was estimated that the program saved $500,000 in Medicaid costs. Unfortunately, as often in the case with innovative programming, the pilot has led to some stumbling blocks. For instance, despite the decrease in costs to Medicaid, the local EMS budget was strained due to reduced reimbursements as premiums are placed on transports to the emergency departments. This becomes a difficult paradox in that transportation directly to the psychiatric facility for treatment is best for the patient in need, yet does not allow for reimbursement most of the related activities (including the increased work of the newly-trained advanced practice paramedics). Although, in the grand scheme of things, this pilot program is better for the emergency medical care system as well – and the system as a whole has been committed to seeing the program work.

The Alternative Destination pilot program appears to be a beneficial option for individuals who experience mental illness symptoms regularly but are not actively in the midst of a crisis. Those that may need a medication adjustment, have not been harmed in any way, and have or were always not in a panic attack or related moment. On a positive note, programs like the Alternative Destination pilot program are beginning to catch the attention of governments and other areas across the nation. The North Carolina state government has recognized the program which has helped to spread information. Similarly, over 260 programs throughout the United States have begun to implement similar protocols.

4.4.4 Community Paramedic Program: Grady EMS (Atlanta)

Meanwhile, in Atlanta, the Grady County EMS (GEMS) Vice President of Operations, Michael Colman began a search for a better option for the mental health calls in the area. Colman was able to identify that about 6%, or 6410, of the 911 calls to GEMS were determined to be psychiatric or suicide related. He reviewed the call volume data and was able to further determine that those that called EMS at least five a month were often made from individuals that had a mental illness. "A financial analysis using a sample of 156 patients from this group determined that it cost Grady EMS over $100 more than they received in reimbursement for each of these transports. In addition, the emergency department spent over $400 more on each patient than they received in reimbursement" (Stanaway, 2016). Consider here, this is the amount is *in addition to* what is already being reimbursed by Medicaid, insurance, et cetera.

In response to this information, Grady EMS implemented a community paramedic project. The California Emergency Medical Services Authority offers fine details about this model:

- Community Paramedicine (CP) is an innovative and evolving model of community-based healthcare designed to provide more effective and efficient services at a lower cost. Community Paramedicine allows paramedics to function outside their traditional emergency response and transport roles to help facilitate more appropriate use of emergency care resources while enhancing access to primary care for medically underserved populations.
- Community Paramedics are licensed paramedics who have received specialized training in addition to general paramedicine training and work within a designated Community Paramedicine program under local medical control as part of a community-based team of health and social services providers. Paramedics are uniquely positioned for expanded roles as they are geographically dispersed in nearly all communities, inner-city and rural; always available; work in home and community-based settings; are trusted and accepted by the public; are trained to make health status assessments; recognize and manage life-threatening conditions outside of the hospital; and operate under medical control as part of an organized, systems approach to care (CEMSA, 2022).

Grady EMS looked to find a solution to help patients experiencing a mental health crisis other than the typical means. Those in crisis "were routinely subjected to unplanned physical restraint, chemical restraint, police restraint and even arrest" (Stanaway, 2016). This is to say that a person experiencing a mental health crisis were often not able to be de-escalated without the use of physical force and/or medication. These are also extra costs as well as safety concerns for all involved.

This pilot program was developed in 2012 and put into operations in early 2013. Grady EMS created a crisis response team which includes a paramedic, a Grady Health System licensed counselor, a Behavioral Health Link clinical social worker, and even, at times, a third-year psychiatry resident. This crisis team responded with the regular EMS staff during the pilot phase of the project. Additionally, the crisis team could be dispatched at the request of those on scene, but did not respond alone and was only available on weekdays. Their part in the on scene process was to provide an assessment and a medical evaluation for the patient in need.

Later, after completion of the pilot phase, the program began implementing the full program. In the full program, the crisis intervention team was then able to respond as an independent unit without regular EMS accompaniment. Further, rather than just the original 40 hours per week availability, the program was expanded to 80 hours to allow for additional services to be provided. GEMS personnel used the Georgia Crisis Action Line (GCAL) in the field when the team was not available:

> GCAL is the 24/7 hotline for accessing mental health services in Georgia. The Georgia Department of Behavioral Health and Developmental Disabilities (DBHDD) provides treatment and support services to people with mental illnesses and addictive diseases, and support to people with mental retardation and related developmental disabilities. (NAMI Georgia, 2021)

Calling GCAL involves a mental health professional the ability to evaluate a patient via phone contact. This evaluation can take place in a matter of minutes and result

Community Paramedicine Pilot Projects, 2018   16 PROJECTS • 12 SITES • 6 CONCEPTS

PD Post-Discharge. Provide short-term, home-based follow-up care for persons recently discharged from a hospital due to a serious health condition to decrease hospital readmissions within 30 days.

TB Directly Observed TB Therapy. Collaborate with local public health services to provide directly observed therapy to persons with tuberculosis (i.e., dispense medications and observe patients taking them to assure effective treatment) to prevent its spread.

HO Hospice. In response to 911 calls, collaborate with hospice agency nurses, patients, and family members to treat patients in their homes, according to their wishes, instead of transporting them to the ED.

EM Frequent EMS Users. Provide case management services to persons who are frequent 911 callers or frequent visitors to EDs to reduce their use of the EMS system by connecting them with primary care, behavioral health, housing, and social services.

Projects approved November 2017. Expected to be operational spring 2018.

Alternate Destinations

MH Mental Health. In response to 911 calls, offer patients who have mental health needs but no emergent medical needs transport to a mental health crisis center instead of an ED.

SC Sobering Center. In response to 911 calls, offer patients who are acutely intoxicated but have no emergent medical needs transport to a sobering center instead of an ED.

The California Health Care Foundation provided support for state-level project management and independent evaluation.

For more information on community paramedicine programs operating today in California, visit www.emsa.ca.gov/community_paramedicine.

Fig. 4.1 Latest Community Paramedicine projects offered by the Emergency Medical Services Authority of California, a leader in community paramedicine innovation

in a number of options with the best interest of the patient upheld. If necessary, the mental health professional could have the paramedics on scene transport the patient directory to a psychiatric facility. Further aiding in the success of the program, Grady EMS created a process that allows 911 dispatchers to transfer some calls directly to the GCAL, if certain criteria are met. GCAL can also call Grady EMS back if an ambulance is in fact needed respond (Fig. 4.1).

Coordinated programs like this one have allowed patients who would otherwise have been arrested or possibly restrained in a most disruptive situation to receive care in a better manner while also saving money and resources. This can be shown by the data, "In 2013, Grady EMS dispatch transferred 175 calls directly to Behavioral Health Line saving Grady EMS about $13,000. The Grady EMS Upstream Crisis Intervention Group responded to 20% of EMD category 25 calls totaling 1,250 responses. The team obtained 275 refusals/no transports. Many of those patients were provided with safety plans and outpatient appointments, which prevented unnecessary emergency department visits totaling about 1,925 bed hours" (Stanaway, 2016). Michael Colman described the financial aspect of the changes within the program and has estimated it to over $140,000 and adding in the referrals that did not require transports savings of $248,000 for 2013. Additionally, "In 2014 the psych unit responded to 1,778 calls, potentially saving EMS over $100,000. In 2015, Grady EMS received 7,668 calls that were psychiatric in nature. Of those, the psych unit handled over 20 percent, again saving EMS over $100,000" (Stanaway, 2016).

Another added benefit of the program is also the job satisfaction increase for Grady EMS. As discussed in another chapter, burnout and compassion fatigue are common occurrences of jobs as first responders often responding to crisis on a regular basis. According to the program director Tina Wright, staff reported a "higher-than-normal" job satisfaction as the program kicked into high gear. Wright discussed that many staff members feel as though they are really making a positive change in their community which has led to a personal sense of satisfaction.

4.4.5   A Survey of Other Approaches Across the Country

There are many more instances of successful and budding programs being sown across the United States. Indeed, there does appear to be progress in the disarray of the current state of the mental health system of care. For example, the State of California is engaging in 13 community paramedicine projects, adopting this model to localized needs (CEMSA, 2017). Madison, Wisconsin is one of six law enforcement-mental health learning sites and serves as a model for other sister jurisdictions (City of Madison, 2015). Statewide efforts have been made in Colorado, Connecticut, Florida, Georgia, Illinois, Maine, Ohio, and Utah to provide specialized training in police responses in cases of mental illness and mental health crises (Bureau of Justice Assistance, 2022). In Alabama, the Birmingham Police Department has a number of programs within their Community Services Division that help to improve the overall relations between the public and law enforcement. These improvements are sought to be done through a variety of community services initiatives. One program specifically works to improve the process of police call outs dealing with individuals with mental illness. The program involved specially trained officers called Community Services Officers (CSOs) that "provide crisis intervention social services through direct service, referral and consultation. Their objective is to stabilize a crisis, attempt to prevent further crises, and enhance their client's well-being. They network and maintain professional relationships with relative community resources and strive to provide exemplary crisis intervention services" (Birmingham Police Department, 2022).

Other communities are adopting a nonlaw enforcement-based team of mental health personnel to respond to crisis calls for service, a mobile crisis intervention program with roots that stretch as far back as 30 years – as is the case for one of the oldest programs of its kind in Eugene, Oregon, called CAHOOTS (Crisis Assistance Helping Out On The Streets). Specifically, CAHOOTS works closely with Eugene Police Department to be the initial contact with individuals in crisis and is the primary mode of transportation of individuals needing nonemergency medical care – handling about 15% of the total calls for service for EPD in 2019, diverting up to 8% of calls completely from the police (Eugene Police Department, 2022).

Much more innovation is occurring in recent years, many of which are smaller pilots that have promise for broader adoption. One thing is for certain, much of the innovation is occurring on the local level, as guided by national resources and broader research trends. While this section does not offer a comprehensive review of the innovations occurring across the country, it is important to note that there has been an explosion of activity of collaborative projects in recent years. This is likely to continue for some years to come. Perhaps in the near future, there will be a clearinghouse of projects similar to other resource databases that have grown popular in recent years.

In 2020, Vera researchers (Beck, Reuland, and Pope) reached out to experts in the field with knowledge of innovations in police–mental health collaborations in search of the most promising approaches across the country. In doing so, they uncovered a typology that ranges on a continuum with police-based responses on one extreme and community-based responses on the other. In the middle of their continuum lies a balanced police-based, coresponse model that encapsulates hybrid approaches. Further, they describe model programs that fit in these domains: (1) for police-based responses, CIT and case management teams are highlighted, (2) for coresponse, primary (when clinicians ride along with police officers) and secondary coresponse teams (clinicians are called to the scene) are highlighted, and (3) community-based responses, crisis lines, peer navigator programs, mobile crisis teams, and EMS-based responses, and 911 diversion programs are highlighted. The Vera study goes on to explore three detailed case studies, including CAHOOTS (described above), the Crisis Response Unit and Familiar Faces programs recently rolled out in Olympia, Washington, and the 911 call diversion to the Crisis Response Network at Phoenix Police Department. Each of these collaborations have deployed evidence-based practices to customize a solution thought to work best for each locale, yet the report highlights some of the hard work to overcome hesitancy to change. For example, the report discusses concerns among Olympia Police Department's officers about civilians having access *and being users* of their police radio frequency. Through collaboration, these fears were overcome through documented successes in dispatching crisis calls to the Crisis Response Unit. Documented successes, such as the ones found in this report, will be crucial for broader buy-in of police–mental health collaborations across the country.

4.5 Conclusion

A persistent issue presented in this chapter is the lack of awareness and training of mental illness among those who currently need it the most, American first responders. This often leads to problematic, and sometimes deadly, police–citizen encounters. While the American public often only learns of the most troublesome of these encounters through the media, bystander accounts and video, and so on, there has been a great deal of innovation to ameliorate the volatility of these encounters through training, partnerships, policy changes, and strategic alterations of systemic responses to potential mental health calls for service. With so much focus placed on law enforcement, it is important to take a step back and take full stock of the collaborative nature among medicine, paramedicine, and law enforcement and understand each role for each of their potential to intervene in mental health crisis events.

These collaborative relationships are critical in one of most comprehensive and promising models to address the consistent problems regarding mental illness today – the persistent contact of individuals with mental illness have with the police and the criminal justice system often without addressing any of the underlying mental health concerns. This model, the Crisis Intervention Team, is increasingly a part of the solution for many communities looking to address the persistent issues discussed in this book. Further, this model tends not to be deployed in absence of other evidence-based solutions to address the underlying problems. Programs such as Mental Health First Aid and Community Paramedicine projects are gaining popularity to add additional layers of awareness and system processes to intercept potential criminal justice concerns with community-based services that typically cost taxpayers much less while offering better outcomes.

Finally, it is important to clearly define the role of probation and parole officers (e.g., community corrections) in regard to serving individuals with mental health concerns. These professionals are often overlooked, just when their role appears to be increasing given the pressures to move away from overutilization of American prisons and to alleviate overcrowding in these facilities. At the time of this writing, community corrections has received far less attention in regards to serving Americans with mental illnesses relative to their first responder counterparts. One exception is the utility of specialized caseloads or units, which seem to offer promising advantages over mixed caseloads for probationers and parolees with mental illness.

Discussion Questions

1. What struggles confront those working on the front lines regarding encounters with justice-involved persons who have mental health concerns? Also, consider other types of frontline workers in this reflection as well, such as counselors, social workers, doctors, nurses, correction officers, etc.
2. How does access to care, or the lack thereof, come into play when discussing police interactions with persons who have mental health concerns?
3. How has COVID-19 impacted how frontline workers interface with persons who have mental health concerns?

4. Consider your future career – how does daily interactions with crisis or negative situations impact a person and their job?
5. How does proper training help first responders interact with the public at large? How does training help with interactions with people with mental illness or who are experiencing crisis?

References

Beck, J., Reuland, M., & Pope, L. (2020). *Behavioral health crisis alternatives*. Vera. https://www.vera.org/behavioral-health-crisis-alternatives. Last accessed: 29 Jan 2022

Begun, A. L., Early, T. J., & Hodge, A. (2016). Mental health and substance abuse service engagement by men and women during community reentry following incarceration. *Administration and Policy in Mental Health and Mental Health Services Research, 43*(2), 207–218.

Birmingham Police Department. (2022). Community Outreach and Public Education. URL: https://police.birminghamal.gov/bureaus/patrol/community-outreach-and-public-education/. Last accessed: 12 Sep 2022.

Borum, R., Williams Deane, M., Steadman, H. J., & Morrissey, J. (1998). Police perspectives on responding to mentally ill people in crisis: Perceptions of program effectiveness. *Behavioral Sciences & the Law, 16*(4), 393–405.

Bureau of Justice Assistance. (2022). Police-mental health collaboration (PMHC) Toolkit. URL: https://bja.ojp.gov/program/pmhc/. Last accessed: 12 Sep 22.

California Commision on Peace Officer Standards and Training. (2022). Mental health training in law enforcement. URL: https://post.ca.gov/mental-health-training-in-law-enforcement. Last accessed: 12 Sep 22.

California Emergency Medical Services Authority. (2018). California pilot project overview. https://emsa.ca.gov/wp-content/uploads/sites/71/2017/07/CP-CommunityParamedicineConceptSheets_v3.pdf. Last accessed: 29 Jan 2022.

California Emergency Medical Services Authority. (2022). Introduction to community paramedicine. URL: https://emsa.ca.gov/community_paramedicine/. Last accessed: 12 Sep 22.

California Legislative Information. (2015). SB11. URL: http://www.leginfo.ca.gov/pub/15-16/bill/sen/sb_0001-0050/sb_11_bill_20150323_amended_sen_v97.htm. Last accessed: 12 Sep 22.

City of Madison. (2015). Crisis intervention & mental health. URL: https://www.cityofmadison.com/news/crisisintervention-mental-health. Last accessed: 12 Sep 22.

Compton, M. T., Demir Neubert, B. N., Broussard, B., McGriff, J. A., Morgan, R., & Oliva, J. R. (2011). Use of force preferences and perceived effectiveness of actions among Crisis Intervention Team (CIT) police officers and non-CIT officers in an escalating psychiatric crisis involving a subject with schizophrenia. *Schizophrenia Bulletin, 37*(4), 737–745.

Crisis Intervention Team International. (2022). What is CIT? URL: https://www.citinternational.org/What-is-CIT. Last accessed: 12 Sep 22.

Dupont, R. T., & Cochran, C. S. (2002). The Memphis CIT model. Serving mentally ill offenders. *Challenges and Opportunities for Mental Health Professionals*, 59–69.

Eugene Police Department. (2022). *CAHOOTS*. https://www.eugene-or.gov/4508/CAHOOTS. Last accessed: 29 Jan 2022.

Fiske, Z. R., Songer, D. M., & Schriver, J. L. (2021). A national survey of police mental health training. *Journal of Police and Criminal Psychology, 36*(2), 236–242.

Fuller, D. A., Lamb, H. R., Biasotti, M., & Snook, J. (2015). *Overlooked in the undercounted: The role of mental illness in fatal law enforcement encounters*. http://www.treatmentadvocacycenter.org/storage/documents/overlooked-in-the-undercounted.pdf. Last accessed: 29 Jan 2022.

Hails, J., & Borum, R. (2003). Police training and specialized approaches to respond to people with mental illnesses. *Crime & Delinquency, 49*(1), 52–61.

Ivory, D., Protess, B., & Bennett, K. (2016). When you dial 911 and Wall Street answers. The New York Times. URL: https://www.nytimes.com/2016/06/26/business/dealbook/when-you-dial-911-and-wall-streetanswers.html. Last accessed: 12 Sep 22.

Lazare, S. & Southorn, D. (2017). How do Chicago Police treat mental health? With SWAT raids. The Intercept. URL: https://theintercept.com/2017/08/06/chicago-police-mental-health-swat-raids-militarized/. Last accessed: 12 Sep 22.

Lopez, G. (2016). How America's criminal justice system became the country's mental health system. Vox. URL: https://www.vox.com/2016/3/1/11134908/criminal-justice-mental-health. Last accessed: 12 Sep 22.

Louisiana Commission on Law Enforcement. (2022). What is POST? URL: https://lcle.la.gov/programs/post/. Last accessed: 12 Sep 22.

Lurigio, A. J. (2001). Effective services for parolees with mental illnesses. *Crime & Delinquency, 47*(3), 446–461.

Jacob, L., & Poletick, E. B. (2008). Systematic review: predictors of successful transition to community-based care for adults with chronic care needs. *Care Management Journals, 9*(4), 154–165.

McIntosh, W. L., Spies, E., Stone, D. M., Lokey, C. N., Trudeau, A. T., & Bartholow, B. (2016). Suicide rates by occupational group — 17 States, 2012. MMWR Morb Mortal Wkly Rep 2016;65:641–645. DOI: http://dx.doi.org/10.15585/mmwr.mm6525a1externalicon. Last accessed: 12 Sep 22.

Mental Health First Aid USA. (2022). Mental health first aid. URL: https://www.mentalhealth-firstaid.org/. Last accessed: 12 Sep 22.

Michelen, W., Martinez, J., Lee, A., & Wheeler, D. P. (2006). Reducing frequent flyer emergency department visits. *Journal of Health Care for the Poor and Underserved, 17*(1), 59–69.

Miller, D. L. (2015). Pilot project trains EMS to bypass the ED with mental health patients. EP Monthly. URL: https://epmonthly.com/article/pilot-project-trains-ems-to-bypass-the-ed-with-mental-health-patients/. Last accessed: 12 Sep 22.

Milner, A., Witt, K., Maheen, H., & LaMontagne, A. D. (2017). Suicide among emergency and protective service workers: A retrospective mortality study in Australia, 2001 to 2012. *Work, 57*(2), 281–287.

NAMI. (2022). Crisis intervention team (CIT) programs. URL: https://nami.org/Advocacy/Crisis-Intervention/Crisis-Intervention-Team-(CIT)-Programs. Last accessed: 12 Sep 22.

NAMI Georgia. (2021). Department of behavioral health and developmental disabilities - Meeting agenda minutes. URL: https://namiga.org/wp-content/uploads/sites/21/2021/09/Georgia-9-8-8-Planning-Coalition-Meeting-Minutes_06.24.2021.pdf. Last accessed: 12 Sep 22.

National Tactical Officers Association. (2018). *SWAT standards for law enforcement agencies.* https://ntoa.org/pdf/swatstandards.pdf. Last accessed: 29 Jan 2022.

New York City Probation. (2017). About probation. URL: https://www1.nyc.gov/site/probation/about/aboutdepartment-of-probation.page. Last accessed: 12 Sep 22.

Plohetski, T. (2008). Mental health patients strain Texas EMS resources. *Journal of Emergency Medical Services.* https://www.jems.com/news/mental-health-patients-strain/. Last accessed: 29 Jan 2022.

Police One. (2019). 7 reasons I'm still a police officer. URL: https://www.police1.com/communitypolicing/articles/7-reasons-im-still-a-police-officer-hpUBprMCIOWZLXj0/. Last accessed: 12 Sep 22.

Rabin, C. (2016). Cop shoots caretaker of autistic man playing in the street with toy truck. *Miami Herald.* http://www.miamiherald.com/news/local/crime/article90905442.html. Last accessed: 1 June 2017.

Rodrigue, A. (2017). *Two attempted suicides-by-cop in two days highlight law enforcement struggle with mental illness.* WWLTV. https://www.wwltv.com/article/news/local/north-shore/two-attempted-suicides-by-cop-in-two-days-highlight-law-enforcement-struggle-with-mental-illness/289-440607429. Last accessed: 29 Jan 2022

Russell, J. (2017). His parents said he just needed sleep. A SWAT team came instead. Boston Globe. URL: https://www.bostonglobe.com/metro/2017/07/15/his-parents-said-just-needed-sleep-swat-team-cameinstead/1sTWdBw2MNqqFGCOUfLnHL/story.html. Last accessed: 12 Sep 22.

Stanaway, N. (2016). Community paramedic program cuts mental health patient volume. EMS1. URL: https://www.ems1.com/community-paramedicine/articles/community-paramedic-program-cuts-mental-health-patientcall-volume-x8RRUvL76VDXSbwC/. Last accessed: 12 Sep 22.

Stewart, C. C. & George-Paschal, L. (2017). Barriers to reentry into society: Listening to parolees' perceptions. *American Journal of Occupational Therapy, 71*(4): 1.

Substance Abuse and Mental Health Services Administration. (2022). Evidence-based practices resource center. URL: https://www.samhsa.gov/resource-search/ebp. Last accessed: 12 Sep 22.

Treatment Advocacy Center. (2017a). TAC reports. http://www.treatmentadvocacycenter.org/evidence-and-research/studies. Last accessed: 1 June 2017.

Treatment Advocacy Center. (2017b). *People with untreated mental illness 16 times more likely to be killed by law enforcement.* http://www.treatmentadvocacycenter.org/home-page/71-featured-articles/2976-people-with-untreated-mental-illness-16-times-more-likely-to-be-killed-by-law-enforcement-. Last accessed: 29 Jan 2022.

Treatment Advocacy Center. (2017c). *Overlooked in the undercounted: The role of mental illness in fatal law enforcement encounters.* http://www.treatmentadvocacycenter.org/evidence-and-research/evidence-and-research/3845. Last accessed: 29 Jan 2022.

Treatment Advocacy Center. (2019). *Road runners: The role and impact of law enforcement in transporting individuals with severe mental illness.* https://www.treatmentadvocacycenter.org/road-runners. Last accessed: 29 Jan 2022.

Tully, T., & Smith, M. (2015). Officer perceptions of crisis intervention team training effectiveness. *The Police Journal, 88*(1), 51–64.

US Department of Justice. (2016). Investigation of the Baltimore City Police Department. URL: https://www.justice.gov/crt/file/883296/download. Last accessed: 12 Sep 22.

Wolff, N., Epperson, M., Shi, J., Huening, J., Schumann, B. E., & Sullivan, I. R. (2014). Mental health specialized probation caseloads: Are they effective?. *International Journal of Law and Psychiatry, 37*(5), 464-472.

Young, L. (2016). Police should rarely be the first responders for those in mental health crisis. *The Baltimore Sun.* http://www.baltimoresun.com/news/opinion/oped/bs-ed-response-team-20161201-story.html. Last accessed: 29 Jan 2022.

Chapter 5
Treatment: Intersection with Criminal Justice

"Well, the part I really don't understand – if you're looking for self-help [books], why would you read a book written by somebody else? That's not self-help, that's help! There's no such thing as self-help. If you did it yourself, you did not help! You did it yourself." George Carlin

When hearing the terms "mental health" or "mental illness," the stereotype is to think of very negative words like "crazy." This stereotypical image is of a person suffering from radical delusions and/or hallucinations, which is also often associated with violence. This common distortion of the realities of mental illness is certainly one leading reason why data collection is important. That is, the best way to combat stereotypes and educate the public on the true face of mental health or mental illness is to gather and deploy factual information. These facts detailing the actual number of people diagnosed with a mental illness help with educating the public of problems in their community. Additionally, friends and families can better understand the needs of their loved ones. Communities can create ways to address the needs of those with a diagnosis or help to prevent symptoms before onset occurs.

This chapter addresses a variety of interventions possible and services available in communities to address mental illness, its symptoms, and the collateral consequences of mental health issues (e.g., family stress and strains, homelessness, unemployment/underemployment, et cetera) – including services that embrace emerging technology and novel approaches. Oftentimes, local social service agencies keep a resource guidebook on hand to assist employees working with clients in connecting people with the resources they may need or serve as a self-help tool for individuals to seek the services which they may feel that they need. The resources and services listed in this chapter serve as a generic blueprint of the core of the majority of these resource guides that every student of crime and mental health should have in their mental rolodex – the essentials of mental health care in American communities. While the below information is not an exhaustive list of treatment options, While the information below is not an exhaustive list of treatment options, the ones highlighted below are intended to spark discussion and give basic understanding of a range of options that may exist in our communities.

© The Author(s), under exclusive license to Springer Nature Switzerland AG 2022 97
J. Hector, D. Khey, *Criminal Justice and Mental Health*,
https://doi.org/10.1007/978-3-031-15338-9_5

5.1   Where Do People Fall Through the Cracks?

Treatment is essential in any health-related area for the overall wellness of an individual and for communities in which they reside. The justice-involved population is certainly no exception and are particularly in need of treatment in several ways as it relates to mental health, and at times, also substance use. The unmet need for treatment is great for persons without a criminal background let alone for individuals with more complex mental health histories; this issue lends itself to the crux part of the problem – how can treatment for all change so everyone can remain healthy? How does a person get help, especially when stigma presents such a roadblock to seeking help in the first place? How does a community overcome the lack of funding and the difficulties often present when citizens try accessing services?

Luckily, conversations regarding change and improvement are happening across the country. As a society, the United States is beginning to acknowledge the need for criminal justice reform; further, many communities have taken decisive strides to address the largest gaps in complex criminal justice systems in which people tend to fall through the cracks without the help they need to succeed in everyday life. Slowly, progress is being made to de-stigmatize mental health and create funding and options for everyone to seek treatment when needed. With that, the idea of working toward more proactive measures to help other concerns with each individual has and will hopefully continue to be part of the discussion. Yet it is important to review the critical lapses in mental health care systems that persist as policymakers and stakeholders move to address these gaps.

As with most politically-relevant topics, especially those critical of government-run or government-related systems, "cracks," fault lines, weak points, and gaps seem inevitable. Specifically, government-run systems and programs often stereotype the beleaguered nature of complex bureaucracies. This is certainly not to say that all bureaucracies are problematic. Yet, even well-run bureaucracies can have secondary problems, such as being difficult to navigate by average citizens unfamiliar with bureaucratic processes. A popular and fitting example is to pick on state Department of Motor Vehicles. One recent case known to the authors speaks volumes:

ATTENTION FLORIDA DRIVERS LICENSE HOLDERS WHO DO NOT HAVE CARS:
I just went to local DMV to transfer FL license to [Pennsylvania]. Could not do it–after three hours of rigmarole–"because my FL license could not be verified by PA. I call FL DMV, they tell me license is "suspended." I ask why. They tell me "for lack of car insurance." I tell them "but I haven't had a car since 2012, and that's why I got rid of car insurance." And I get silence on the phone.

Then I ask how/when was I notified of this suspension, and I get silence on the phone. They tell me they can fix it on phone since "it has been longer than three years," but that it takes 24–48 hours to update system. I ask them if they can send confirmation to PA DMV, they say yes, we'll fax it. 45 minutes later, no fax.

This is on top of ridiculous PA …ID requirements which include the following documents to be presented in order to transfer license:

Passport, or raised seal birth certificate–note photo ID from Florida NOT acceptable for ID at PA DMV

TWO of following: tax records, current gun permit, mortgage, lease, w2, utility bill in my name

ALL addresses must match.

AND social security card

So, gotta hit DMV again in "24–28 hours" I guess (Khey, unpublished research).

Imagine trying to navigate these issues if you did not feel physically well. Similar comparisons could be made to trying to navigate these issues when not feeling mentally well.

In addition, bureaucracies are certainly not easy to change; adjustments to federal, state, and local law/policy require time, systems need to lay out how to address these changes to stay in compliance with the law/policy, and these plans require action that may take a while to perfect. While the intent of this text is not to delve into complexities of public administration, it may be helpful to highlight some of the issues in civic processes to answer questions like "why doesn't someone just change it?" Of course, the answer is that this is easier said than done, but it helps to remind ourselves why. State legislatures, for example, operate in sessions in which new bills or amendments to bills can be introduced. One problem lies in the amount of time it takes for legislation to be reviewed and the number of hands it must pass through to get approved. This process could take weeks or months and still fail in the end. Further, it could take years to even develop into a bill worthy of bringing to the legislature in the first place, let alone the issues of political gridlock and partisanship, the influence of special interests, and so on.

Governmental processes aside, one persistent "crack" in mental health care systems lies more in the control of the communities they reside; specifically, and simply, access to care – and further, quality care – has been a core issue since the early development of mental health care. Accessibility issues can be borne from seemingly simple barriers, such as the lack of transportation options to seek treatment or a consumer's ability to pay. Alternatively, appropriate treatment options for mental health and substance use disorder patients, much less those that are justice-involved, may not be readily available in some areas yielding long waits, or even not available at all. While outlining these issues, the former director of the National Institute of Mental Health (NIMH), Thomas Insel, released a report in 2010 discussing the changes needed in the treatment of serious mental illness. The report notes:

> There are several facts about mental illness in the United States that always seem to surprise those who are not directly involved:
>
> - Each year, there are nearly twice as many suicides (33,000) as homicides (18,000) (as reported by Insel in 2010, which remains the case into the late 2010s, see Morgan et al., 2018)
> - The life expectancy for people with major mental illness is 56 years (the average life expectancy in the U.S. is 77.7 years, as reported by Insel in 2010 and confirmed by a World Health Organization (2022) report concluding that, worldwide, individuals with severe mental illness tend to die 10–25 years sooner)

- Mental disorders and substance abuse are the leading cause of disability in the United States and Canada

To this list we can now add another statistic – according to the Treatment Advocacy Center, and based on an analysis of data provided by the Substance Abuse & Mental Health Services Administration, **people with mental illness are three times more likely to be in the criminal justice system than hospitals**. In some states, such as Nevada and Arizona, the ratio is closer to 10 times more people with mental illness in jails and prisons (Insel, 2010).

As mentioned earlier in this text, there has been a drastic decrease (about 90%) in the number of state hospital beds over the past 50 years. Yet, the number of Americans with mental illness continues to increase as the population expands. Policy changes have significantly impacted the number of individuals with mental illness being sent to jails and prisons. As discussed earlier, people with mental illness are more likely to also have a substance abuse problem. Keeping this in mind, mandatory sentencing requirements for drug crimes means that these individuals are now being incarcerated without any (or, at minimum with little) consideration to the underlying mental health concerns in fueling drug-related offending. "Most of all, however, [the] statistic [above] reveals a failure to provide alternatives in the mental health care system for people requiring hospitalization" (Insel, 2010).

Individuals with mental health concerns begin to fall through the cracks in the systems of care in American communities. Recall that the National Alliance on Mental Illness commonly cites an important National Institute of Mental Health statistic – typically, it takes an average of eight to ten years after the onset of mental health symptomatology to *begin to* formally address these mental health concerns (NAMI, 2017a). This does not take into consideration any gender or cultural differences that may even further delay the time it takes to seek help. Rhetorically, it appears as though the popular perception of mental illness in the form of a "crazy," "delusional," and "violent" individual aggravates this delay in seeking help; or alternatively, the lack of mental health awareness blunts our ability to detect mental health concerns until mental health symptomatology reaches some critical mass. As addressed in other chapters, these types of ideas only fuel the stigma surrounding mental health. This critical mass could present itself when an individual winds up homeless, in an emergency room, or as a jail inmate; it does seem that, many times, these costly issues to remedy tend to be a starting point in addressing underlying mental health concerns. The following section takes a deeper look into mental health safety net and its continued inherent problems.

5.2 Common Problems

One leading and pervasive problem is access to services within a local area, particularly among the most vulnerable individuals in our communities. Ex-offenders reentering society postincarceration certainly fall among this broader class of vulnerable individuals. Simple gaps in access can be just transportation (*reliable* transportation) to get to treatment services, participate in group and support meetings, travel to the pharmacy or doctor's office to obtain medication (even if they were affordable or free), and so on. Depending on the location in which a person resides, (e.g., rural versus urban), there may be insufficient to nonexistent public transportation services available. As such, the lack of transportation can be a primary barrier to treatment, services, and employment. Fortunately, some treatment facilities and new programs (including grant-funded programs and program streams), are adding in the funding to supply clients with transportation options, such as taxi reimbursement, gas cards, transit "tokens" or preloaded cards, et cetera (Fraze et al., 2016). For example, a recent workshop of the National Academies of Sciences, Engineering, and medicine recently evaluated the available data and metrics on the value of connecting patients to transportation services. Of particular value, the experts present at the workshop opined on the return on investment of these services:

> There is stiff competition for limited transportation resources, Ed Christopher said, and Congress requires justification for the spending of public money to ensure that the money spent achieves a positive return.... He observed that return on investment is viewed differently by different stakeholders. For transportation access to care, he said, the questions revolve around whether the efforts are making people healthier. Lefler noted that return on investment is difficult to ascertain in health care because it depends on illness, age, income level, and other factors of the many individuals involved. The ultimate question is whether quality of life is being improved.... Cronin highlighted the need for new and innovative cross-discipline research and stressed the need to "speak the language" of those you are trying to convince. He described some of his early work on return-on-investment calculations for medically related transportation services. One approach is to calculate cost avoidance (as a result of, for example, reduced ED visits, hospitalizations, or missed days of work). He said that much of the work at that time was based on assumptions about relationships between transportation and care (e.g., how many trips to care might correlate with avoidance of a 1-day in-hospital stay). He agreed that medical trips are about quality of life improvement, but he added that those controlling the funding (i.e., the tax dollars) want to show that they are generating a financial return (NASEM, 2016).

Often, transportation can be one of the costliest parts on a treatment budget, and this can have an impact on the treatment quality given the high cost of gasoline, insurance (including liability), motor pool maintenance, and so on; Some care providers may be a great distance from clients, particularly in suburban and urban areas. Or, there may be only one provider in a large area because the funding and options are based on population rather than size of the area. In these cases, creativity is needed to ensure proper treatment. For example, some programs offer treatment providers to go to the clients (e.g., make house calls) rather than the other way around. This is part of the benefit of "assertive community treatment," described more in depth in an upcoming section within this chapter (Table 5.1).

With ongoing budget cuts and political barriers, mental health and substance use services have become increasingly scarce in many communities across the United States. Less public facilities, less providers (and less quality providers), and less beds/space available continue to be a primary concern among mental health care leaders. Statistics show that behavioral health needs are increasing but the

Table 5.1 Summary of the main points of speakers of the workshop on the value of connecting patients with treatment services, National Academies of Science, Engineering, and Medicine

Inclusive planning is a key element of success. It is important to directly engage the people who will be served by community transportation in the planning process and to understand what their specific needs are.
Education can improve transportation. Transportation providers might not understand what accommodations the patient needs; health care providers often do not know the transportation options available and therefore cannot advocate for patients; and patients are often unaware of or do not understand how to use the transportation that is available in the community.
Different stakeholders view return on investment differently, depending on their individual goals.
Cross-sector collaboration will be aided by developing a shared vocabulary and shared metrics.
There is an immediate need to make the business case that investing in transportation to care is of economic value, and there is also a need for longer-term research that demonstrates improvement in quality of life and the impacts of prevention.

availability of treatment is decreasing. This leads to the major focus of this text: the obstacles described here lay the foundation of the key problem that has existed for years. Now more than ever, more individuals are using (or being forced to use since there are no other options) jails and prisons to sober up from substances. Families and friends are also encouraging this idea since there are no other options. Ironically, for those suffering from a mental illness, "getting clean" can increase the possibility of mental health concerns surfacing – leading to a particularly vulnerable moment in people's lives.

5.2.1   Medical Coverage

An obvious obstacle to seeking treatment is the lack of insurance, particularly access to Medicaid, to cover the cost of care. "Medicaid is the single-most important financing source of mental health services in the [United States], covering nearly 27% of all mental health care in [the country] and nearly half of the public mental health spending, according to SAMHSA" (NAMI, 2017b). Further, if a person is unable to acquire gainful and *meaningful* employment due to a criminal background, they are often unable to secure private health insurance of any kind. Without health insurance, the options for treatment are very limited, require the most severe symptoms before consideration, often have considerable waitlists, or completely unavailable. Fortunately, some states have been moving forward with plans to help people leaving prison; This change typically comes in the form of adopting Medicaid expansion under the Affordable Care Act. Yet, "[even] with increased spending for Medicaid because of the Affordable Care Act, the share of Medicaid budgets spent on treating [mental illness and and substance use disorder] is expected to decline. In 2009, 10.4% of Medicaid spending went for [mental health] treatment; by 2020, that share is expected to fall to 7.9%" (SAMHSA, 2014).

Louisiana offers a recent example. In 2016, after a long period of resisting Medicaid expansion, a bipartisan effort was spearheaded to join over thirty states who have expansion in place. This policy shift allows for ex-prisoners to be eligible for Medicaid upon release, with the potential of having benefits the moment these individuals leave prison facilities. The goal is to initiate and complete the process to receive Medicaid (as well as other relevant benefits) in the months leading up to release. To do so, the Louisiana Department of Health (LDH) is collaborating with the Department of Public Safety and Corrections (DOC) to develop the ability to maintain a "suspended" status on Medicaid benefits that can be activated on a particular date (e.g., a release date). To date, it is routine to simply cancel benefits, forcing individuals to handle reapplication on their own upon re-entry; as an interim process, sporadic reentry programs across the state employ case managers who assist with the application process. Allowing inmates to gain access to health benefits will hopefully allow improvements in health and decrease in returns to prison. "LDH and DOC implemented phase one of the pre-release enrollment initiative in January for offenders in the seven DOC state facilities. As of February 27, 2017, 230 offenders have been linked to a health plan, and it is expected that approximately 2,800 offenders will qualify for coverage annually, with about 30 percent of these former offenders being eligible for case management" (Louisiana Department of Health, 2017). As of this writing, efforts to expand Medicaid access to all reentering persons are ongoing with a focus of aiding individuals serving time in facilities managed by sheriffs and private corporations – another note on how progress can occur slowly when instituting change in large, complex bureaucracies. Author discussions with insiders have revealed that the majority of facilities are capable of processing enrollment; however, the system is facing some logistical challenges preventing full enrollment before individuals are released back to their communities.

With the Affordable Care Act, and Medicaid for that matter, in peril due to loud calls for reform in the current political discourse, it is very difficult to anticipate how these trends will continue into the intermediate or distant future regarding individuals with a criminal record (particularly, felons). While it is easy to cast political opponents of Medicaid expansion as adversaries of mental health, bipartisan political forces seem to be sending mixed messages. For example, the 21st Century Cures Act continues to receive bipartisan support. Any movement to defund Medicaid may be supplanted with the support embedded in the 21st Century Cures Act to some extent. Since the fates of the Affordable Care Act and Medicaid are still being debated, and the policy changes of the 21st Century Cures Act are being put into place, positive gains in mental health infrastructure appear to be secure in the foreseeable future, with the distant future having a murkier outlook.

5.2.2 Medical Records

Electronic Health Records (EHR) or Electronic Medical Records are digital copies of an individual's clinical history. Hospitals are working to adopt these electronic records for many reasons. First, ease of use is highly beneficial in most medical settings. A doctor can use a laptop or iPad throughout the hospital to have a patient's current medical information in seconds. Additionally, the information can be much more accurate and in real time since staff can input information immediately. EHRs allow for less use of resources since there is less need for storage, copies and physical transfers of information. On a bigger scale, EHRs can offer access to information among many facilities, across many areas. If a person moves out of state, their electronic file can be easily obtained by the new treating physician to maintain care without any gaps. Perhaps the most important reason of any listed here, EHRs have become required for any organization to seek Federally funded research dollars.

The use of EHRs can be vital in working with individuals with mental illness. Maintaining accurate history regarding physical issues, medications, or even family contacts can be difficult with some who suffer from a mental health diagnosis. Additionally, individuals who have a mental health diagnosis and begin medication management often stop taking their medication once they "feel better." Having issues such as these well-documented can empower each provider, stakeholder, and/ or partner to engage in informed decision-making with their patient/client. In other words, EHRs can be vital in maintaining a continuum of care for an individual, especially those with mental illness and in the criminal justice system (particularly, those who are passing from one system to the other and vice versa). Often with mental illness, and not unlike other illnesses, treatment may not be immediate. Individuals can use resources like medication management and other therapies to help treat their diagnosis. Using electronic medical records, other doctors and treatment professionals can understand the medical history of the individual being treated. Understanding a person's medical history can help treatment professionals identify best practices and hopefully prevent future setbacks. Ideally, jails and prisons will also move toward the use of electronic medical records to also ensure the best care for individuals involved in the criminal justice system with a mental health diagnosis. With this process, the hopes would be to eliminate further "cracks" in treatment.

SAMHSA discusses the use of health records for patients and their families. Often, over the course of care, an individual will coordinate with multiple different providers including doctors, mental health professionals and other service providers. The use of EHRs will allow for less information to be lost, resulting in better overall wellness. SAMHSA explains using health information technology, "Health IT also offers you these benefits:

- Secure access to your personal health information
- Easy care coordination between providers
- Access to remote care from your home
- Self-management tools for you and your caregivers" (SAMHSA, 2017).

While the concept of EHRs is far from new, the issue is that health care systems have been slow to adopt this tool or have yet to fully integrate this tool into all facets of each system (Palabindala et al., 2016). Yet, much progress has been made in the wake of the Health Information Technology for Economic and Clinical Health Act (2009). Data on EHR adoption can be found at the Office of the National Coordinator for Health Information Technology (https://healthit.gov), which details that most American physicians using some form of EHR (86% in 2017) and over 90% of critical access hospitals of various sizes throughout the country. In addition, all nonfederal acute care hospitals had obtained health IT certification by 2017. Thus, at this point, the issue is not whether or not the tool is in use, but *how* it is used. As providers gain more experience using EHRs, the benefits of using these systems – improved clinical decision-making, better communication among providers and between providers and patients, and reducing medication errors – can be fully realized. In addition, and of critical value for mental health professionals, the quality of case notes placed in EHRs can vary from provider to provider. While having access to medical histories can provide a rich resource to current providers, an abundance of poor case notes within an EHR may present a lost opportunity to make use of previous treatment encounters. For example, a recent review of a local agency providing mental health services in Louisiana showed considerable variation in the quality of case notes entered into a popular EHR. One provider working at the agency tended to use very brief, and often repetitive narratives to describe his/her interactions with clients. As such, the case notes did not offer any individualized narratives for each client. This finding was shared with the agency's quality assurance manager as it is highly unlikely that all clients are presenting the same circumstances, experiences, and symptoms in the same way (Khey, unpublished research).

At this time, it is unclear just how much of the narrative-type of information placed in EHRs can be considered valuable and usable. What is clear is that medication histories have been reliable, and EHRs have a proven track record of reducing medication errors relative to medication errors of patients in systems not using EHRs. This medication history can also offer mental health professionals some clues as to prior treatment decisions, and in conjunction with even moderate-quality case notes, can continue to be invaluable for making contemporary decisions. As these systems continue to flourish, their capacity to aid patients will certainly continue to grow.

5.2.3 Barriers of Public Housing

Often, individuals with mental illness and/or a criminal background have difficulty finding housing. This can be because of either or both "classifications" – the mentally ill or the criminal. Family and loved ones may not have the resources necessary to care for a person with higher needs, or may not want to help, particularly with the cumbersome and/or expensive process of securing housing. Additionally, with stigma for both mental health and crime, shame and guilt can be factors influencing the involvement of loved ones. Housing difficulties are often the result of criminal history:

> **Public Housing Occupancy Guidebook provided by the United States Department of Housing & Urban Development**
>
> Ineligibility Because of Criminal Activity (24 CFR § 960.204) PHAs are required to prohibit admission of families with members:
>
> Who were evicted from federally assisted housing for drug related criminal activity for three years following the date of eviction (unless the family can demonstrate that the person who engaged in the drug related activity has been rehabilitated or is no longer a member of the household); or
>
> Who are currently engaging in illegal use of a drug; or
>
> Who have shown a pattern of use of illegal drugs that may interfere with the health, safety, or right to peaceful enjoyment of the premises by other residents; or
>
> Who are subject to a lifetime registration requirement under a State sex offender registration program; or
>
> Whose abuse of alcohol or pattern of abuse of alcohol would interfere with the health, safety or right to peaceful enjoyment of the premises by other residents; or
>
> Who have ever been convicted of drug-related criminal activity for manufacture of methamphetamine on the premises of federally assisted housing.

The Guidebook goes on to discuss in more detail what would eliminate a person from eligibility:

> Involvement in Criminal Activity on the Part of Any Applicant Family Member that Would Adversely Affect the Health, Safety or Right to Peaceful Enjoyment of the Premises by Other Tenants (24 CFR § 960.203(c)(3) and 960.204) PHAs are required to check an applicant's history of criminal activity for a history of crimes that would be lease violations if they were committed by a public housing resident. **Before the screening steps are examined, consider that certain actions and behaviors require a rejection of an applicant:**[emphasis added] · Persons evicted from federally assisted housing for drug-related criminal activities may not be admitted for three years from the date of eviction. In cases where the statute prohibits admission for a certain period of time, PHAs may now set a longer period of time for the prohibition (24 CFR § 960.203 (c) (3) (ii)). - Where the regulations specify a prohibition period for certain behavior, PHAs can consider the mandatory period and any extension of the discretionary period. - The discretionary time period for prohibition of admission can vary based on the type of activity. For example, a PHA may have a policy that an eviction where the applicant was manufacturing or dealing drugs results in a 5-year prohibition. In the case of life-time sex offender registrants, a PHA may establish long periods or a lifetime ban. · Persons engaging in the illegal use of a drug.... (U.S. Housing and Urban Development, 2017).

Solutions to housing restrictions are described below in the following section.

5.3   Common Resources

Outside of incarcerated settings and in the "free world," there are number of treatment options for and resources available to individuals suffering from mental health concerns. Traditional treatment options often include individual or group therapy, and even family therapy. Individual therapy featuring regular one-on-one sessions with a licensed mental health professional, on its own, offers a lightweight and effective treatment option for common mental health symptomatology. Also known as counseling or psychotherapy, individual therapy sessions often occur weekly in the therapist's office or in virtual settings (over a secure Internet/cellular connection). Therapists can be licensed professional counselors, licensed clinical social workers, and psychologists, and ideally, these mental health professionals would work in conjunction with a psychiatrist who could potentially prescribe medication to the patient, if/as needed. Each session generally lasts around one hour, with the length depending on the needs of the client. Sessions can discuss an array of topics including social skills, coping skills, and relationships, to name a few.

On the other hand, Assertive Community Treatment (ACT) is considered one of the most intensive treatment options available for severe mental illness that demands an "all-hands" approach. ACT is a team-based model designed to treat individuals on a 24-hour-a-day, 7-day-a-week basis while the patient remains in the community. Described in detail below, an ACT team features professionals across several disciplines and perspectives that can aid treatment provision. Thus, there are many different types of treatment that vary depending on the severity of illness, time available, and as always, funding. Further, treatment options include a variety of settings, each with advantages to consider when customizing a patient's individualized treatment plan.

Additionally, group therapy can be beneficial for some individuals. Group therapy consists of a therapist and a group of clients. The ideal number for a successful group should be less than twelve clients, but this can vary in different settings. Also, groups can be topic based as well and range from grief to substance abuse to parenting and beyond. Often, group therapy is most readily available to most mental health "consumers" due to its relative low cost and effectiveness. More frequently, support groups are also leveraged for the same reasons. In many circumstances, support groups lack the lead of a trained clinician; however, and more often, support groups feature peer support specialists that can aid individuals with mental illness and/or substance use disorder cope with their disease, learn more about their triggers, and heal through shared experiences.

Each of these modalities are described below, along with other resources available in the community to help individuals with mental illness heal, learn to live with their illness, live comfortably, and live life to the fullest extent possible.

5.3.1 Detox

Some substance use disorders must be treated immediately with medically monitored detoxification, or "detox." In this process, the patient will be forced into withdrawal from their drug(s) of choice in the safest way possible, which many times requires medication to moderate the discomfort of withdrawal symptoms, to stabilize vital signs, and to protect a patient from harm and death directly due to withdrawal or indirectly due to the psychological effects of withdrawal. Medical detox is most important for the cessation of chronic alcohol, barbiturates, and opioids; in particular, the withdrawal syndromes produced by chronic alcohol and/or barbiturates consistently produce life-threatening effects.

To be specific, SAMHSA defines detoxification as "a set of interventions aimed at managing acute intoxication and withdrawal. It denotes a clearing of toxins from the body of the patient who is acutely intoxicated and/or dependent on substances of abuse" (SAMHSA, 2006). Typically, the detoxification process takes place within an inpatient setting to allow for the proper monitoring of the person by trained medical staff around the clock. "During inpatient detoxification, a person is monitored 24/7 by a trained medical staff for up to 7 days. Inpatient detoxification is generally more effective than outpatient for initial sobriety. This is because inpatient treatment provides a consistent environment and removes the person battling addiction from exposure to people and places associated with using" (NAMI, 2017c). Importantly, detoxification alone is not sufficient in the treatment and rehabilitation of substance use disorders (Table 5.2).

It is further helpful for individuals unfamiliar with the inner workings of detoxification services to note its principles for care as promulgated by SAMHSA. These nine principles are often mantra-like in the industry, a phenomenon that occurs often in the treatment business: (1) detox is not a cure for substance abuse or

Table 5.2 Guiding principles and assumptions of detoxification and substance abuse treatment (SAMHSA, 2006)

1. Detoxification alone is not sufficient treatment for substance dependence but it is one part of a continuum of care for substance-related disorders.
2. The detoxification process consists of the following three components: • Evaluation • Stabilization • Fostering patient readiness for and entry into treatment A detoxification process that does not incorporate all three critical components is considered incomplete and inadequate by the consensus panel.
3. Detoxification can take place in a wide variety of settings and at a number of levels of intensity within these settings. Placement should be appropriate to the patient's needs.
4. Persons seeking detoxification should have access to the components of the detoxification process described above, no matter what the setting or the level of treatment intensity.
5. All persons requiring treatment for substance use disorders should receive treatment of the same quality and appropriate thoroughness and should be put into contact with a treatment program for substance use disorders after detoxification.
6. Ultimately, insurance coverage for the full range of detoxification and follow-up treatment services is cost-effective. If reimbursement systems do not provide payment for the complete detoxification process, patients may be released prematurely, leading to medically or socially unattended withdrawal.
7. Patients seeking detoxification services have diverse cultural and ethnic backgrounds as well as unique health needs and life situations. Organizations that provide detoxification services need to ensure that they have standard practices in place to address cultural diversity.
8. A successful detoxification process can be measured, in part, by whether an individual who is substance dependent enters, remains in, and is compliant with the treatment protocol of a substance abuse treatment/rehabilitation program after detoxification.

substance use disorder. Instead, it is likely to be a first step into drug recovery (and a recovery orientation) and can be the first entry point into an array of treatment events in one's life; (2) substance use disorder can be treated, and patients can have hope to progress into recovery; (3) substance use disorder is a chronic brain disease that often features relapse. This disease should not be mistaken for moral weakness; (4) patients are to be treated with respect and in a dignified manner; (5) further, patients are to be treated supportively and without judgment; (6) individualized treatment plans should be made in partnership with the patient and, as warranted, with his or her support network (e.g., family, friends, partners, and/or employers); (7) all treatment personal should promote rehabilitation and maintenance activities at all times, as appropriate, and should be prepared to link the patient with subsequent services immediately after discharge from detox; (8) active participation and involvement of a patient's support system should be encouraged when appropriate while ensuring patient's privacy, confidentiality, and HIPPA rights; and (9) treatment professionals must consider differences in background, culture, preferences, sexual orientation, disability, vulnerabilities, and strengths of each patient when providing care (SAMHSA, 2006). Emphasis must be placed on the fact that detox often serves as an entry event that begins the path to recovery (also known as a treatment "career"), but also may be necessary several times across one's substance use "career."

5.3.2   Inpatient Treatment Services

Inpatient treatment can be beneficial and possibly necessary for a person experiencing serious mental illness and/or severe substance abuse. The inpatient setting allows for 24/7 care for both physical and/or mental health medical needs. Individuals often receive a multitude of complementary treatments, supports, and care while in an inpatient treatment center. An individual receives social support, medication management, medical care, individual therapy, group therapy, at times recreational therapy, and possibly art therapy. All facets work together with the overall goal of recovery from mental illness and substance use. This comprehensive treatment approach can also work to aid in overcoming past trauma or other underlying causes of the mental illness or substance use, yet is the costliest of options (outside of incarceration; NAMI, 2017c).

The popular culture references to 28-day programs, particularly for substance use disorder treatment, often colors our perception of inpatient treatment services. In reality, inpatient treatment is very diverse and includes several types of facilities, including hospitals. Further, duration of inpatient services is often dictated by ability to pay and insurance coverage, while also considering a patient's underlying mental illness. According to a recent report by Owen and her colleagues (2019), inpatient stays to principally address mental health and substance use disorders costs $7,100 per stay and averages 6.4 days. Even for severe mental illness, such as schizophrenia, stays tend not to stretch beyond two weeks on average – in the case

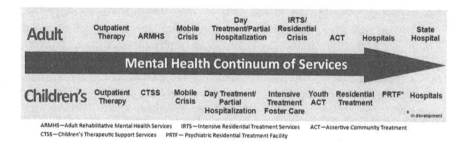

Fig. 5.1 Continuum of mental health services, courtesy of the Minnesota Department of Human Services (2017)

of schizophrenia, Owen et al. found patients who primarily sought treatment for this condition averaged 11 days inpatient (the second longest average in their study, only behind eating disorders) with an average cost of $8,900 per stay. As has been discussed throughout this text, the capacity to offer inpatient treatment services has been sharply decreased relative to past decades. Thus, these services are reserved for severe illness and for mental health crises that require these services (see Fig. 5.1 for a range of options that address mental illness with increasing severity).

5.3.3   Intensive Outpatient (IOP) Treatment

Intensive Outpatient Treatment or IOP is akin to "partial hospitalization" in that a person receives treatment on a regular basis in a medical setting, but returns home each night (NAMI, 2017e). In an IOP program, an individual has multiple treatment sessions each week. This type of treatment is often used in a transition after inpatient and leads to a step down to outpatient treatment. It can also be coordinated with a sober or halfway house for a fuller range of treatment support. Some programs differentiate between IOP and partial hospitalization in that the former is the less intensive version of the latter, but essentially, both require attendance during the day for several days a week and will release patients into the community in the afternoon or late afternoon.

5.3.4   12 Steps – AA/NA and Alternatives, Such as SMART Recovery

Alcoholics Anonymous and Narcotics Anonymous (AA/NA) are group *support* meetings, not therapy, that take place with a community-like approach to support recovery from alcohol and drugs. These meetings are run and attended by individuals that suffer from addiction. Meetings can be open to the public or closed, specific groups. Additionally, some meetings can be segregated to just women only. The purpose of AA/NA meetings is to hold members accountable for their processing of the 12 steps of the program. As the title implies, group members remain anonymous in that what is discussed in the meeting is not discussed outside in public.

Twelve-step programs like Alcoholics Anonymous have become ubiquitous in all treatment systems in the United States and are widely adopted worldwide, in general. Overall, this support group orientation is effective in promoting recovery: individuals who attend twelve-step programs are twice as likely to remain abstinent relative to those who do not and more frequent attendance of twelve-step meetings are statistically correlated with higher rates of abstinence (Kaskutas, 2009). Further, and perhaps most critically, these programs are incredibly cheap to run (ostensibly, free). These support groups should always be part of a broader individualized treatment plan; however, individuals using AA/NA as their sole source of support and "treatment" have been successful in improving their progress in recovery.

It should be noted that many AA/NA programs have varying levels of religious and/or spiritual focus, which may pose as a barrier to some people seeking help who do not see themselves as such. In recent years, several support programs have been developed for this population – the most popular being Self-Management And Recovery Training (SMART). "Self-Management And Recovery Training (SMART) is a global community of mutual-support groups. At meetings, participants help one another resolve problems with any addiction (to drugs or alcohol or to activities such as gambling or over-eating). Participants find and develop the power within themselves to change and lead fulfilling and balanced lives guided by our science-based and sensible 4-Point Program®" (SMART Recovery, 2022). Further, SMART features a broad online presence, allowing for broad access to online meetings (over 50 available each week at the time of this writing, an online chat tool that is managed around the clock every day, and a message board. SMART primarily operates in the United States, the United Kingdom, and Australia, with programming is available in English and Spanish languages. Figure 5.2 provides the principles of both AA and SMART recovery for comparison.

5.3.5 Assertive Community Treatment (ACT) Teams

Assertive Community Treatment (ACT) is a multidisciplinary team-based approach that provides around the clock care to patients *in situ* (that is, where the patients are in the community and not at any particular facility; NAMI, 2017d). Rather than a work through referral process, ACT provides treatment directly to clients by offering a team of professionals to handle any would-be referral among the team and not "refer out." In other words, any service a patient may need can be handled among team members immediately, cutting out any "middlemen" of treatment provision. ACT operates as a 24/7 treatment team just like inpatient services; however, ACT services are provided at the location of the client rather than in a hospital/inpatient

THE TWELVE STEPS OF ALCOHOLICS ANONYMOUS

1. We admitted we were powerless over alcohol—that our lives had become unmanageable.

2. Came to believe that a Power greater than ourselves could restore us to sanity.

3. Made a decision to turn our will and our lives over to the care of God as we understood Him.

4. Made a searching and fearless moral inventory of ourselves.

5. Admitted to God, to ourselves, and to another human being the exact nature of our wrongs.

6. Were entirely ready to have God remove all these defects of character.

7. Humbly asked Him to remove our shortcomings.

8. Made a list of all persons we had harmed, and became willing to make amends to them all.

9. Made direct amends to such people wherever possible, except when to do so would injure them or others.

10. Continued to take personal inventory and when we were wrong promptly admitted it.

11. Sought through prayer and meditation to improve our conscious contact with God as we understood Him, praying only for knowledge of His will for us and the power to carry that out. 12. Having had a spiritual awakening as the result of these steps, we tried to carry this message to alcoholics, and to practice these principles in all our affairs.

4-Point Program® of SMART Recovery

1. Building and maintaining the motivation to change.

2. Coping with urges to use.

3. Managing thoughts, feelings, and behaviors in an effective way without addictive behaviors.

4. Living a balanced, positive, and healthy life.

Fig. 5.2 The twelve steps of Alcoholics Anonymous (Alcoholics Anonymous, 1981) and 4-Point Program® of SMART Recovery (SMART Recovery, 2022)

setting. The team members are trained on multiple areas of topics including nursing, substance abuse, social work, psychiatry, and vocational counseling.

According to NAMI, assertive community treatment began in 1972 as the brain-child of Arnold Marx, Leonard Stein, and Mary Ann Test at Mendota State Hospital in Wisconsin. ACT was initially meant to serve as a support system for patients reentering the community from state hospitals during the early stages of the deinstitutionalization movement. In particular, these mental health professionals noted that many gains in mental health quickly tended to devolve after patients return back into their communities. As ACT services is reaching its half-centennial of existence, its proven success has earned it the distinction of being an evidence-based service by SAMHSA.

The key features of ACT are: 1) "**Treatment**: psychopharmacologic treatment, including new atypical antispyschotic and antidepressant medications individual supportive therapy mobile crisis intervention hospitalization substance abuse treatment, including group therapy (for clients with a [co-occurring disorder] of substance abuse and mental illness)," 2) **Rehabilitation**: behaviorally oriented skill teaching (supportive and cognitive-behavioral therapy), including structuring time and handling activities of daily living supported employment, both paid and volunteer work support for resuming education," and 3) "**Support services**: support, education, and skill-teaching to family members collaboration with families and assistance to clients with children direct support to help clients obtain legal and advocacy services, financial support, supported housing, money-management services, and transportation" (NAMI Minnesota, 2017).

5.3.6 The Value of Compulsory Treatment

Specialty courts are discussed in a different chapter within this book, but there are other ways that treatment can be required for those involved in the criminal justice system. In fact, *compulsory treatment* often leads to the most successful treatment experiences among patients, particularly when evaluating the likelihood of treatment completion. Importantly, successful completion of treatment is correlated with lasting success in recovery and healthy lives.

With court mandated treatment, the added "benefit" of legal ramification with treatment noncompliance helps to keep patients on the path to successfully complete treatment regimes, often giving them the best chances of future success. Further, treatment can be an option in lieu of incarceration or prosecution, which also aids in giving people reason to stay clean, compliant, and out of trouble. According to the NIDA, "most studies suggest that outcomes for those who are legally pressured to enter treatment are as good or better than outcomes for those who entered treatment without legal pressure. Individuals under legal pressure also tend to have higher attendance rates and remain in treatment for longer periods, which can also have a positive impact on treatment outcomes" (2017).

5.4 Treatment Settings

Treatment can be provided in a number of settings and locations. The settings depend on the goals and recovery process of the individual seeking treatment. The benefit of multiple options is that there can be multisystemic approach. In other words, what works for one person may not work for another so trying different settings to find the "right fit" may be best.

Private practice for a therapist is similar to a doctor's office. Often a therapist has their own office or is with a group in a building. This setting lends to a more open environment that is designed and decorated by the therapists themselves rather than a more hospitals type vibe. Typically, if in a group, each therapist has their own office in which to meet with clients. Insurance can be used in private practice settings to help offset the cost of sessions. Individual, family, and group sessions can take place in private practice offices. The following sections offer a review of other treatment settings available to patients in the community setting.

5.4.1 Community Mental Health Centers

Community Mental Health Centers (CMHC) provide mental health services to the public. Generally, those visiting a community mental health center receive Social Security disability and/or Medicaid benefits (Centers for Medicare & Medicaid Services, 2017). Local governments of the parish or county operate these centers, which offer a variety of services to the public. Those services can include outpatient treatment, group therapy and/or support groups, medication management, case management and some offer specific substance abuse addiction services. CMHCs can be very helpful in that they can offer referrals to other treatment providers and useful programs in the community. Most people who seek help at an CMHC experience a severe impact of symptoms on their activities of daily living. This can range between a variety of needs which result in a variety of referrals from day programs to longer term inpatient supportive housing.

5.4.2 Emergency Rooms and Hospitalization

As with certain medical situations, there are times when an emergency arises and immediate treatment is needed for mental health as well. Additionally, in times of suicidal ideations or homicidal ideations, seeking emergency help is in the best interest for safety of the individual and/or others. A person can be brought to the Emergency Room for immediate attention for a mental health concern. As NAMI describes, "Situations that might require a trip to the emergency room include: a suicide attempt, assault or threatening actions against another person, hearing voices, paranoia, confusion, et cetera, or drugs or alcohol escalating to a person's mental health issue" (2017e). Often, going to an emergency room, whether voluntarily or involuntarily (loved one, ambulance, law enforcement, et cetera) can be the first step in beginning the process of treatment. Luckily, many emergency rooms in major metropolitan areas have psychiatric areas specifically used to treatment emergent situations with a mentally ill person. Also, the staff is trained to handle a psychiatric crisis and make the best decision for continued care.

5.4.3 Group Homes

At times, a group home may be a necessary type of supportive housing for a person who needs more attention and care. For individuals in need of medication management, but not in mental health crisis, a group home can be an option (NAMI, 2017f). As SAMHSA describes, "research literature documents that persons with serious mental illnesses, and substance use disorders die younger than the general population – mainly due to preventable risk factors (e.g., smoking) and treatable conditions (e.g., cardiovascular disease and cancer)" (SAMHSA, 2012: 7). Part of the measures taken to work to overcome these risk factors include improving access to primary care. In some cases, that care can be provided "in-house" while a person is living in a group home or supportive housing, in collaboration with medical partners in the community. Individuals who are chronically ill can have access to both medical and mental health treatment within the setting of the group home or be transported by the group home to attend appointments for these services in the community. Additionally, individuals can live with other peers and work toward social improvements. Group homes often offer the opportunity to learn skills and activities all with the extra care.

5.4.4 Transitional Housing and Recovery Residences: Halfway Houses, Sober Houses, and Three-Quarter Houses

For some leaving prison or a secure medical facility, a "halfway house" or other form or transitional housing is a great option (often, the only tangible option) that allows an individual to learn how to re-enter society. This type of housing helps to slowly reacclimate to everyday life, learn life skills, coping skills, and begin the process of recovery on solid footing alongside others who can benefit from the group therapy dynamic. An individual begins to regain their independence while also maintaining structure and support to ensure ease in the most difficult transition time. This type of housing is seen as a "step down" from previous, more restrictive treatment efforts and attempts to bridge the gap between inpatient and home.

The vernacular for transitional housing varies across the country. Broadly speaking, transitional houses – or recovery residences – refers to an array of housing options that offer various levels of rule-strictness, obligations to attend treatment, and structure. For example, halfway houses have stricter rules, often have requirements of attending AA/NA or other twelve-step (or similar) meetings and engage in drug testing to ensure abstinence in comparison to three-quarters houses. In addition, halfway houses may place restrictions on residents in their ability to leave the house freely as they wish. In reality, a variety of transitional housing resources exist throughout the country with varying levels of rules, restrictions, and resources; the goal would be to find a resource that would match the facility to the needs of the client with the overarching goal, in most cases, to gradually step-down the restrictions on this client until he or she can live independently, healthy, and engage in broad pro-social behaviors.

5.4.5 Safe Haven, Behavioral Health Solutions Center, and Other "Centralized" One-Stop Facilities

One innovation recently gaining broader adoption and expansion across the United States is an initial catchment point could be set up with first responders to capture individuals with potential mental illness *before* they go to jail. In other words, for individuals who are having a mental health crisis, but may not be engaging in illegal behavior, first responders should have a resource available to them to affect an intervention. While various iterations of "community crisis centers" have existed for quite some time, these efforts stand out in their approach to tackle crises broadly by including diverse partnerships of stakeholders to ensure success.

A model called Safe Haven, developed in San Antonio, serves as a leading model across the country for this very situation. Safe Haven has been developed to be a centralized hub and shelter for the care of individuals in crisis, with staffing by key agencies and personnel most apt to help – mental health professionals (including substance use), housing specialists, law enforcement (including probation and parole), education and career development professionals, among others. While originally intended to serve the homeless, a Safe Haven can offer screening and assessment with referral out to services just like a jail can, yet at an earlier point of intercept (e.g., before arrest or hospitalization is imminent). Jails should often be included as a partner in these projects as data sharing can become critical. For example, if an individual released from jail and ends up homeless, any effort to connect this individual to treatment or any screening and assessment performed by the jail may be extremely valuable to a Safe Haven.

This sort of model has recently been replicated in Denver (Canady, 2021), opening its doors to serve the public in May 2021. The Behavioral Health Solutions Center – offers a 24/7 operation staffed by clinicians, nurses and nurse practitioners, peer support specialists, counselors, and other support staff to offer triage care and referral services, crisis stabilization services (for up to 5 days) with a 16 bed capacity, and provide transitional shelter for up to 30 adults for 30 days. The focus of this facility is to keep individuals in crisis who do not necessarily need emergency care out of emergency departments while also ensuring that these individuals do not end up in jail if their crises remain unattended to. In the case of Denver's model, community stakeholders also expanded the use of a mobile "wellness" unit – called Wellness Winnie (based out of an RV) – that seeks to provide connectivity with the Behavioral Health Solutions Center while also providing a broader array of services such as peer support care and navigation to community-based resources, education, hypodermic needle disposal, behavioral health screening and assessment, distribution of essential care items, and Narcan® distribution (Denver, 2022). This unit can also serve as a mobile cooling and hydration center or a warming center in extreme weather conditions.

Key to each of these emerging innovative centers to serve those in crisis is a multidisciplinary, comprehensive collaborative stakeholder model that embraces a true community effort to tackle the systemic lapses in care facing communities around the world.

5.5 Federal/National Resources

The federal system for criminal justice and health care changes with each change in administration. These changes can be both good and bad. First, the instability on the system and all involved every four to eight years can be a struggle. Additionally, each administration can vary wildly in their views and ways to handle the needs of the country, including by setting priorities and funding schemes to match these priorities (particularly among major federal grant-funding agencies). Fortunately, or unfortunately, each state in the United States operates differently on some systems. There are federal standards to adhere to for hospitals and levels of treatment, but with other matters, policies can be changed or adjusted by state government. Further, the issue of treating mental health as a separate issue, allows for more "flexibility" with treatment and funding at the state level. State governments make decisions about the allocation of money to each different entity, like public run hospitals. If a state is in need of making financial adjustments, they can choose to defund those programs and even hospital. The following sections feature nationwide or federal resources that offer support to the issues documented in this book.

5.5.1 SAMHSA

The Substance Abuse and Mental Health Services Administration (SAMHSA) is a federal government agency that oversees many programs related to both mental health and substance abuse. Under the umbrella of SAMHSA include many different programs, campaigns, and initiatives including: advisory councils to lead behavioral health policymaking, strategic initiatives "to help provide treatment and services for people with mental and substance use disorders [and support their family]," social media campaigns, literature for professionals, individuals, and families, and current data on substance use and abuse as well as mental illness. Additionally, SAMHSA offers opportunity for funding via grants for state governments, local governments, and other related agencies (NAMI for example). These grants can offer opportunities for agencies, localities, and states to develop and expand existing programs or innovate to create new programs (Table 5.3).

Table 5.3 SAMHSA-funded programs (2017–2022)

Grant program	Program description
State Pilot Grant Program for Treatment for Pregnant and Postpartum Women	"Supports family-based services for pregnant and postpartum women with a primary diagnosis of a substance use disorder, including opioid disorders; 2) help state substance abuse agencies address the continuum of care, including services provided to women in nonresidential-based settings; and 3) promote a coordinated, effective and efficient state system managed by state substance abuse agencies by encouraging new approaches and models of service delivery."
Cooperative Agreements for Expansion and Sustainability of the Comprehensive Community Mental Health Services for Children with Serious Emotional Disturbances	"This cooperative agreement will support the provision of mental health and related recovery support services to children and youth with SED and those with early signs and symptoms of serious mental illness (SMI), including first episode psychosis (FEP), and their families…The SOC Expansion and Sustainability Cooperative Agreements will build upon progress made in developing comprehensive SOC across the country by focusing on sustainable financing, cross-agency collaboration, the creation of policy and infrastructure, and the development and implementation of evidence-based and evidence-informed services and supports."
State Targeted Response to the Opioid Crisis Grants	"The program aims to address the opioid crisis by increasing access to treatment, reducing unmet treatment need, and reducing opioid overdose related deaths through the provision of prevention, treatment and recovery activities for opioid use disorder (OUD) (including prescription opioids as well as illicit drugs such as heroin)."
Cooperative Agreement for the Provider's Clinical Support System – Medication Assisted Treatment Supplement	"Program purpose is to expand on the Drug Addiction Treatment Act (DATA) of 2000 and continue SAMHSA's currently funded PCSS-MAT initiative…This supplement will provide additional support to the current PCSS-MAT grantee by enhancing/expanding medication assisted treatment (MAT) training and educational resources to health professionals on evidence-based practices for preventing, identifying, and treating opioid use disorders."
Promoting Integration of Primary and Behavioral Health Care	"The purpose of this cooperative agreement is to: (1) promote full integration and collaboration in clinical practice between primary and behavioral healthcare; (2) support the improvement of integrated care models for primary care and behavioral health care to improve the overall wellness and physical health status of adults with a serious mental illness (SMI) or children with a serious emotional disturbance (SED); and (3) promote and offer integrated care services related to screening, diagnosis, prevention, and treatment of mental and substance use disorders, and co-occurring physical health conditions and chronic diseases."
Grants for the Benefit of Homeless Individuals	"The purpose of this program is to support the development and/or expansion of local implementation of a community infrastructure that integrates behavioral health treatment and services for substance use disorders (SUD) and co-occurring mental and substance use disorders (COD), permanent housing, and other critical services for individuals (including youth) and families experiencing homelessness."

(continued)

Table 5.3 (continued)

Grant program	Program description
Cooperative Agreement for the Historically Black Colleges and Universities Center for Excellence in Behavioral Health	"The purpose of this program is to continue to enhance the effort to network the 105 HBCUs throughout the United States to promote behavioral health, expand campus service capacity, and facilitate workforce development. The HBCU-CFE seeks to address behavioral health disparities among racial and ethnic minorities by encouraging the implementation of strategies to decrease the differences in access, service use, and outcomes among the racial and ethnic minority populations served and trained by the program. The goals of the HBCU-CFE are to promote student behavioral health to positively impact student retention; expand campus service capacity, including the provision of culturally and linguistically appropriate behavioral health resources; facilitate best practices dissemination and behavioral health workforce development; and increase awareness of the early signs of emotional distress and resources for early intervention."
Comprehensive Addiction and Recovery Act: Building Communities of Recovery	"The purpose of this program is to mobilize resources within and outside of the recovery community to increase the prevalence and quality of long-term recovery support from substance abuse and addiction. These grants are intended to support the development, enhancement, expansion, and delivery of recovery support services (RSS) as well as promotion of and education about recovery."
Grants to Expand Substance Abuse Treatment Capacity in Family Treatment Drug Courts	"The purpose of this program is to expand and/or enhance substance use disorder (SUD) treatment services in existing family treatment drug courts, which use the family treatment drug court model in order to provide alcohol and drug treatment (including recovery support services, screening, assessment, case management, and program coordination) to parents with a SUD and/or co-occurring SUD and mental disorders who have had a dependency petition filed against them or are at risk of such filing. Services must address the needs of the family as a whole and include direct service provision to children (18 and under) of individuals served by this project."
The Substance Abuse and HIV Prevention Navigator Program for Racial/Ethnic Minorities Ages 13–24 Cooperative Agreement	"The purpose of this program is to provide services to those at highest risk for HIV and substance use disorders, especially racial/ethnic males ages 13–24 at risk for HIV/AIDS including males who have sex with other males (MSM). The program will place a particular emphasis on those individuals who are not in stable housing in communities with high incidence and prevalence rates of substance misuse and HIV infection. It will provide opportunities to enhance outreach to the population of focus and assist them in receiving HIV medical care."
Resiliency in Communities After Stress and Trauma	"The purpose of this program is to assist high-risk youth and families and promote resilience and equity in communities that have recently faced civil unrest through implementation of evidence-based, violence prevention, and community youth engagement programs, as well as linkages to trauma-informed behavioral health services. The goal of the ReCAST Program is for local community entities to work together in ways that lead to improved behavioral health, empowered community residents, reductions in trauma, and sustained community change."

(continued)

Table 5.3 (continued)

Grant program	Program description
Cooperative Agreements to Implement the National Strategy for Suicide Prevention	"The purpose of this program is to support states in implementing the 2012 National Strategy for Suicide Prevention (NSSP) goals and objectives focused on preventing suicide and suicide attempts among adults age 25 and older in order to reduce the overall suicide rate and number of suicides in the U.S. nationally."
Grants for the Benefit of Homeless Individuals	"The purpose of this program is to support the development and/or expansion of local implementation of a community infrastructure that integrates behavioral health treatment and services for substance use disorders (SUD) and co-occurring mental and substance use disorders (COD), permanent housing, and other critical services for individuals (including youth) and families experiencing homelessness."
Cooperative Agreement for the Historically Black Colleges and Universities Center for Excellence in Behavioral Health	"The purpose of this program is to continue to enhance the effort to network the 105 HBCUs throughout the United States to promote behavioral health, expand campus service capacity, and facilitate workforce development. The HBCU-CFE seeks to address behavioral health disparities among racial and ethnic minorities by encouraging the implementation of strategies to decrease the differences in access, service use, and outcomes among the racial and ethnic minority populations served and trained by the program. The goals of the HBCU-CFE are to promote student behavioral health to positively impact student retention; expand campus service capacity, including the provision of culturally and linguistically appropriate behavioral health resources; facilitate best practices dissemination and behavioral health workforce development; and increase awareness of the early signs of emotional distress and resources for early intervention."
Comprehensive Addiction and Recovery Act: Building Communities of Recovery	"The purpose of this program is to mobilize resources within and outside of the recovery community to increase the prevalence and quality of long-term recovery support from substance abuse and addiction. These grants are intended to support the development, enhancement, expansion, and delivery of recovery support services (RSS) as well as promotion of and education about recovery."
Grants to Expand Substance Abuse Treatment Capacity in Family Treatment Drug Courts	"The purpose of this program is to expand and/or enhance substance use disorder (SUD) treatment services in existing family treatment drug courts, which use the family treatment drug court model in order to provide alcohol and drug treatment (including recovery support services, screening, assessment, case management, and program coordination) to parents with a SUD and/or co-occurring SUD and mental disorders who have had a dependency petition filed against them or are at risk of such filing. Services must address the needs of the family as a whole and include direct service provision to children (18 and under) of individuals served by this project."

(continued)

Table 5.3 (continued)

Grant program	Program description
The Substance Abuse and HIV Prevention Navigator Program for Racial/Ethnic Minorities Ages 13–24 Cooperative Agreement	"The purpose of this program is to provide services to those at highest risk for HIV and substance use disorders, especially racial/ethnic males ages 13–24 at risk for HIV/AIDS including males who have sex with other males (MSM). The program will place a particular emphasis on those individuals who are not in stable housing in communities with high incidence and prevalence rates of substance misuse and HIV infection. It will provide opportunities to enhance outreach to the population of focus and assist them in receiving HIV medical care."
Resiliency in Communities After Stress and Trauma	"The purpose of this program is to assist high-risk youth and families and promote resilience and equity in communities that have recently faced civil unrest through implementation of evidence-based, violence prevention, and community youth engagement programs, as well as linkages to trauma-informed behavioral health services. The goal of the ReCAST Program is for local community entities to work together in ways that lead to improved behavioral health, empowered community residents, reductions in trauma, and sustained community change."
Cooperative Agreements to Implement the National Strategy for Suicide Prevention	"The purpose of this program is to support states in implementing the 2012 National Strategy for Suicide Prevention (NSSP) goals and objectives focused on preventing suicide and suicide attempts among adults age 25 and older in order to reduce the overall suicide rate and number of suicides in the U.S. nationally."
Project AWARE	"The purpose of this program is to build or expand the capacity of State Educational Agencies, in partnership with State Mental Health Agencies (SMHAs) overseeing school-aged youth, and with three local education agencies (LEAs) to (1) increase awareness of mental health issues among school-aged youth; (2) provide training for school personnel and other adults who interact with school-aged youth to detect and respond to mental health issues; and (3) connect school-aged youth who may have behavioral health issues (including serious emotional disturbance [SED] or serious mental illness [SMI]), and their families, to needed services."
Assisted Outpatient Treatment Program for Individuals with Serious Mental Illness	"This four-year program is intended to implement and evaluate new AOT programs and identify evidence-based practices in order to reduce the incidence and duration of psychiatric hospitalization, homelessness, incarcerations, and interactions with the criminal justice system while improving the health and social outcomes of individuals with a serious mental illness."
Harm Reduction Grant Program	"The purpose of the program is to support community-based overdose prevention programs, syringe services programs, and other harm reduction services."

5.5.2 National Alliance on Mental Illness

The National Alliance on Mental Illness or NAMI is a mental health organization created to help improve the lives of people suffering from mental illness. The goals of NAMI include educating and advocating on topics related to mental illness. Additionally, the organization works to promote awareness with events including NAMIWalks as well as offer help and support with the NAMI HelpLine. For colleges and universities, NAMI on Campus is a campus club that works to end the stigma associated with mental illness as well as help to make connections for services and needs for students on campus. NAMI offers a startup packet and support to create a club on campus for those interested.

As an example of a NAMI local office, NAMI New Orleans offers a prime example of a vibrant NAMI operation working in collaboration with community partners to advance its mission. NAMI New Orleans operates two offices in the greater New Orleans area and provide a variety of services for the community. Adults living with severe mental illness in the area can receive services like, Counseling, Community Psychiatric Support and Treatment (CPST), Permanent Supportive Housing Services, Psychosocial Rehabilitation Skills Training (PSR), and even a Drop-In Center.

The Drop-In Center provides groups weekly as well as educational courses that last for 10 weeks regularly. These groups are run by peers trained by the NAMI Peer-to-Peer program. "The Peer-to-Peer program helps [an individual]:

- Create a personalized relapse prevention plan
- Learn how to interact with healthcare providers
- Develop confidence for making decisions and reducing stress
- Stay up-to-date on mental health research
- Understand the impact of symptoms on the person's life
- Access practical resources on how to maintain the journey toward recovery" (NAMI, 2017g).

Programs like these are important in that an individual with mental illness can receive support and help from others who understand their situation. Additionally, and importantly, individuals can learn to advocate for themselves in their own lives, especially in relation to medical needs. Ultimately, support and confidence can aid in the overall recovery and wellness for the person with mental illness.

In addition to services provided directly to the individuals in need in the community, NAMI also provides programming for family members and caretakers of those with mental illness. These programs can be beneficial to understand the illness of a loved one, understand their role in recovery and wellness, help to reduce stigma and boost awareness, and finally aid in reduction of burnout and compassion fatigue. NAMI New Orleans provides Mental Health First Aid, Mental Healthcare Navigation Team, Family Education and Support, Peer Education and Support, Advocacy and Community Education, and Advance Directive for Mental Health Treatment.

The Family Education and Support programs vary from structured multiweek courses taught by trained professionals to the Survivors of Suicide Loss support group which "is a free peer-led support group for adults whose lives have been impacted by the loss of a loved one to suicide, whether recently or in the past" (NAMI New Orleans, 2017).

5.6   Example of Innovation in Available Resources and Emerging Technology – Mobile Health (mHealth) and Telehealth Options

The use of applications or apps by many has grown for all sorts of options. From shopping to language skills and everything in between "there's an app for that." Now, there's also apps for therapy and treatment. Talkspace is a web-based treatment platform that can be used on a computer or cell phone. The process involves an initial assessment, then a matching process (not unlike online dating) to establish a positive relationship between therapist and potential client. Users can denote special needs like LGBTQ friendly or Veteran knowledge to assure their needs are met in future therapy session. Though application and web-based treatment options are nontraditional, they do provide options and help for those who may not otherwise have access or not seek treatment. The use of electronic devices can make the argument of both a help and a hindrance since there have been many studies regarding the limits on screen time or being present rather than glued to a phone, but that is a different book entirely.

The American Psychiatric Association (APA) has taken notice of the use of technology in treatment and is working to ensure best practices are used. The APA provides a process for rating apps by professionals. As well as rating, professionals can use the App Evaluations Model on the APA's website to review and identify the best apps for their clients. The model is founded in the idea of "do no harm."

The four areas comprising the model (beyond gathering basic background information) are:

1. Safety/Privacy
2. Evidence (i.e., effectiveness)
3. Ease of Use
4. Interoperability (American Psychiatric Association, 2017).

mHealth options are now available for individuals with any level of mental health need. Any person can benefit from speaking with a licensed and trained mental health professional, increasingly more often from the comfort of their own space with the benefit of telehealth. Generally, industry analysis of telehealth usage has seen increases close to 80 times higher from a prepandemic baseline (McKinsey, 2021), with usage stabilizing at 38 times higher over prepandemic utilization into 2021. That translates somewhere between 10% and 20% of all office visits, varying by medical specialty. In fact, psychiatry (broadly defined) and substance use disorder treatment services continue to dominate telehealth utilization by measure of outpatient and office visit claims by specialty (McKinsey, 2021) – with 50% of psychiatry and 30% of substance use disorder outpatient and office visit claims utilizing telehealth services in February 2021.

For-profit companies, such as Talkspace, Better Help, and Cerebral being the most visible at this time, offer on-demand mental health services using telehealth as its primary business model. Such services may prove to be crucial in addressing critical shortages in care across many swaths of the country, if not beyond. "For example, 56% of counties in the United States are without a psychiatrist, 64% of counties have a shortage of mental health providers, and 70% of counties lack a child psychiatrist. This kind of access may also be an opportunity to expand community, payer, and provider partnerships" (McKinsey, 2021). This sort of access is crucial in expansive rural areas where options are few and far between. Perhaps the most useful feedback provided by industry analysis of telehealth usage has been the consumer feedback. Most notably, only 1 in 10 consumers utilized telehealth options before the pandemic, compared to about 3 in 4 consumers who show interest in using these services in the future. The landscape is changing rapidly, and we are only now starting to understand the implications of these monumental shifts in how consumers receive care.

5.7   A Canary in the Shaft – American Mental Health Troubles Seen Abroad

Unfortunately, the struggles to treat mental illness are more widespread than the United States, particularly when discussing the issues of justice-involved individuals with mental health issues. In Italy for example, there were recent changes in government and funds which resulted in the closing of the forensic hospitals. This means that all individuals in the hospital that were previously being treated were either transferring to a regular hospital, put into a traditional jail/prison setting, or released. As a result, the health care system, criminal justice system, and community are all affected. In 2015, Italy finally closed their six remaining forensic psychiatric hospitals (Barbui & Saraceno, 2015; Casaccia et al., 2015):

> In 2012, a new law (Law 9/2012) established that new residential facilities had to be developed to better meet the needs of providing intensive and high-quality mental healthcare to socially dangerous individuals with mental disorders under proper secure conditions. These small-scale facilities (no more than 20 individuals, up to 4 patients per bedroom) are intended to replace admissions to forensic psychiatric hospitals.... As expected, the new law has activated a heated debate among Italian mental health professionals. As a general point it should be emphasized that this reform has been approved without clear cut evidence of its cost-effectiveness. Similarly, the results of studies describing the outcomes of patients discharged from forensic psychiatric hospitals are unavailable, and no recent and reliable information on the clinical characteristics and care needs of forensic psychiatric patients have been collected.... [A]nother critical consideration is the extra burden that community services will face. Several facilities in Italy are presently understaffed and in the past few years economic resources have been cut, to a varying degree, across the country. Additional resources will also be needed to increase the competence of mental health professionals working in community services in treating criminal offenders with mental disorders (Barbui & Saraceno, 2015: 445).

It appears that the American experience is not exclusive nor unique. As such, American students and professionals should be aware of other systems under stress and observe differences (and similarities) to other approaches to navigate these problems as a learning device. Further, growth from shared experiences works for mental health patients; why should it not be helpful for mental health professionals as well?

5.8 Conclusion

In the conversation about treatment, specifically for justice involved individuals, there is both good news and bad news. There are new innovations and technology being created daily to aid in allowing access to treatment for persons who otherwise may not have had any help. Additionally, federal grant funding allows for counties, parishes, and states to incorporate successful models that have been proven to work but would not have been a possibility due to funding. That being said, there continues to be strife in the realm of treatment for many states. The point here is that individuals experiencing symptoms of mental illness need treatment, not unlike any other illness. If a person needs treatment, then why are they often incarcerated? The answer – a system that continues to be broken. The entrenched dysfunction of the system of care sees some progress, yet progress is slow.

Those with severe mental illness are more likely to be homeless. If they are homeless, they may be out in public experiencing delusions and/or hallucinations. As mentioned before, the stigma and stereotype with mental illness lead the public and sometimes first responders (who may not be properly trained) to believe these individuals are violent or cause a public threat. In reality, most of these individuals are not violent but are in dire need of help and care. Taking a person to jail who is hearing voices or is severely paranoid is not the answer. Jail will not help because it is not treatment. Not only that, if they are paranoid or in the midst of a delusion or hallucination being taken against their will only to be locked up will most likely escalate the situation. Imagine being locked away and not understanding why or fearing harm. This compromises the safety of the individual, the first responders, the public, and those inside the jail/prison system.

This brings back the conversation regarding jail and prison staff and their safety. Without treatment, illnesses get worse and in this case those illnesses lead to further delusions or hallucinations. Often, this results in self-harm, possibly suicide. Then, consider those witnessing these acts and attempting to help. Incarceration does not cure mental illness.

Even further, the cost of incarcerating an individual comes into play. Keeping a person in jail or prison for days, weeks, months, or even years gets expensive. Alternatively, treatment can be provided and may be shorter and cost less.

Obviously, some violent crimes are the exception to the treatment instead of incarceration argument. There is a reality of those who commit horrible, violent crimes due to a mental illness and incarceration is part of the sentence for those crimes.

Humanity should be considered in all situations. No one would ever think to lock up a person with diabetes or cancer so why should bipolar disorder or schizophrenia be any different. Even consider nonpsychotic disorders like depression and anxiety. If a person experiencing clinical depression is incarcerated without treatment, how is that person expected to recovery? If they are released, how can society expect success? Also, as mentioned before, these individuals tend to return time and time again to jail. Each time costs money and each time does nothing to help the person with mental illness. Therefore, time and money are wasted, and the person's illness gets worse. Then, the person may seek medical attention as well. Thus, costing more money from the health care system. This benefits no one including the taxpayer.

Changes should be made at all levels of interaction local, state, and federal. On one side, there are taxpayers and government officials often discussing the fiscal side of the argument. The other side includes individuals with mental illness, their loved ones, and health professionals. It may appear to have a simple solution – send those with mental illness to treatment rather than jail or prison. It saves the local county/parish money, state, and federal government and helps the person. Ideally, that is simple, but the obstacles and barriers involved can be overwhelming, time consuming and shrouded with fear and misunderstanding often crippling the system and halting any change.

Many people know of someone with mental illness or a substance abuse problem. Whether it be a close friend or family member or a distant relative or coworker, these concerns do exist and are prevalent. Now, considering that person, do they not deserve treatment to help them recover?

First responders often struggle with the reality of the broken system as well. As discussed before, their job (and often identity) is to help others in need. Keeping that in mind, imagine the difficulty of repeated attempts to help individuals encountered on a regular basis. How does a first responder keep faith in the system? In their job? Further, the local/state/federal government? These issues all lead to burnout and mental health struggles for those on the front line. Not to mention, the growing frustration of the lack of help being provided to those in need. Visually seeing people deteriorate regularly cannot be easy.

Furthermore, for the individual inside the system, hope and positivity can be difficult to find. Fear of incarceration may be reason alone for a person to avoid seeking help when needed. Leading to hopelessness and again, worsening symptoms. Without a proper support system, this fear may also lead to grave consequences with suicide. Add in the stigma of mental illness, substance abuse, and criminal history and the results are a trifecta of negativity. It can seem impossible to change or even begin steps to recover, sobriety and wellness. Those in need of help may also not know the resources available to them or even worse, may not have access to seek out said resources.

Thinking of loved ones, the importance of education and support is also essential here. Families can play a crucial role in helping a person change for the better after a mental illness crisis or even just a diagnosis. Also, those with substance abuse and criminal history are in dire need of education and support. Those who live with the individual in need can learn to understand the signs and symptoms of their illness(es). Learning these can aid in proactive measures to possibly prevent further issues or from an eruption of symptoms. Additionally, support after treatment can be beneficial to possibly prevent further issues (Fig. 5.3).

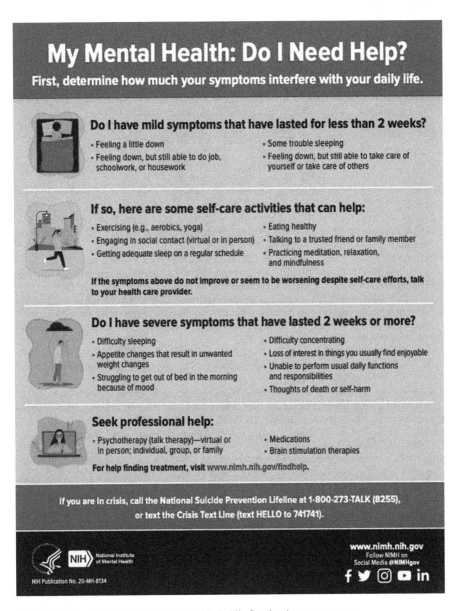

Fig. 5.3 National Institute of Mental Health, Public Service Announcement

Discussion Questions

1. What types of coverage do most U.S. medical insurance plans offer for mental health treatment (talk therapy, outpatient, inpatient, substance use, etc.)?
2. How do countries address mental health treatment? In particular, compare the United States with a country that has universal health coverage.
3. Explain how the use of electronic records ensures the continuity of mental health care.

References

Alcoholics Anonymous. (1981). *The twelve steps of Alcoholics Anonymous.* URL: https://www.aa.org/assets/en_US/smf-121_en.pdf. Last accessed: October 27, 2017.

American Psychiatric Association. (2017). *App evaluation model.* URL: https://www.psychiatry.org/psychiatrists/practice/mental-health-apps/app-evaluation-model. Last accessed: 27 Oct 2017.

Barbui, C., & Saraceno, B. (2015). Closing forensic psychiatric hospitals in Italy: A new revolution begins? *The British Journal of Psychiatry, 206*(6), 445–446.

Canady, V. A. (2021). New program to address solutions for people in a BH crisis. *Mental Health Weekly, 31*(20), 3–4.

Casacchia, M., Malavolta, M., Bianchini, V., Giusti, L., Di, V. M., Giosuè, P., Ruggeri, M., Biondi, M., & Roncone, R. (2015). Closing forensic psychiatric hospitals in Italy: a new deal for mental health care? *Rivista di psichiatria, 50*(5), 199–209.

Centers for Medicare & Medicaid Services. (2017). *Community mental health centers.* URL: https://www.cms.gov/Medicare/Provider-Enrollment-and-Certification/CertificationandComplianc/CommunityHealthCenters.html. Last accessed: 31 Oct 2017.

Denver, the Mile High City. (2022). *Wellness Winnie.* URL: https://www.denvergov.org/Government/Agencies-Departments-Offices/Agencies-Departments-Offices-Directory/Public-Health-Environment/Community-Behavioral-Health/Behavioral-Health-Strategies/Wellness-Winnie. Last accessed: 3 Feb 2022.

Fraze, T., Lewis, V. A., Rodriguez, H. P., & Fisher, E. S. (2016). Housing, transportation, and food: How ACOs seek to improve population health by addressing nonmedical needs of patients. *Health Affairs, 35*(11), 2109–2115.

Insel, T. (2010). *Turning the corner, not the key, in treatment of serious mental illness.* URL: https://www.nimh.nih.gov/about/directors/thomas-insel/blog/2010/turning-the-corner-not-the-key-in-treatment-of-serious-mental-illness.shtml. Last accessed: 25 Oct 2017.

Kaskutas, L. A. (2009). Alcoholics Anonymous effectiveness: Faith meets science. *Journal of Addictive Diseases, 28*(2), 145–157.

Khey, D. N. Unpublished research – Findings from an audit of a local Louisiana mental health provider.

Khey, D. N. Unpublished research – unnamed informant.

Louisiana Department of Health. (2017). *Department of health and department of corrections team up to provide health care coverage for newly released offenders.* URL: http://new.dhh.louisiana.gov/index.cfm/newsroom/detail/4170. Last accessed: 27 Oct 2017.

McKinsey & Company. (2021). *Telehealth: A quarter-trillion-dollar post-COVID-19 reality?* URL: https://www.mckinsey.com/industries/healthcare-systems-and-services/our-insights/telehealth-a-quarter-trillion-dollar-post-covid-19-reality. Last accessed: 7 Feb 2022.

Minnesota Department of Human Services. (2017). *First episode psychosis.* URL: https://mn.gov/dhs/people-we-serve/adults/health-care/mental-health/programs-services/first-episode-psychosis.jsp. Last accessed: 27 Oct 2017.

Morgan, E. R., Rowhani-Rahbar, A., Azrael, D., & Miller, M. (2018). Public perceptions of firearm-and non–firearm-related violent death in the United States: a national study. *Annals of Internal Medicine, 169*(10), 734–737.

National Academies of Sciences, Engineering, and Medicine. (2016). *Connecting patients to transportation: Incentives and return on investment.* URL: https://www.ncbi.nlm.nih.gov/books/NBK402427/. Last accessed: 27 Oct 2017.

National Alliance on Mental Illness. (2017a). *Mental health by the numbers.* URL: https://www.nami.org/Learn-More/Mental-Health-By-the-Numbers. Last accessed: 25 Oct 2017.

National Alliance on Mental Illness. (2017b). *Medicaid.* URL: https://www.nami.org/Learn-More/Mental-Health-Public-Policy/Medicaid. Last accessed: 27 Oct 2017.

National Alliance on Mental Illness. (2017c). *Dual diagnosis.* URL: https://www.nami.org/Learn-More/Mental-Health-Conditions/Related-Conditions/Dual-Diagnosis. Last accessed: 27 Oct 2017.

National Alliance on Mental Illness. (2017d). *Psychosocial treatments.* URL: https://www.nami.org/Learn-More/Treatment/Psychosocial-Treatments. Last accessed: 27 Oct 2017.

National Alliance on Mental Illness. (2017e). *Treatment settings.* URL: https://www.nami.org/NAMI/media/NAMI-Media/Images/FactSheets/Treatment-Settings-FS.pdf. Last accessed: 27 Oct 2017.

National Alliance on Mental Illness. (2017f). *Securing stable housing.* URL: https://www.nami.org/Find-Support/Living-with-a-Mental-Health-Condition/Securing-Stable-Housing. Last accessed: 27 Oct 2017.

National Alliance on Mental Illness. (2017g). *NAMI Peer-to-Peer.* URL: https://www.nami.org/Find-Support/NAMI-Programs/NAMI-Peer-to-Peer. Last accessed: 27 Oct 2017.

National Alliance on Mental Illness Minnesota. (2017). *Fact sheet: Assertive Community Treatment (ACT).* URL: http://www.namihelps.org/assets/PDFs/fact-sheets/General/Assertive-Community-Treatment.pdf. Last accessed: 27 Oct 2017.

National Alliance on Mental Illness New Orleans. (2017). *Survivors of suicide loss support group (Uptown).* URL: https://namineworleans.org/event-registration/. Last accessed: 27 Oct 2017.

National Alliance on Mental Illness St. Tammany. (2017). *Resources.* URL: http://namisttammany.org/resources/. Last accessed: 25 Oct 2017.

National Institute on Drug Abuse. (2017). *Principles of drug abuse treatment for criminal justice populations - A research-based guide.* URL: https://www.drugabuse.gov/publications/principles-drug-abuse-treatment-criminal-justice-populations/legally-mandated-treatment-effective. Last accessed: 27 Oct 2017.

Office of the National Coordinator for Health Information Technology. (2017). *Dashboard.* URL: https://dashboard.healthit.gov. Last accessed: 27 Oct 2017.

Owens, P. L., Fingar, K. R., McDermott, K. W., Muhuri, P. K., & Heslin, K. C. (2019). *Inpatient stays involving mental and substance use disorders, 2016.* URL: https://www.hcup-us.ahrq.gov/reports/statbriefs/sb249-Mental-Substance-Use-Disorder-Hospital-Stays-2016.pdf. Last accessed: 30 Jan 2022.

Palabindala, V., Pamarthy, A., & Jonnalagadda, N. R. (2016). Adoption of electronic health records and barriers. *Journal of Community Hospital Internal Medicine Perspectives*, 6(5). URL: http://www.tandfonline.com/doi/full/10.3402/jchimp.v6.32643. Last accessed: 27 Oct 2017.

Substance Abuse and Mental Health Services Administration. (2006). *Detoxification and substance abuse treatment.* Treatment improvement protocol (TIP) Series, No. 45. URL: https://store.samhsa.gov/shin/content/SMA13-4131/SMA13-4131.pdf. Last accessed: 27 Oct 2017.

Substance Abuse and Mental Health Services Administration. (2012). *People with mental health & substance use conditions: The core clinical features.* URL: https://www.integration.samhsa.gov/clinical-practice/CIHS_Health_Homes_Core_Clinical_Features.pdf. Last accessed: 27 Oct 2017.

Substance Abuse and Mental Health Services Administration. (2014). *Projections of national expenditures for treatment of mental and substance use disorders, 2010–2020.* URL: https://store.samhsa.gov/sites/default/files/d7/priv/sma14-4883.pdf. Last accessed: 30 Jan 2022.

Substance Abuse and Mental Health Services Administration. (2017). *Health IT for patients and families*. URL: https://www.samhsa.gov/health-information-technology/patients-families. Last accessed: 27 Oct 2017.

United States Department of Housing and Urban Development. (2017). *Public housing occupancy guidebook*. URL: https://www.hud.gov/sites/documents/DOC_10760.PDF. Last accessed: 27 Oct 2017.

World Health Organization. (2022). *Premature death among people with severe mental disorders*. URL: https://www.who.int/mental_health/management/info_sheet.pdf. Last accessed: 30 Jan 2022.

Chapter 6
Jails

You never really understand a person until you consider things from his point of view…until you climb into his skin and walk around in it – Harper Lee

The fact that jails have become a key focal point for mental illness over the years is not inherently the central problem. This may be a semantical point, but it is an important one to think over. As discussed earlier, the history of caring for those with mental illness is fraught with horrors, stigma, abuse, and misunderstanding. Shifting the primary location of care for patients from the asylum to the communities they reside was quite intentional and, in part, driven by humanitarian interests. The perception of this shift is remarkable. What better way exists to "fix" a broken system than destroying it and freeing the tortured souls bound up in its clutches? Truly, these are almost identical interests that drove the creation of asylums in the first place just a generation before – recall our discussion of Dorothea Dix and her advocacy for these very reforms. While it is tempting to simply suggest that jails are no place for individuals with mental illness, the broader truth is that jails can perform a vital role in the continuum of treatment when tailored evidence-based programs are put into place. This brings us to *the* central problem: jails are utilized as the *de facto* focal point for mental illness largely without process, decisive action, and dedicated programing. Thus, shifting the responsibility of care effectively did little to solve the underlying issue of a broken continuum of care, with the operational word being *care*.

6.1   Know the Role

As a legal matter, the standard of care rests in how we have come to define a constitutionally acceptable level of care. What this boils down to, in most circumstances, is defining the absolute minimum level of care required to run a legally compliant jail. Yet, even this standard can be quite costly. For example, a Southwestern Louisiana jail administrator speculated that her costs run upwards to $100 per day to care for an individual with mental illness at this standard. In all actuality, this estimate runs on the cheaper end of the spectrum across the United States; for example, an often cited report in *The Miami Herald* estimated that care for individuals with mental illness in the Broward County, Florida jail, is about $130 per day compared to the $80 for an "average" inmate back in 2007 (Miller & Fantz, 2007). A Vera Institute report updated in 2014 has compiled similar situations across the country. In Harris County (Houston), Texas, the annual expenditure for mental health care reached $24 million dollars per year. In Northeast Ohio, over half of a jail's medical budget was spent on psychotropic drugs alone (Vera Institute, 2014). Again, most of these tallies cover just the bare necessities as required by the constitution.

This institutional mentality is beginning to thaw as justice professionals are increasingly acknowledging the failing logic of providing short-term care that only covers basic needs. Largely driven by the desire to tamp down cost, justice administrators have recently sought out ways to adapt their forced role of primary mental health care providers for an at-risk population by partnering diverse array of community stakeholders to formulate a stronger continuum of care (and dispersing the costs involved to a wider range of players). As this innovation is taking place, the vast majority of jurisdictions are slow to respond, if at all. Major court decisions have driven reform in the past, and even these pressures brought about change slowly.

6.1.1   Constitutionally Acceptable Level of Care: The Status Quo

The basis for defining a "legal" level of care began with litigating perceived protections of incarcerated persons under the Eighth Amendment – "Excessive bail shall not be required, nor excessive fines imposed, nor cruel and unusual punishments inflicted." In 1974, a prisoner in Texas named J.W. Gamble filed a civil rights action under 42 U.S.C. § 1983 by handwritten petition. While it seems that Gamble's primary objective was compensation for maltreatment, his case instead defined the first set of constitutional obligations of medical care for the incarcerated. Gamble's complaint described a back injury he sustained in 1973 while unloading a truck full of cotton bales as a part of his prison work duties. He continued to work, but soon reported his discomfort to prison staff and was granted a pass to the medical unit at the facility. Gamble was evaluated by a medical assistant (with prescribing capabilities) for a hernia and was initially sent back to his cell. He continued to have problems and was able to go back to the medical unit – this time being seen by a nurse and a doctor. At this point, he obtained some medication for pain. The next day, he returned to the medical unit and was seen by another doctor, Dr. Astone, received a diagnosis of a lower back strain, and was placed on a treatment plan consisting of medication and cell restriction requiring Gamble to remain in his cell with the only exclusion of showering. A few days later, Dr. Astone extended this treatment plan after reevaluation, and further ordered that Gamble be assigned to a bottom bunk (an order the prison staff did not enforce). This sort of treatment carried on throughout the month of November under Dr. Astone's care, seemingly without improvement.

It was at this point things seemed to shift for Gamble. On December 3, 1974, Dr. Astone removed Gamble's cell restrictions, which also approved him for light work, despite continued pain and discomfort. As staff assigned work duties to him, his complaints to supervisory staff landed him in segregated housing as punishment. This issue was heard by a disciplinary committee days later resulting in a recommendation to be seen by medical staff; but, they insisted that he be seen by a different physician. Dr. Gray treated Gamble for high blood pressure and pain, prescriptions were lost and delayed, and he remained in segregation for the entire month. This treatment stretched into January and came to a head in February. At this point, Gamble reported chest pains and "blank outs," yet staff were slow to respond, taking all day on February 4th to move him from segregation to the medical unit. He was hospitalized that evening and diagnosed with an arrhythmia, yet, soon sent back to segregation. When his symptoms reappeared, staff refused to bring him back to the medical unit – Gamble asked several times on February 7th and 8th, and he was turned down repeatedly. Finally, on February 9th, he was again treated for his heart condition, and he wrote his petition to the courts on February 11th.

Initially, the district court dismissed his petition as the presiding judge did not view his case to have a clear legal claim. Typically, a judge at this level is trained to evaluate if a plaintiff can argue concrete, tangible harms have occurred and have been clearly documented. The appeals court was not moved by this logic and reinstated the complaint based on their finding of an insufficient levels of medical treatment. Soon, the Supreme Court would weigh in with an 8 to 1 decision:

> We therefore conclude that deliberate indifference to serious medical needs of prisoners constitutes the "unnecessary and wanton infliction of pain," *Gregg v. Georgia, supra,* at 173 (joint opinion), proscribed by the Eighth Amendment. This is true whether the indifference is manifested by prison doctors in their response to the prisoner's needs [n10]or by prison guards in intentionally denying or delaying access to medical [p105] care[n11] or intentionally interfering with the treatment once prescribed. [n12] Regardless of how evidenced, deliberate indifference to a prisoner's serious illness or injury states a cause of action under § 1983.

At first glance, it seems as though the Court was moved by Gamble's handwritten petition. Perhaps Gamble was able to lay out a claim based on the repeated times he was denied care, or his accounts of how his prescriptions were lost, or when the prison staff interfered with his treatment when they put him back to work or punished him by sending him to a segregation unit. The truth is that the case is much more complicated than it appears:

> This conclusion does not mean, however, that every claim by a prisoner that he has not received adequate medical treatment states a violation of the Eighth Amendment. An accident, although it may produce added anguish, is not on that basis alone to be characterized as wanton infliction of unnecessary pain….in the medical context, an inadvertent failure to provide adequate medical care cannot be said to constitute "an unnecessary and wanton infliction of pain" or to be [p106] "repugnant to the conscience of mankind." Thus, a complaint that a physician has been negligent in diagnosing or treating a medical condition does

not state a valid claim of medical mistreatment under the Eighth Amendment. Medical malpractice does not become a constitutional violation merely because the victim is a prisoner. In order to state a cognizable claim, a prisoner must allege acts or omissions sufficiently harmful to evidence deliberate indifference to serious medical needs. It is only such indifference that can offend "evolving standards of decency" in violation of the Eighth Amendment.

As it turns out, the Court believed the district court judge was correct in that Gamble did not have a § 1983 claim, at least against the medical director Dr. Gray. The majority opinion cited the repeated instances of treatment Gamble received by the prison medical staff – whether it was "good" treatment was not to be decided in this venue. Further, since the lower court of appeals' decision focused on the care of the physicians and medical staff under Dr. Gray, their decision outlining the lack of civil rights violations was limited to these individuals (particularly, absolving Dr. Gray). Instead of deciding the fate of the other litigants mentioned in the petition, like the warden of the prison and the Texas Department of Corrections leadership, the Supreme Court decided to push this back down to the lower courts to decide in light of their recent clarifications of the Eighth Amendment in this situation. The level of care may have amounted to malpractice, which would need to be litigated differently; however, the decision rendered that incarcerated persons were constitutionally protected against "wanton infliction of unnecessary pain." Gamble may have lost, but his case surely caused ripples in correctional medical care.

This was the legal foundation for all cases involving standards of medical care for incarcerated people that will follow; however, there has not been a landmark case on the level of Estelle v. Gamble to directly address mental health care for justice-involved individuals. One key exception exists from a stream of action in California. Advocates there took a different approach to address the emerging mental health deficiencies in jails and prisons beginning in the 1990s – focus on increasing sparseness of resources and personnel given an expanding incarceration population. It was these broadening deficiencies in adequate care that triggered § 1983 civil rights violations, infringing upon inmates' constitutional rights under the Eighth Amendment. The momentum for this conflict began to surge when a magistrate certified a class "consisting of 'all inmates with serious mental disorders who are now or who will in the future be confined within the California Department of Corrections'" (with limited exceptions) who together had volumes of stories of neglect and maltreatment. After years of litigation, this case – *Coleman v. Wilson* – was initially resolved in 1995 by appointing a special master to oversee a remediation plan to remedy the conditions in California prisons. Importantly, this special master was charged with holding the California Department of Corrections accountable for six components of mental health treatment to meet minimal constitutional requirements:

The six components are: (1) a systematic program for screening and evaluating inmates to identify those in need of mental health care; (2) a treatment program that involves more than segregation and close supervision of mentally ill inmates; (3) employment of a sufficient number of trained mental health professionals; (4) maintenance of accurate, complete and confidential mental health treatment records; (5) administration of psychotropic medication only with appropriate supervision and periodic evaluation; and (6) a basic program to identify, treat, and supervise inmates at risk for suicide. *Balla v. Idaho State Board of Corrections,* 595 F.Supp. 1558, 1577 (D.Idaho 1984)

This case references precedent that originated out of Texas (*Ruiz v. Estelle,* 503 F.Supp. 1265 (S.D.Tex.1980)), which was expanded upon further in a case against the Idaho Department of Corrections in 1984. These six components defining the minimal constitutional level of mental health care would eventually become further tested at the Federal District Court level when California failed several times to resolve Coleman v. Wilson under the appointed special master. This new case, Coleman v. Brown, sought to bring California into compliance with Coleman v. Wilson almost 10 years later in 2013. Yet again, a judge sided with the plaintiffs, arguing that California needed to continue to provide relief to the class of mentally ill inmates under the care of the California Department of Corrections.

These key features of legal precedents, as many others across the country, can also be found interwoven in the accreditation standards of the corrections industry. In fact, the evolution of best practices (again, geared to ensure a *minimal* array of services to be constitutionally acceptable) can be easily gleaned from each edition of industrial standards released by the American Correctional Association (ACA) and the National Commission on Correctional Health Care (NCCHC). For example, the ACA Performance Based Standards for Adult Community Residential Services (2001) mandate the following: round-the-clock emergency health care with onsite crisis intervention, emergency rooms or other appropriate health facilities, and on-call mental health professional services with an emergency health facility is not located nearby (Standard 4-ACRS- 4C-03), a training program to be in place for *care worker* staff to recognize signs and symptoms of mental illness, substance use disorder, and intellectual disability (Standard 4-ACRS- 4C-04), mental health screening by trained professionals that covers mental health problems and suicide attempts/ideation, substance abuse, and direct observation of behaviors (Standard 4-ACRS- 4C-06), a written suicide prevention and intervention program with dedicated training that covers all staff who supervise inmates. These standards have become commonplace throughout American corrections. Yet, given the fact that more individuals with mental illness remain untreated rather than receive treatment in jails should give us pause. Perhaps these standards provide a safety net for the most seriously ill; however, it appears that they are ineffective for the vulnerable population en masse.

6.1.2   Common Interactions

For generations now, vocations that care for individuals with mental illness have suffered from a lack of prestige, pay, desirability, and so on. Jobs within jails certainly fall in this category. A quick search for information on these jobs reveals high turnover, issues with burnout, and, at times, a lack of further career opportunities.

Yet, as mentioned earlier, jails have become a critical focal point for mental health crises – roughly 15% of male and 30% of female jail inmates have a serious mental illness and the vast majority do not receive any treatment (NAMI, 2017). Further, most correctional officers have little training in mental health and substance abuse awareness and treatment (Stohr et al., 1992). A majority of jails across the country thus heavily depend on their treatment staff to identify mental illness, develop a treatment plan, and help to ensure the six components of mental health care are provided to meet constitutional standards.

Jail correctional officers, in particular, play a critical role in promoting a healthy environment for both fellow staff and inmates. The recent stories brimming from the Orleans Parish Prison (the New Orleans Jail ran by the Orleans Parish Sheriff's Office) and Riker's Island Prison Complex (the New York City jail ran by New York City Correction Department) offer allegories as to the serious behavioral health consequences of staffing issues among other organizational failures. For example, in New Orleans, just months after opening a state-of-the-art jail complex, the Orleans Parish Sheriff's Office reported 200 inmate-on-inmate altercations, 44 instances of use of force on inmates by state, 16 assaults on staff, 3 rapes, 29 inmates transferred to the hospital for injury or sickness, and 16 suicide attempts – all within the first 3 months (McCampbell et al., 2017; Sledge, 2017). In New York, tales of correctional staff retaliating against inmates who attempt suicide at Riker's Island have surfaced, depicting just how brutal the jail environment has become (Rayman, 2016). Both failing jails are now notorious for high turnover, leading to the stagnation of the critical changes needed to promote a safe and therapeutic environment. While these are extreme cases, it is important to note that line correctional officers are often only equipped to identify suicide risk by a matter of policy and receive little more training pertaining to mental health. Their jobs are wrought with low job satisfaction, little autonomy, and inadequate pay. Mental health seems to be a low priority for line officers who spend the most interface time with inmates, by far.

The key players involved in the post-arrest phase of a potential justice-based intervention include jail intake and medical/treatment staff, line correctional officers, public defenders, prosecutors, and judges, with the heaviest burden on intake and medical/treatment staff to flag potential inmates for services and assistance. Robust research has only begun to evaluate the systemic breakdown in counties and parishes across the country to successfully capture mental illness and explore effective interventions. As such, we do not have a deep understanding of the everyday interactions of these key players and inmates with mental illness. Of particular importance here, the Stepping Up Initiative (2022) is the leading movement for change at the local level. This Initiative is a partnership of The National Association of Counties, The Council of State Governments Justice Center, and the American Psychiatric Association Foundation, which partnered to offer a structured guide, training, and seed funding to reduce the number of people with mental illness in jails beginning in 2015. As of this writing, 537 counties (up from 365 in 2017) have passed resolutions through local leadership to join this initiative, the first step of which is to engage in a comprehensive system-wide evaluation of just how individuals with mental illness are processed and captured (or not captured) by the current system. The Initiative also serves to assist localities in building a diverse partnership of key stakeholders who have been deemed essential to creating successful models for change.

6.1.3   Common Problems

As the Stepping Up Initiative prepared to launch, its advertising campaign to counties and parishes identified the following common-place problems in jails across the United States: 1) prevalence of serious mental illness was three to six times higher in jails relative to the general population, 2) three out of four of these individuals have co-occurring disorders, 3) once in jail, these individuals tend to experience longer stays in jail relative to individuals without mental illness, and 4) these individuals are at a much higher risk of recidivism upon release relative to individuals without mental illness (Council of State Governments Justice Center, 2014). Certainly, this list is not exhaustive, but it captures the failing logic of the current systems in place across the country – it depicts a system that has recurring failures as an intervention for people with mental illness. The analogy to a revolving door has become apt.

Perhaps the systemic failure is most punctuated by an examination of suicide ideation, attempts, and completions in jails; As indicated earlier in this text, the risk of suicide tends to be the highest in jails. According to the Bureau of Justice Statistics, suicides among jail inmates have been on the rise, with the most current rate being 49 per 100,000 inmates as of 2019 (Noonan, 2015; Carson, 2021). Compare this to a national average of roughly 13.9 per 100,000, the difference in jails is about four times higher than the general population (Centers for Disease Control and Prevention, 2021). Existing data on suicide ideation and attempts among jail inmates is scant and much older. However, the underlying patterns of crisis still emerge.

One of the first briefs coming from the Stepping Up Initiative leadership summarizes a growing body of knowledge on what, exactly, our failures are in the jail setting. It begins by outlining the changes that have occurred in services for individuals with mental illness over the last decade: a mass proliferation of specialized police response teams and programs, specialized programming to divert low-level offenders with mental illness from the mainstream justice system, broader use of specialty courts, and enhanced mental health services in jails to name a few. Even with these innovations in place, the brief describes four barriers preventing gains. First, and primarily, most locales suffer from the lack of adequate data to identify a targeted population and monitor it effectively. For example, having access to basic information such as the total number and identities of individuals with mental illness arrested and who currently in the local jail is important. Additional relevant information about this population is also crucial, such as the length of stay in jail, bond status, whether individuals have previously received treatment or are currently being treated, and the ability to follow rearrest. Without adequate data tools, developing a system-wide response to any underlying problem becomes problematic. Second, many programs that are in place lack an evidence-based services, tools, and programming, and critically, "community-based behavioral health care providers are rarely familiar with (or skilled in delivering) the approaches that need to be integrated into their treatment models to reduce the likelihood of someone offending" (Haneberg et al., 2017). Third, due to scarce resources, innovation has been small in scope and scale, thus blunting any ability to create sustained systemic changes. Finally, and related to the first barrier, many innovations have lacked adequate tracking to determine their impact. Did the initiatives reduce arrests for individuals with mental illness, reduce the length of time these individuals spend in jail, and/or increase treatment options, connections, and adherence to treatment regimes? These barriers translate into underdiagnosis/lack of diagnosis, continued exasperated behavioral problems, overpopulation through recidivism, and continued vulnerability for individuals with mental illness in potentially problematic and unhealthy jail environments.

The services offered to inmates within jails continue to be in line with constitutional minimums, yet change is afoot. Oftentimes, only one mental health professional is dedicated to providing services for an entire jail of hundreds of inmates. While prisons offer programs for education, vocational training, etc. that help with mental health and behavioral change, jails have consistently lacked the same breadth of scope of programs for inmates in many jurisdictions. Further, jail inmates usually serve a shorter sentence than those in prison; this lack of time does not afford the chance for long-term treatment services or programming. Thus, this highlights the importance of a collaboration between jails, courts, probation, and community players to shore up a continuum of care to break this cycle. This is exactly what the Stepping Up Initiative lays out.

6.1.4 Preventable Tragedies

Unfortunately, death of inmates inside jails and prisons are real possibilities. Even further, inmates with mental illness are more likely to suffer harm while incarcerated according to many studies. One report published by The University of Texas School of Law Civil Rights Clinic (2016) called "Preventable Tragedies" discusses the deaths of ten different inmates in county jails, all with mental health concerns – such as Terry Borum in Swisher County Jail, Gregory Cheek in Nueces County Jail, and Amy Lynn Cowling in Gregg County Jail. The first part of the report describes each of the deaths in personal detail to highlight the "cracks" in the county jail system in Texas and its real impact on human lives. An interesting point to note here is that each of these deaths took place under very different circumstances and in different county jails. These tragedies were all easily preventable in many ways. This report also goes on to provide 12 recommendations for Texas county jails based on national standards to help improve care for inmates with mental illness, which the authors truly believe would serve to prevent each of the tragedies listed in this study.

Similar recommendations were also provided by the Stanford School of Law in their study on mental health in jail inmates (more on this study in Chapter 8; Steinberg, Mills, & Romano, 2017).

Each of the stories provided in the "Preventable Tragedies" report sheds light on a different problem with the county jail system, specifically in Texas. Earlier in this text, the statistics on jail settings were discussed which included the elevated number of inmates, increasing number with mental health diagnoses, lack of funding, lack of access to care, etc. The trends that these statistics depict also are typical in Texas, and the evidence supporting this claim is provided with each case in this report. For example, the story of Terry Borum is alarming in that his severe alcoholism was known prior to his incarceration by jail staff and the Sheriff, but no action was taken to care for him until his case became an emergency situation. Terry had a history of depression that resulted in his alcoholism, and when a minor altercation led him to the county jail, his symptoms reached a breaking point. His past suicide attempt complicated his mental health history and should have been one of the first reasons to prioritize medical treatment to ensure his care was appropriate. As the report details the story, treatment did not happen at all, and after he went into delirium tremens that included hallucinations and seizures, he fell inside his jail cell causing a serious head injury. It was at this point that medical care was initialized and Borum was fully evaluated. Yet, it was too late; due to the lack of nutrition, the haphazard care provided, and the jail's unwillingness to use their medical care budget on Terry, he was not able to survive a survivable injury and died in a nearby hospital.

In another case within the "Preventable Tragedies" report, Gregory Cheek was arrested after breaking into a home and painting the walls blue and yellow. At the time of his arrest, he was covered in blue paint and suffering from delusions. Despite this, his intake assessment reported no medical issues, no mental health issues, and no medications prescribed at the time. Gregory was seen by the jail's psychiatrist who recommended he be transferred to the state hospital on more than one occasion. Additionally, a magistrate judge ordered that Gregory be transferred to the state hospital, but none of these instructions were followed. After suffering the beginning signs of hypothermia, Gregory died in jail from a bacterial infection that was left untreated. A review of his case after his death reveals that the jail psychiatrist ignored reports from the medical staff to follow up on Gregory's medication while inadequate medical care and follow-up attention was paid to a worsening physical condition. It turns out that Gregory succumbed to Waterhouse-Friderichsen syndrome – a severe bacterial infection of the adrenal glands causing gland failure and bleeding. In this case, neither Gregory's physical or mental health were attended to, which can be surprising to some as his mental health symptoms were severe and readily recognizable, as was his signs of his failing physical health, specifically his rapid weight loss and chronic hyperthermia in days nearing his death.

Amy Lynn Cowling's story was similar to Terry Borum above in that her death is attributed to the complications of withdrawal. Yet in Cowling's case, several prescriptions meant to treat her mental health illnesses (Seroquel and Xanax) and substance use disorder (methadone) were discontinued due to the Gregg County Jail's strict policy on drugs in the jail. While the jail's physician would have ordered an alternative course of medical treatment to fit the jail's policy and keep Amy's treatment from slipping, she never had the chance to see the doctor. The reason – the doctor only makes visits to the jail on Wednesdays and Amy was booked on a Friday. After her medication was discontinued, Amy's physical and mental health rapidly decompensated and she was moved to an isolation cell with orders to be closely watched. Yet, the correctional officers on watch that evening decided to falsify the observation logs and could not account for why Amy was found unresponsive on the day she died.

These stories are just three of the many across the country of individuals with mental illness dying in county jails. The stories of Terry and Gregory are different, but both show the results of improper care while incarcerated. Terry's illness was known to jail officials, but they chose to ignore his needs as well as use the budget of the jail as an excuse not to seek medical treatment. In Gregory's case, he was initially treated as though he was perfectly healthy and later evaluated. Upon evaluation, the mental health professionals and even a judge decided he needed more treatment than the jail could offer, but no one chose to uphold the orders. It seems like a comedy of errors has led to the deaths of these ten people – Terry Borum, a 53-year-old grandfather who lived by and maintained traditional country values; Gregory Cheek, a young artist and surfer, husband and father to a young girl; and Amy Lynn Cowling, a 33-year-old mother of three who was in recovery for her opioid addiction.

The stories of deaths in county jails are alarming and unsettling, and they happen with a frequency that surely can be reduced. Yet, this seems difficult when considering the level of care inherent in what is deemed as constitutionally acceptable. The authors offer the following areas of improvement to aid in reform while maintaining this very same standard: 1) increase diversion from jail for low-risk individuals with mental illness, 2) improve screening and assessment tools to ensure adequate care and informed decision-making, 3) arm the judiciary with the results of screening and assessment to aid in diversion, whenever appropriate, 4) evaluate and refine suicide prevention programs with partnerships that include mental health professionals, 5) increase and strengthen collaborations with mental health professionals and local agencies, 6) ensure the ability to continue medication treatment regimens with appropriate medications or their alternatives, 7) develop and update medical detoxification programming, 8) consider adding peer support specialists, 9) improve monitoring programs and ensure that jail staff are accountable for monitoring inmates with mental health concerns, 10) reduce the use of restraints and isolation cells, and 11) limit the use of force and consider the use of force only as a last resort. While these steps are a good start for jail administrators, these recommendations remain quite inward-looking and fail to address some of the broader concerns that impact the jail that are outside of its control. The following section addresses some of the most promising approaches in recent years to address the issues the "Preventable Tragedies" report unearths.

6.2 Evidence-Based Solutions

The state-of-the art for local, system-wide reform has deftly been outlined by the Stepping Up Initiative materials, to be customized to each location through local partnerships all focused on providing better care for individuals with mental illness (Haneberg et al., 2017). The initial call to action outlines six steps to structure progress: (1) assemble a team of local leadership across multiple agencies and key stakeholders and decision-makers throughout the community committed to change, (2) invest in an ability to identify individuals with mental illness and gauge their risk of recidivism, and further, identify the needs of these individuals, (3) assess treatment and service capacity in the local area, (4) create a plan with measurable outcomes, (5) implement an approach with a scientific research design to ensure quality assurance and accountability of each partnership, and (6) track the progress using data and make data-informed decisions to ensure continued success. Each step along the way, any interested county/parish partnership can access a large resource pool supported by the National Alliance on Mental Illness, Major County Sheriffs' Association, National Association of County Behavioral Health and Developmental Disability Directors, National Association of State and Drug Abuse Directors, National Association of State Mental Health Directors, National Council on Behavioral Health, National Sheriffs' Association, and Policy Research Associates, among many more.

The first step provides the backbone of change. It requires a wide range of stakeholders to "put skin in the game" to address the problems of justice-involved mental health individuals. Typically, each entity signs onto a memorandum of understanding defining its commitment to this team, its role, and its responsibilities. Primarily, this gets all the key players in the same room to begin discussing strengths and weaknesses, resources and gaps, and problems and solutions. A key advantage of having these partnerships is that it helps to avoid blind spots in planning; each partner brings a unique perspective and experiences to aid in building a strategy to problem solve.

6.2.1 Step Two: Latest Generation Assessment and Screening Tools and Data Capacity

After assembling a team, many localities realize that their tools for identifying individuals with mental illness being processed through the justice system are old, outdated, and perform poorly, and jails are often at the center of this process. Further, the team may also realize that their local jails do not have a definition of mental illness and serious mental illness consistent with the state and/or local health officials' definitions – a serious issue if these jails are the primary centers for mental health screening for the area. This lack of definition would critically pose problems when trying to connect individuals to care in the community for follow-up care.

Following the establishment of a consistent definition of mental illness across the local system (including substance use disorders), the team can move on to select validated screening tools for mental illness and substance use disorders to proficiently flag individuals with potential mental illness and substance abuse disorders that fit this definition (see Table 6.1). Subsequent to screening, any flagged concerns must be further evaluated by mental health professionals using validated and reliable assessment techniques. Just like the instruments embedded into the population surveys of jail and prison inmates that are used to identify individuals with mental illness, the tools described in Table 6.1 provide reliable and accurate information about potential mental health and substance use disorder diagnoses. In fact, these tools were designed to be given by any trained personnel, not just mental health professionals or sworn officers.

Importantly, screening and assessment does not equate to a diagnosis or diagnoses that can, in turn, inform treatment. All flagged individuals must then be seen by a mental health professional to confirm or refute the screening result and, if appropriate, begin an individualized treatment plan. Many times, the mental health professional assessment is done after release, thus requiring communication and data sharing between the jail and community mental health partners. Or, as mentioned earlier, initial mental health assessments may require follow-ups to continue to define and/or refine diagnoses. In other words, not all diagnoses are black or white... often, gray areas exist. For some, diagnosis requires time and more than one evaluation, or a second option for another doctor. For others, mental illness develops slowly over time so it may not be an easy diagnosis right away, or a change may need to be made. Either way, the screening and assessment tools described in

Table 6.1 Evidence-based screening tools, adapted from SAMHSA

Mental disorders	Substance use disorders	Co-occurring disorders	Motivation and readiness	Trauma history and PTSD	Suicide risk
Brief Jail Mental Health Screen (BJMHS) Correctional Mental Health Screen (CMHS-F or CHHS-M) Mental Health Screening Form-III (MHSF-III)	Texas Christian University Drug Screen-V (TCUDS-V) Simple Screening Instrument (SSI) Alcohol, Smoking, and Substance Involvement Screening Test (ASSIST)	Mini International Neuropsychiatric Interview Screen (NINI-Screen) BJMHS combined with TCUDS-V CMHS-F or CMHS-M combined with TCUDS-V	Texas Christian Motivation Form (TCU-MotForm) University of Rhode Island Change Assessment Scale-M (URICA-M)	Trauma History Screen (THS) Life Stressor-Checklist (LSC-R) Life Events Checklist for DSM-5 combined with Posttraumatic Stress Disorder Checklist for DSM-5 (PCL-5)	Interpersonal Needs Questionnaire (INQ) combined with Acquired Capacity Suicide Scale (ACSS) Beck Scale for Suicide Ideation (BSS) Adult Suicidal Ideation Questionnaire (ASIQ)

Table 6.1 can be performed expeditiously, with the intent that it can easily be integrated with jail intake.

Further, latest generation risk and need assessment tools provide users with the ability to prioritize treatment for individuals who, after screening, are identified as high risk and high need. In other words:

> With mounting research that demonstrates the value of science-based tools to predict a person's likelihood of reoffending, criminal justice practitioners are increasingly using these tools to focus limited resources on the people who are most likely to reoffend. At the same time, mental health and substance use practitioners are trying to prioritize their scarce treatment resources for people with the most serious behavioral health needs....when [a] person is assessed as being at moderate to high risk of reoffending, connection to treatment is an even higher priority, along with interventions such as supervision and cognitive behavioral therapy to reduce the risk of recidivism. (Haneberg et al., 2017)

Thus, having a well-defined screening and assessment process, equipped with the latest generation actuarial tools (many of which are in the public domain and free to use), introduces vast improvements in the efficiency of mental illness interventions. This makes a broad catchment system possible and is the foundation for change, while preserving precious resources for optimal results. While the ideal goal for each locale would be to provide services for each individual with a mental health diagnosis, a realistic goal would be to provide an individualized treatment plan for each individual while providing direct services for those with the highest risk and needs.

Having such a process also enables local partnerships to monitor change. For example, while planning its local Stepping Up Initiatives, the partnerships in Bexar County, Texas (e.g., San Antonio), realized they did not have a reliable accurate count of just how many individuals in the Bexar County Jail have mental illness on any given day. Their solution was to explore and establish a universal screening process for mental illness together as a partnership. Other important baseline data may be sought during this planning stage, such as length of stay, connectivity to treatment after release, and a reliable method to measure recidivism. All these metrics rely on the ability to accurately and reliably identify individuals with mental illness and need to be put into place to measure successes and inefficiencies in the system being put into place.

The Stepping Up Initiative literature identifies four key data tools that need to be constructed for optimal success: (1) a tool to track the number of people with mental illness (and/or serious mental illness) passing through intake at the jail (e.g., being booked); (2) a tool that tracks the length of stay all individuals, with the ability to compare the length of stay of those with mental illness (and/or serious mental illness) to the overall average, or more importantly, to individuals without mental illness; (3) a tool that tracks connections to treatment, in particular, *successful* connections to treatment; and (4) a tool that tracks recidivism based on an accepted definition by the team. A reflection on these data tools suggests that jail staff and leadership shoulder the effort to create and maintain these resources; in the team context, any barriers the jail leadership may face in development and maintenance of these tools can, indeed, be troubleshooted by the team in good faith. However, the jail remains a core conduit of change.

6.2.2   Defining a Sequential Intercept Model and Notating Gaps in Services

A tool that has promulgated in counties/parishes considering change is the Sequential Intercept Model. Initially developed by Mark Munetz and Patricia Griffin (2006), the Sequential Intercept Model is a visualization of the flow of individuals with mental illness into and out of the criminal justice system, beginning with law enforcement and first responder contact and entry into jail, and follows each the various pathways of criminal justice processing through eventual release and termination of justice-involvement (Griffin et al., 2015). These models are customized to each locality, with the emphasis of finding what Munetz and Griffin call points of interception at which an intervention can be developed for qualifying individuals; these intervention points commonly occur at initial contact with first responders, at initial detention and preliminary hearings, during a stay in jail, interface with the courts (e.g., public defenders, prosecutors, and judges), or upon psychiatric evaluation, at reentry back into the community, and with interface with community corrections (e.g., probation and parole officers). As this is a visual tool, an example can be found with Fig. 6.1.

The Stepping Up Initiative literature states that local teams should look beyond the Sequential Intercept Model and include an exhaustive community model for mental health crisis. This extra step will allow for proactive measures to be taken to potentially intervene before justice-involvement even begins. After each point of interception has been defined, teams can then evaluate local resources available to intervene at each point, identify the training necessary for the players involved at point to effectively intervene, perhaps identify additional personnel who can make intervention possible, and so on. For example, if a law enforcement agency has the capacity to train its officers to differentiate potential misdemeanor cases involving individuals experiencing potential mental health symptoms (see above), then there stands a chance to divert potential mental health consumers out of the criminal justice system before criminal processing begins. In this case, the intervention involves not only players in the criminal justice system, but providers in the community that can work cases brought to them by law enforcement while ensuring public safety.

In other words, the Sequential Intercept Model, or a broader, detailed process analysis, gives the ability to map out failures or inefficiencies in the system that require priority attention by the team. Here is an example – a Stepping Up Initiative team discovered that a large number of individuals with serious mental illness were being processed for probation revocations due to technical violations and new crimes. Upon this discovery, the team (including representatives from probation) identified that did not have any specialized probation supervision services available for individuals with severe mental illness and high risk of recidivism. Solutions can be designed, installed, measured, and further refined, if necessary.

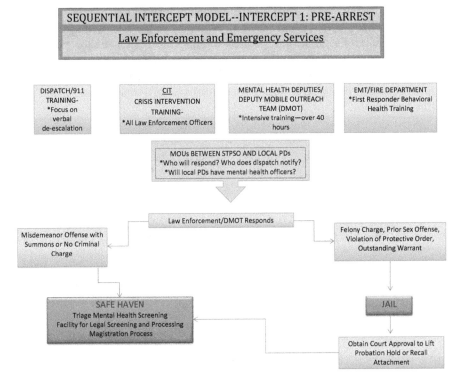

Fig. 6.1 The refined Sequential Intercept Model, Pre-Arrest, for the 22nd Judicial District Court of Louisiana and its local partners. Courtesy of Judge Peter J. Garcia and Diane Dicke

6.2.3 Prioritize and Implement New Policies, Practices, and Improvements and Then Track Progress

After a complete introspection of local needs, strengths, and gaps, the team can begin prioritizing improvements to the local system. For jails, emphasis is typically placed on ensuring successful reentry back into the community as well as connectivity to treatment and/or court programs customized for individuals with mental illness (specifically, customized for different types of individuals based on risk and need). As mentioned earlier, jails shoulder the burden of developing and maintaining the data tools to inform decision-making in a data-driven way – and most importantly – serve as the hub for mental health screening and assessment. These initiatives often are identified as an immediate goal by the group; the Stepping Up Initiative literature also recommends for each locale to prioritize further goals into short-term and long-term categories, based on an agreed upon logic (e.g., need and/or initiatives that hold promise for broad impacts). After the foundational tools and processes have been put into place during the planning period, the team is free to work with one another to determine its priorities; recommendations are available by the

Stepping Up partnerships; however, determinations should be driven by local decision-making. It is likely that one or a few parties on the team will take lead on one of several chosen initiatives, perhaps forming subcommittees for each task/ implementation plan. Thus, regular progress updates should occur as a team that includes robust evaluation components to determine impact and to identify room for improvement and quality assurance. Strong communication and partnerships are key to success.

Finally, each initiative *must* be monitored to track progress. For example, the team may ask, is training needed? If so, was the training successful? To determine success, the team may partner with a local university and/or researcher to study the knowledge gained from training and/or ability to successfully put training into use. This may require a pre-test, post-test design – giving trainees an exam before they are trained and upon successful completion of training to determine knowledge gained; and/or it may require observation of trainees after successful completion of training to determine whether someone who received training is using the skills and knowledge gained in their jobs. Each evaluation should be customized to the location, its partners, the situation, and so on. However, the key point here is that each initiative should be devised in a way that allows for adequate evaluation with a robust research design to ensure wise investment of funds and optimal success.

6.3 Bureau of Justice Assistance: A Source of Support

The Bureau of Justice Assistance, a child agency within the US Department of Justice (Office of Justice Programs), has been the leading funding agency to support Stepping Up Initiatives across the country. Key funding streams for jail initiatives include opportunities under the Second Chance Act such as Targeting Adults with Co-occurring Substance Abuse and Mental Health Disorders, Adult Mentoring, and Adult Offender Reentry Demonstration; as well as opportunities under the Mentally Ill Offender Treatment and Crime Reduction Reauthorization and Improvement Act of 2008, primarily the Justice and Mental Health Collaboration Program. Historically, these funding streams have aided jails in adopting, piloting, and troubleshooting screening assessment tools and processes, provided training, and have aided local partnerships in developing and adopting *evidence-based* programs and services with the intent that these initiatives are sustainable if deemed successful.

6.4 Evidence-Based Practices Resource Center and Crime Solutions

The Evidence-Based Practices Resource Center (formerly the National Registry of Evidence-Based Programs and Practices, or NREPP) is an extremely useful resource created in 1997 by SAMHSA. While it continues to evolve, the Resource Center provides practitioners with a bounty of literature featuring scientifically vetted programs and services (as well as programs/services not quite making the cut) to serve as a guide for potential solutions for initiatives calling for mental health and substance use interventions. In previous years, the NREPP has provided independent assessments, by certified assessors, of the existing research on each intervention since its inception. Each assessment is designed to generate easy-to-use ratings (currently being effective, promising, ineffective, and inconclusive) of various components of the intervention to summarize the volumes of research examined an assessment team. In July of 2017, the NREPP hosted 466 interventions, with the ability to narrow potential programs/services by easy-to-use criteria based on the target population to receive this program/service. Yet, policy-makers realized that the science and evidence guiding our understanding of these programs and services continues to evolve, at times rapidly. This led to the modern day Resource Center:

> This new Evidence-Based Practices Resource Center aims to provide communities, clinicians, policy-makers and others in the field with the information and tools they need to incorporate evidence-based practices into their communities or clinical settings. The Resource Center contains a collection of scientifically-based resources for a broad range of audiences, including Treatment Improvement Protocols, toolkits, resource guides, clinical practice guidelines, and other science-based resources. The retooled EBPRC neither accepts open submissions from outside program developers nor rates individual programs. (SAMHSA, 2022)

For example, a jail professional can use the Resource Center search tools to look for interventions by specific target audience, in this case, people in the criminal justice system – which narrows down the field to 11 resources currently available. One of these resources, Medication-Assisted Treatment (MAT) for Opioid Use Disorder in Jails and Prisons: A Planning and Implementation Toolkit, offers "correctional administrators and health care providers recommendations and tools for implementing medication-assisted treatment (MAT) in correctional settings." The toolkit is coupled with two recent webinars (February and July 2020) featuring experts that span across discipline (e.g., health and corrections). These dynamic resources are able to aid in broad dissemination to reduce the barriers of adopting these solutions in practice.

Similar to the NREPP's original approach, Crime Solutions, developed by the National Institute of Justice and launched in mid-2011, offers repository of independently assessed programs and practices to aid in informed initiative development and implementation – just with exclusive focus on programs with justice-involved individuals and with a slightly more simplistic *overall* rating scale (e.g., effective, promising, and no effects, with only one finding per program and practice). As of January of 2022, 650 programs (e.g., "a specific set of activities carried out according to guidelines to achieve a defined purpose" – up from 471 in 2017) and 116 practices (e.g., "a general category of programs, strategies, or procedures that share similar characteristics with regard to the issues they address and how they address them" – up from 58 in 2017) have been assessed by CrimeSolutions.gov. Diving deeper, if an end user were to search for specific programs tailored specifically to individuals with mental illness in correctional facilities (excluding substance use disorder), Crime Solutions displays just one effective program, three promising programs, and no practices for review (as of January 2022). At this time, the identified effective program was the Mentally Ill Offender Community Transition Program in Washington state.

Thus, a great deal of work needs to be done to explore meaningful interventions in jails and within partnerships with jails. Part of the point of the Stepping Up Initiative is for counties/parishes to take bold steps to implement initiatives that can build on our collective knowledge of what works, what is promising, and what is flat out ineffective or counterproductive. As of this writing, more than 600 awards have been given by the Bureau of Justice Assistance under the Second Chance Act programs and 568 awards under the Justice and Mental Health Collaboration Program; many of these funded projects will aid in furthering our knowledge, which will expand the information found in the EBPRC and Crime Solutions.

6.5 The Role of Jails in the Future

The original core intent of jails are twofold: (1) to *strategically* hold individuals in confinement awaiting trial, with public safety as the chief concern when considering decisions to detain, and (2) as a sentencing option for minor offenses that do not require prison time. For a litany of reasons, but primarily due to the lack of evidence-based data tools, jails have not been able to aid in strategically holding individuals who pose a public safety risk while helping to release individuals who do not. Further, jails do not have the capacity or have limited capacity to offer the necessary services to help individuals with mental illness, which will remain to be the case in the foreseeable future. Jail professionals are increasingly accepting their roles within a broader partnership of local community stakeholders to best serve individuals with mental illness, with key emphasis remaining on services rendered in the community. This ideal, to deliver care in the least restrictive environment, has become renewed with an understanding that jails are a critical catchment point to *begin* or *restart* behavioral health interventions.

For example, a recent study by Holliday and her colleagues revealed that most of the jail mental health population of Los Angeles County Jail in 2019 – 61% – were suitable candidates for diversion and alternative programs, with another 7% being possible candidates given some additional individualized scrutiny among stakeholders (Holliday et al., 2021). This finding was from a direct review of the assessments performed by a brand-new department within the Los Angeles County Department of Health Services launched in 2015 called the Office of Diversion and Reentry Division. To be able to appropriately identify suitable candidates, Holliday and her research team work diligently with district attorneys, public defenders, sheriff's representatives, and clinicians to customize legal and clinical criteria for alternative programming. Yet, this was only one piece to a broader restructuring of effort to serve this population. In their study, the researchers describe a collaborative effort led by the Los Angeles County Board of Supervisors that began in 2018 to further explore alternatives to incarceration, with a focus on justice-involved persons with mental illness. This soon led to a mandated development of a diversion road map that included identifying paths to treatment options as well as guided stakeholders to explore strategic investments to expand of these options. One central piece of these developments was replacing the Men's Central Jail (run by corrections professionals) with a brand new Consolidated Correctional Treatment Facility. Yet, upon further study, stakeholders wanted to tackle this issue by increasing their ability to serve this population in community-based facilities rather than in a secure setting – and soon cancelled their plans to replace the Men's Central Jail. Sure enough, Holliday and her colleagues concluded that the vast majority of those who would have been served by the new Consolidated Correctional Treatment Facility – originally scaled to treat 3,800 incarcerated persons with mental illness – were suitable for treatment in community settings. By numbers, Holliday found that in 2019, 3,368 individuals were suitable for community-based alternative programing while 1,762 were not appropriate. The race was now on to be sure that eligible persons are connected with alternative programming, with central focus on the partnership between the new Office of Diversion and Reentry Division and local criminal justice partners, particularly the Los Angeles County Jail.

Therefore, jails of the future will need be better connected with community and agency partnerships, particularly relating to shared communication and critical data sharing. Jails will become a primary referral service for individuals, with an emphasis on connecting individuals with evidence-based care tailored to their needs. Jail professionals will take the lead on identifying the vast majority of individuals needing care in these improved local catchment systems. Therefore, they will become a major player and have a central for implementing change. Individuals who have historically needed care and have been cycling through the justice system due to lack of care, being underserved, or just receiving services proven to have no evidence to effect change will begin to get the care they deserve.

6.5.1   Drain the Jail: Customized Specialty Courts

One intervention option for jails is to establish a partnership with the local criminal court in the creation of a mental health court, particularly if individuals with mental illness tend to have longer jail stays relative to those without mental illness. Mental health courts, which will be expanded on in the next chapter, allow for individuals with mental illness to be released from jail into a program supervised by a team – typically, a judge, case manager, treatment provider, probation officer, prosecutor, and defense attorney. The court then takes lead in connecting their clients with appropriate evidence-based treatment, monitor progress, treatment compliance, and setbacks, and ensuring public safety.

The jail continues to be a key partner in two primary ways. First, jail professionals continue to take in identifying individuals who may have mental illness to be potential clients. Ideally, this should be accomplished through validated screening and assessment tools; however, if the jail simply does not have the resources to upgrade their data tools, mental health court case managers can be trained to go into jails to provide these services to identify potential clients. If the latter workflow is chosen, the jail-court partnership may invest in training of key staff to better identify signs and symptoms of mental illness (e.g., Mental Health First Aid) in order to assist case managers in identifying individuals to be screened and assessed as often individual case managers will not have the capacity to review every individual booked into jail. While not ideal, it is a step in the right direction in the absence of a central screening and assessment process.

Second, jails often serve as a behavior modification tool for mental health courts. Specifically, these programs commonly employ jail sanctions for noncompliance with program rules or treatment protocols, with this sanction type being the most punitive short of dismissal from the program. Typically, this happens when a client fails a drug screen, repeatedly misses treatment sessions, and so on. There is a stream of research that attempts to estimate the number of days jail sanctions should last for positive change in light of non-compliance; it should be noted that too lengthy of a stay can backfire and cause problems, so great care must be taken in partnership with the jail to ensure the success of this measure.

6.5.2 Avoid the Jail: One-Stop Crisis Mental Health Facilities

Instead of intercepting individuals as they pass through jail as described above, and partnering with the court as a primary referral source, many communities have chosen to heavily invest their resources into creating a robust one-stop mental health crisis center – such as Safe Haven and the Behavioral Health Solutions Center. This contrasts slightly with the approach Los Angeles has taken, which emphasizes a strong partnership with jails to ensure those experiencing mental health crises and need acute care for substance use disorders are screened, assessed, referred to services, and subsequently connect with care customized to their needs. Typically one-stop centers require broad buy-in from and robust training of frontline public safety and emergency medical personnel to ensure the target population is being routed to these facilities – as, oftentimes, they serve as the primary referral and transportation mechanism for individuals in crisis. Thus, special consideration must be made among communities that continue to place the primary burden of screening and identification on jails or, instead, rely on frontline public safety and emergency medical personnel. There is emerging evidence to support both use cases; however, for each to be successful, stakeholders will need to invest in the resources and support each system needs to thrive and succeed.

6.5.3   Use the Jail: Expand Available Services, Case Management, and Use of Re-entry Plan

Jails with resources may have the ability to adopt evidence-based programs and services to act on the findings of screening and assessment immediately. This becomes important for inmates serving time in a jail. In fact, recent research suggests that individualized treatment that begins prior to release and continue into aftercare post-release are most likely to be successful (Travis & Visher, 2005; Osher, 2006; Osher, 2007). As such, jail reentry programs will continue to grow and proliferate in the upcoming years. Also, recall from the Los Angeles study by Holliday above – a small, but sizeable proportion of people passing through jails will be ineligible for community-based treatment – largely due to legal ineligibility, perhaps because of the seriousness of the charges pending in their cases. These individuals deserve suitable treatment, in this case in a secure facility. Yet, the quality of care available in jails across the country can vary widely. One recent study by Comartin and her colleagues (2021a, b) evaluated potential differences in outcomes borne from individuals receiving mental health services from for-profit versus non-profit organizations. Their findings were compelling – each system was able to utilize screening tools with equal success, yet further assessment and identification for severe mental illness was significantly lower in the facilities with for-profit providers. The same pattern follows for connecting individuals referred to mental health services and the provision of care across facilities with for-profit and non-profit providers (with the largest gap in the latter). Specifically, 73.4% of individuals referred to services in facilities with non-profit providers were successfully linked up with services versus only 39.7% of individuals in facilities with for-profit providers – these are marked differences. While these results may not be representative, they surely put a spotlight on potential differences in following best practices being at the root of this divide in care.

Thus, researchers must engage in mixed-methods studies that allow for qualitative assessment of the programming rendered to help us contextualize potential differences in the quality of care. Study designs must look into whether evidence-based treatment programs and services are available, delivered to those who would benefit, and delivered with high fidelity to a model program of its type. For example, Seeking Safety is one such program designed for individuals (men and women) with post-traumatic stress disorder symptoms or diagnosis co-occurring with substance use disorder (Najavits, 2001). This flexible program is designed to provide clients with effective coping skills and psychoeducation. To do so, the program focuses on defining safety as one's primary goal in one's relationships, thinking patterns, behaviors, and emotions while addressing PTSD symptoms along with substance use simultaneously. The Hampton Roads Regional Jail in Portsmouth, Virginia, is currently piloting this program with local funding with hope to expand on its evidence-based in the local area through external grant funding. Many jails across the country are engaging in similar strategies as they search for a pool of funding to rely on to sustain these initiatives. The trick is to find out whether facilities like Hampton Roads Regional Jail are rolling out such programming in a way that is optimal. Further research must be responsive to these concerns to help make progress in improving the provision of care at the local level.

Holistic reentry programs designed to treating substance use disorder, not specifically mental illness, are much more commonplace and routinely funded. One excellent example is the Allegheny County Jail-Based Reentry Specialist Program. This program begins in the jail with 5 or more months of programming that includes case management, education (literacy and GED classes, tutoring, basic education, and pre-apprenticeship training), structured job readiness classes, relapse prevention, cognitive behavioral therapy, and gender-specific drug treatment for substance use disorder, housing support services, parenting classes, and much more. Upon release, clients can receive up to twelve additional months of programming, with many of the same offerings available in the community. This model is becoming increasingly popular, and jails are increasingly working with community partners to ensure the continuity of programing and services upon release. At some point in the near future, this model will be customized for individuals with mental illness to provide services for individuals that must serve time in jail and who may not be a good fit for alternative programs available, such as diversion or mental health court.

One final note on the roles of jails – a study by Comartin and her colleagues (2021a, b) reveals that screening tools alone are insufficient in identifying individuals at jail intake who may have mental health concerns, particularly if there is not a distinct plan in place to help guide decision-making based on screening results. This study points out that recently developed best practices promulgated by the American Psychiatric Association recommends *both* utilization of a validated screening tool and staff observation to help flag individuals for further assessment to help determine treatment need and eligibility for alternative programming. This study sought to compare jails who utilize staff observation to jails who solely rely on screening tools and found that individuals observed and flagged by jail staff tended to be connected to jail- and community-based treatment services more often than those persons screened with screening suggesting further assessment is required. Even more, the results of the screens in the study indicated that the group receiving only screens tended to have much more behavioral health risks than those who were identified by staff observation. This study concluded that both elements were crucial – and that jail staff need to be properly trained in robust observational skills to identify signs and symptoms of both mental illness and suicide risk for optimal outcomes.

6.5.4 Out of the (Pizza) Box Innovations

Chicago's Cook County Jail is using a new and innovate approach to fund programming within the jail (Babwin, 2017; Janssen, 2017). Rather than using taxpayer dollars to fund their version of a work release program called "Recipe for Change," they have turned to an internal solution. The inmates at Cook County Jail are creating and selling pizzas inside the jail. According to media interviews, jail staff are using the pizza system as a means to treat inmates humanely while affording inmates an opportunity to learn skills that may be helpful upon release from jail. Additionally, this pizza program is used as a behavior incentive. If any inmate is involved in disruptive behavior, they are immediately transferred out Division 11 cell block where the Recipe for Change program is housed – thus, resulting in the loss of pizza privileges.

Participating inmates attend classes 5 days each week, just like many other jail culinary program. Classes are taught on different topics related to the foodservice industry, such as food safety and sanitation, as well as preparation techniques and cooking skills. There is a set menu daily, which always includes a pizza that uses fresh ingredients from the nearby Cook County Sheriff's garden (Freeman, 2017).

Sheriff Tom Dart suggests that this program has already begun to show an immediate positive impact on inmates. The plan in the future is to obtain a food truck so that the pizzas can be sold to a nearby courthouse, creating additional revenue to self-fund this training program. The Recipe for Change program is just one small step in positivity within the jail system and the community. Jail inmates are finding a bit of humanity among good food. Upon return to their community, their skills in the kitchen are transferable. Yet, it should be noted that it seems as though the program lacks an evidence-based for broad impact. The out-of-the-box revenue generation concept of the program can fund solutions to resolve this gap. At times, solutions such as these are easier to come by as taxpayers are often wary of increasing their burden.

6.6 Conclusion

In the United States our jail system continues to be a large provider of mental health services. This fact is both alarming and concerning in that, there is a need to have those services be both adequate and documented. Budget cuts and funding concerns have led to understaffing and overcrowding in most local jails. Additionally, recidivism and lack of alternative resources in community only help to fuel the fire of increased inmates and struggles. Slowly, communities are coming together to work toward a better way to handle these issues for those in their area. In later chapters, some of those resources will be discussed with the hopes of bringing to light success stories. Those success stories can continue to the process of creating change.

As it stands now, there is a lack of adequate research on the jail system and how inmates are treated both physically and mentally. Additionally, on that note, there exists a lack of baseline knowledge about training of corrections officers from one state to another, much less within the counties/parishes in each state. This is significant because lack of information does not allow for proper comparisons. Without proper comparison, there is no evidence to support positive or negative outcomes. In this, the struggle of improving becomes nearly impossible. For instance, taking into consideration jails within major cities like Los Angeles and New York. If there does not exist standardized information on training of corrections officers, how would a researcher be able to compare? If officers in both California and New York were required to have a specific certificate, research could be done to establish success or failure. Additionally, comparisons could be made to say that certain trains or methods work better than others, thus improving the system as a whole. All in all, these changes could allow for a more comprehensive approach to overcoming obstacles within the jail system and the treatment of those incarcerated.

Moving on, as discussed many times with recidivism, typically a person who is incarcerated without programming to help in change, will return to jail or prison. Going along with that thought, it could be safe to say that those in these jail systems, may very well enter the prison system eventually. Why is this important? Research about short-term stays within the jail system could lead to significant information as it relates to the prison system. Therefore, having states work together for better standards or even just within a state system could vastly change outlooks for the criminal justice system of the United States.

Another note regarding the lack of research, if a community has no information on the number of individuals with mental illness within their jail system, then there would be no initiative to treat those individuals. Often these jails have known that there were individuals within the system with mental health, but no knowledge was known of the extent of the number. Luckily, this has prompted some communities to take action.

Discussion Questions

1. How can jails innovate to improve outcomes considering limited funding?
2. How can a mental health screening process in a local jail impact a criminal justice system?
3. This chapter describes several evidence-based solutions that have been vetted through years of research. Which evidence-based solutions discussed would work in your local area? Why?
4. What reforms to policies and practices must be explored by stakeholders when trying to adopt evidence-based solutions?

References

28 F.Supp.3d 1068 - COLEMAN v. BROWN, United States District Court, E.D. California.
42 U.S.C. § 1983. Civil action for deprivation of rights.
503 F.Supp. 1265. Ruiz v. Estelle, United States District Court, S.D Texas.
595 F.Supp. 1558. Balla v. Idaho State Board of Corrections. United States District Court. D. Idaho.
933 F.Supp. 954 – COLEMAN v. WILSON, United States District Court, E.D. California.
Estelle v. Gamble. 429 US 97.
American Correctional Association. (2001). *Performance-based standards for adult community residential services.*
Babwin, D. (2017). *Chicago inmates can order fancy Italian pizza made in jail.* US News. URL: https://www.usnews.com/news/best-states/illinois/articles/2017-05-26/chicago-inmates-can-order-fancy-italian-pizza-made-in-jail. Last accessed: 1 June 2017.

Carson, E. A. (2021). *Suicide in local jails and state and federal prisons, 2000-2019 – Statistical Tables*. Bureau of Justice Statistics. URL: https://bjs.ojp.gov/sites/g/files/xyckuh236/files/media/document/sljsfp0019st.pdf. Last accessed: 30 Jan 2022.

Center for Disease Control and Prevention. (2021). *Changes in suicide rates*. URL: https://www.cdc.gov/mmwr/volumes/70/wr/mm7008a1.htm. Last accessed: 30 Jan 2022.

Comartin, E. B., Milanovic, E., Nelson, V., & Kubiak, S. (2021a). Mental health identification practices of jails: The unmet needs of the "silent" population: special issue: Criminal justice and community psychology: Our values and our work. *American Journal of Community Psychology, 67*(1-2), 7–20.

Comartin, E., Nelson, V., Hambrick, N., Kubiak, S., Sightes, E., & Ray, B. (2021b). Comparing for-profit and nonprofit mental health services in county jails. *The Journal of Behavioral Health Services & Research, 48*(2), 320–329.

Council of State Governments Justice Center. (2014). *Stepping up: A national initiative to reduce the number of people with mental illnesses in jails*. URL: https://csgjusticecenter.org/wp-content/uploads/2014/12/SteppingUpInitiative.pdf. Last accessed: 1 June 2017.

Freeman, S. (2017). *A Chicago chef is rehabilitating inmates one pizza at a time*. Vice. URL: https://munchies.vice.com/en_us/article/53q3ba/a-chicago-chef-is-rehabilitating-inmates-one-pizza-at-a-time. Last accessed: 1 June 2017.

Griffin, P. A., Heilbrun, K., Mulvey, E. P., DeMatteo, D., & Schubert, C. A. (Eds.). (2015). *The Sequential Intercept Model and criminal justice: Promoting community alternatives for individuals with serious mental illness*. Oxford University Press.

Haneberg, R., Fabelo, T, Osher, F., & Thompson, M. (2017). *Reducing the number of people with mental illnesses in jail: Six questions county leaders need to ask*. URL: https://stepuptogether.org/wp-content/uploads/2017/01/Reducing-the-Number-of-People-with-Mental-Illnesses-in-Jail_Six-Questions.pdf. Last accessed: June 1, 2017.

Holliday, S. B., Pace, N. M., Gowensmith, N., Packer, I., Murrie, D., Virani, A., Han, B., & Hunter, S. B. (2021). Estimating the Size of the Los Angeles County Jail Mental Health Population Appropriate for Release into Community Services. *Rand Health Quarterly, 9*(2).

Janssen, K. (2017). *Cook County jail inmates can order hot pizza delivered to their cells*. Chicago Tribune. URL: http://www.chicagotribune.com/news/chicagoinc/ct-pizza-in-jail-0510-chicago-inc-20170509-story.html. Last accessed: 1 June 2017.

McCampbell, S.W., Grenawitzke, H.E., Patterson, R.F., Greifinger, R.B., Frasier, M.L., Hardyman, P.L., & Hodge, D.R. (2017). *Report No. 7 of the independent monitors*. URL: http://www.nolajailmonitors.org/uploads/3/7/5/7/37578255/_7_compliance_report.pdf. Last accessed: 15 July 2017.

Miller, C.M. & Fantz, A. (2007, November 15). *Special "psych" jails planned*. Miami Herald.

Munetz, M. R., & Griffin, P. A. (2006). Use of the sequential intercept model as an approach to decriminalization of people with serious mental illness. *Psychiatric services, 57*(4), 544–549.

Najavits, L. M. (2001). *Seeking safety: A treatment manual for PTSD and substance abuse*. Guilford Press.

National Alliance on Mental Illness. (2017). *Jailing people with mental illness*. URL: https://www.nami.org/Learn-More/Public-Policy/Jailing-People-with-Mental-Illness. Last accessed: 1 June 2017.

National Institute of Justice. (2017). *Crime solutions*. URL: https://www.crimesolutions.gov. Last accessed: 1 June 2017.

Noonan, M. (2015). *Mortality in local jails and state prisons, 2000–2013 – Statistical tables*. Bureau of Justice Statistics: Washington, D.C. URL: https://www.bjs.gov/content/pub/pdf/mljsp0013st.pdf. Last accessed: 1 June 2017.

Osher, F. C. (2006). *Integrating mental health and substance abuse services for justice-involved persons with co-occurring disorders*. National GAINS Center.

Osher, F. C. (2007). *Short-term strategies to improve reentry of jail populations: Expanding and implementing the APIC model*. American Jails. URL: https://www.bja.gov/Publications/APIC_Model.pdf. Last accessed: 1 June 2017.

Rayman, G. (2016). *Rikers inmate moved to isolation cell after suicide attempt*. New York Daily News.   URL: http://www.nydailynews.com/new-york/rikers-inmate-moved-isolation-cell-suicide-attempt-article-1.2531720. Last accessed: 1 June 2017.

Sledge, M. (2017). *Report: New Orleans jail has 'regressed' under new administrator, with 'unacceptable' violence*. The New Orleans Advocate. URL: http://www.theadvocate.com/new_orleans/news/courts/article_d281246a-3059-11e7-9c76-abc1dd0205eb.html. Last accessed: 1 June 2017.

Stepping Up Initiative. (2022). *Stepping up: A national initiative to reduce the number of people with mental illnesses in jails*. URL: https://stepuptogether.org/. Last accessed: 30 Jan 2022.

Stohr, M. K., Self, R. L., & Lovrich, N. P. (1992). Staff turnover in new generation jails: An investigation of its causes and prevention. *Journal of Criminal Justice, 20*(5), 455–478.

Substance Abuse and Mental Health Services Administration. (2017). *National registry of evidence-based programs and practices*. URL: http://nrepp.samhsa.gov/landing.aspx. Last accessed: 1 June 2017.

Substance Abuse and Mental Health Services Administration. (2022). *Evidence-based practices resource center*. URL: https://www.samhsa.gov/resource-search/ebp. Last accessed: 12 Sep 22.

Travis, J., & Visher, C. (Eds.). (2005). *Prisoner reentry and crime in America*. Cambridge University Press.

University of Texas School of Law Civil Rights Clinic. (2016). *Preventable tragedies: How to reduce mental health-related deaths in Texas jails*. URL: https://law.utexas.edu/wp-content/uploads/sites/11/2016/11/2016-11-CVRC-Preventable-Tragedies.pdf.   Last   accessed: 1 June 2017.

Chapter 7
Court Programs

> *We should not be held back from pursuing our full talents, from contributing what we could contribute to the society, because we fit into a certain mold – because we belong to a group that historically has been the object of discrimination – Ruth Bader Ginsburg.*

The dawn of widespread court intervention for mental health concerns truly began with the drug court concept developed in Dade (now Miami-Dade) County, Florida, at the conclusion of the 1980s in direct response to Miami's infamous drug scene. The darker aspects of popular culture depictions of drugs impact on Miami – *Scarface, Cocaine Cowboys, Miami Vice*, to name a few – were in plain view on a daily basis for local judges, public defenders, and prosecutors. Specifically, these key players grew wary of witnessing the same offenders appear before the court under the same or incredibly similar circumstances, sparking the concept of drug court (Goldkamp & Weiland, 1993). Later named a problem-solving court, specialty court, or therapeutic court, the innovation of drug court centers on its holistic approach of combining aspects of treatment, providing general care by leveraging community resources (e.g., housing, healthcare, food banks, transportation, etc.), and judicial oversight to enable its participants a chance to break the drugs-crime-criminal justice pattern in their lives (Carey et al., 2012). In years to come, this concept was reinforced and fine-tuned with emerging evidence-based practices to ensure the lasting success and pro-social gains of participants, and a vast array of research would be published to support the successes of a fully operational drug court steeped in evidence-based practices (Gottfredson et al., 2003; Rossman & Zweig, 2012; Wilson et al., 2006). Soon, this model would be redeveloped to cater to individuals with the mental health-(drugs)-crime-criminal justice pattern in their lives – called mental health court, or behavioral health court. These specialty courts lie at the forefront of local court innovations to intervene on behalf of individuals with mental illness being processed by the criminal justice system.

7.1 Know the Role: Drug Court

According to the National Drug Court Resource Center (2022), there are 1755 adult drug courts (up from 1558 in 2015) and 308 juvenile drug courts (down from 409 in 2015) in operation as of December 2020, with at least one in operation in each of the United States. While variability in the program exists, the core operation in each appears to be consistent. This core begins with defining the appropriate target population to serve, which, in this case, should be adults or juveniles (not both) with a known substance use disorder (Eckholm, 2008). To ensure that this target population is indeed being targeted by the program, evidence-based screening and assessment tools *must* be adopted. A notable criticism of drug courts is that, historically, programs have generally defined eligible participants as nonviolent, probation-eligible individuals who have committed a drug offense or a drug-related offense, which may widen the criminal justice net to include individuals without a substance use problem (Drug Policy Alliance, 2011). In doing so, much of the previous research may have been overly optimistic in their rates of success. Follow-up research continues to support the success of drug court when (1) validated screening and assessment tools are in place, and when (2) evidence-based programming with success in the target population is used. However, it is difficult to determine just how many of the 1755 adult drug courts and 308 juvenile drug courts operate with fidelity to these two prerequisites for success.

Generally speaking, prospective drug court *clients* must enter a guilty plea to their charges if determined to be eligible for the program. The drug court team – consisting of a presiding judge, case manager, prosecutor, defense attorney, treatment professional, and probation officer – will consider each client for admittance on a case-by-case basis. The program itself is set up in phases, which begin at a high intensity of programming and hands-on participation and eventually eases until independence can be established (Adult Drug Court Research to Practice Initiative, 2017). For example, Phase 1 often requires an intensive weekly schedule of mandatory drug treatment hours that may include counseling, intensive outpatient (IOP) drug treatment, several sessions of group therapy (likely, Alcoholics Anonymous or Narcotics Anonymous), and routine randomized drug screening. It also includes a weekly status meeting with the judge and the drug court team to monitor progress, reward compliance and success, attend to potential emerging problems, and meaningfully correct any relapse, noncompliance, or misbehavior. As a client is successful in the program, each requirement of the program eases – less time spent in treatment, lower number of group therapy meetings required (although additional attendance is still encouraged), fewer status meetings in court each month, and less frequent drug testing. In all, drug courts typically have three to five phases which can last 12, 18, or 24 months with an added aftercare phase to aid in a prosocial, drug- and crime-free lifestyle (Lowenkamp et al., 2005).

As this program has matured, the National Association of Drug Court Professionals has been key in promulgating best practices and standards for the continued optimal success of drug courts. Its seminal "Ten Key Components of Drug Courts," published over a year ago, establishes the core elements indicative of successful programs after years of introspection and research (see Table 7.1).

Table 7.1 Ten key components of drug court

Key components
1. Drug courts integrate alcohol and other drug treatment services with justice system case processing.
2. Using a nonadversarial approach, prosecution and defense counsel promote public safety while protecting participants' due process rights.
3. Eligible participants are identified early and promptly placed in the drug court program.
4. Drug courts provide access to a continuum of alcohol, drug, and other related treatment and rehabilitation services.
5. Abstinence is monitored by frequent alcohol and other drug testing.
6. A coordinated strategy governs drug court responses to participants' compliance.
7. Ongoing judicial interaction with each drug court participant is essential.
8. Monitoring and evaluation measure the achievement of program goals and gauge effectiveness.
9. Continuing interdisciplinary education promotes effective drug court planning, implementation, and operations.
10. Forging partnerships among drug courts, public agencies, and community-based organizations generates local support and enhances drug court program effectiveness.

National Association of Drug Court Professionals. Drug Court Standards Committee, and United States. Drug Courts Program Office (1997). Defining drug courts: The key components. US Department of Justice, Office of Justice Programs, Drug Courts Program Office

The overall successes of a well-run drug court, based on whether or not these courts can stay true to these ten key components, are substantial. Reductions of crime range from 8 to 26 percent, cost savings have been estimated at $2 to $27 dollars per every dollar invested into drug court, and drug court participants are consistently more likely to reduce drug use relative to non-participants.

7.1.1   Drug Court Adaptations for Special Populations

As soon as criminal justice practitioners realized the promise of drug courts, forward thinkers began to adapt the core structure of drug court to other target populations that become commonly involved with the criminal justice system (Brennan et al., 2011; Festinger et al., 2015; Halper, 2014; Marlowe, 2010; Morse et al., 2014; Tiger, 2012). In June 2015, the National Association of Drug Court Professionals recognized and tabulated the following therapeutic courts (with tabulations updated using the National Drug Court Resource Center data, whenever available): family court (also known as family preservation court, designed to aid a drug dependent mother, father, or both in maintaining custody of their children and healing familial strains and dissolution due to drug abuse – 312 in 2015; 634 in 2020), veterans court (designed to focus on the special needs of former military members, often by addressing traumatic experiences of combat – 313 in 2015; 952 in 2020), sobriety court (also known as DUI or DWI court, designed specifically for alcoholism in conjunction with driving under the influence – 284 in 2015; 546 in 2020), tribal court (designed to focus on American Indians – 138 in 2015), mental health court (also called co-occurring or behavioral health court, designed to focus primarily on mental health diagnoses with secondary focus on substance use disorder – *366 reported by the GAINS Center* in 2015; 938 in 2020), re-entry court (designed to focus on the experiences common to individuals returning to the community from incarceration – 29 in 2015; 128 in 2020), and campus courts (also known as back on TRAC, designed to focus on college students – 3 in 2015). Each customization often taps additional team members with expertise in the targeted "special" population to ensure success. For example, for a veterans court, the team may expressly search for case managers, probation officers, and treatment professionals with a military background to aid in better understanding client behaviors and to have better success in building better rapport for best outcomes. Further, former military members in recovery may serve as better peer support specialists and/or mentors with veteran court clients than those without military experience. These differences can assist clients in tamping down feelings of isolation and any "us versus them" sentiment compared to enduring a traditional drug court experience. The same arguments can be made for tribal court and campus court. Research on these adaptations is ongoing, but show promise in effecting change for each targeted population.

7.1.2   Mental Health Courts

According to a Bureau of Justice Assistance report in 2000, mental health court was pioneered in four very different jurisdictions, beginning in Broward County (Fort Lauderdale), Florida, and King County (Seattle), Washington, Anchorage, Alaska, and San Bernardino, California. In each of these jurisdictions, the mental health court team commonly faced defendants with issues related to homelessness, persistent lapses of the community mental health care system, jail overcrowding, and unabated drug abuse. To address these issues, the traditional drug court program was equipped with treatment, including psychiatric and counseling services, geared for co-occurring disorders, stronger ties to housing assistance, and team members familiar with mental health disorders and individuals with mental illness.

Additionally, drug courts are, by and large, steeped in an abstinence-based orientation. Mental health courts, by necessity, must alter this long-standing tradition to accept required medication regimes to treat clients' underlying mental illness. Often, these therapeutic courts work with treatment professionals to find medications that may minimize substance use disorder symptomatology. For example, clients diagnosed with anxiety disorders may have historically been treated with medications known to be commonly abused, such as Xanax. In the context of mental health court, if a client has a pattern of substance use disorder co-occurring with an anxiety disorder, the mental health court team may work with treatment providers to find the treatment protocol for this case. Commonly, final treatment decisions remain with treatment providers.

Another key difference exists when comparing traditional drug courts and mental health court as it pertains to defining and measuring success. For drug court clients, success is easier to conceive – pro-social drug- and crime-free living, as indicated by clients passing drug tests, successfully complying and completing treatment, paying all restitution and fees, and so on (BJA, 2000). Mental health court clients, on the other hand, strive for optimal functionality given their lifelong mental health diagnoses, and this level of functioning will vary from client to client. Thus, success will vary across mental health court clients. With this in mind, outcome studies have shown promising reductions in recidivism and violence (McNiel & Binder, 2007; Moore & Hiday, 2006). The most recent meta-analysis of mental health court confirms sufficient evidence supportive of this program's ability to reduce recidivism rates across 20 robust studies (Loong et al., 2019). This study also found that case management and supportive housing was crucial to programmatic success.

The proliferation of mental health courts has also created a demand for a customized set of key components derived from the drug court model (Council of State Governments Justice Center, 2007; summarized in Table 7.2). Just like drug court, these components guide the creation, implementation, and continued success of mental health courts and provides a foundation for a standardized orientation.

Thompson et al. (2008)

7.1.3 The 22nd Judicial District Behavioral Health Court of Louisiana

The Behavioral Health Court (BHC) in the 22nd Judicial District Court of Louisiana (Covington), only one of three in the state, was designed as a win-win for stakeholders and clients alike. For clients, individuals receive both professional drug treatment and mental health services while remaining in the community in lieu of potential incarceration with little chance of receiving anywhere near this level of care, with the goal of treatment continuation. For stakeholders, rehabilitation presents an opportunity to disrupt established drug-crime trajectories; its success thus holds the key to produce increases in local public safety and vast cost savings to the local justice and health care system.

The BHC program began in November of 2011 with each member of the BHC team volunteering their time during the lunch hour. Founded by District Judge Peter Garcia (in memorium), BHC partnered with the local National Alliance on Mental Illness outpost and the Florida Parishes Human Services Authority to offer linkages to community services such as housing, transportation, co-occurring group therapy, food assistance, and assistance in obtaining public benefits, as well as mental health and substance use treatment services. While the Judge Garcia and his team were building capacity to provide the best care possible for current and future clients, the State of Louisiana had moved forward with a plan to privatize mental health services and divest a large portion of public funds to aid this effort. This resulted in a widespread closure of local, state-run behavioral health clinics and hospitals, leaving the criminal justice system as the only likely source of mental health care. This action further weakened the ability of the Florida Parishes Human Services Authority to provide optimal care for individuals with co-occurring disorders. At this time, Louisiana ranks 43rd out of the 50 states for per capita expenditures on

Table 7.2 Ten key components, or "essential elements," of mental health court

Key components
1. Planning and Administration: A broad-based group of stakeholders representing the criminal justice, mental health, substance abuse treatment, and related systems and the community guides the planning and administration of the court.
2. Target population: Eligibility criteria address public safety and consider a community's treatment capacity in addition to the availability of alternatives to pretrial detention for defendants with mental illness. Eligibility criteria also take into account the relationship between mental illness and a defendant's offenses, while allowing the individual circumstances of each case to be considered.
3. Timely participant identification and linkage to services: Participants are identified, referred, and accepted into mental health courts, and then linked to community-based service providers as quickly as possible.
4. Terms of participation: Terms of participation are clear, promote public safety, facilitate the defendant's engagement in treatment, are individualized to correspond to the level of risk that the defendant presents to the community, and provide for positive legal outcomes for those individuals who successfully complete the program.
5. Informed choice: Defendants fully understand the program requirements before agreeing to participate in a mental health court. They are provided legal counsel to inform this decision and subsequent decisions about program involvement. Procedures exist in the mental health court to address, in a timely fashion, concerns about a defendant's competency whenever they arise.
6. Treatment supports and services: Mental health courts connect participants to comprehensive and individualized supports and services in the community. They strive to use – and increase the availability of – treatment and services that are evidence-based.
7. Confidentiality: Health and legal information should be shared in a way that protects potential participants' confidentiality rights as mental health consumers and their constitutional rights as defendants. Information gathered as part of the participants' court-ordered treatment program or services should be safeguarded in the event that participants are returned to traditional court processing.
8. Court team: A team of criminal justice and mental health staff and service and treatment providers receives special, ongoing training and helps mental health court participants achieve treatment and criminal justice goals by regularly reviewing and revising the court process.
9. Monitoring adherence to court requirements: Criminal justice and mental health staff collaboratively monitor participants' adherence to court conditions, offer individualized graduated incentives and sanctions, and modify treatment as necessary to promote public safety and participants' recovery.
10. Sustainability: Data are collected and analyzed to demonstrate the impact of the mental health court, its performance is assessed periodically (and procedures are modified accordingly), court processes are institutionalized, and support for the court in the community is cultivated and expanded.

mental health; Florida Parishes Human Services Authority further receives less funding per capita than most of its sister districts, leaving the 22nd Judicial District Court vulnerable citizens even more vulnerable (Miller & Khey, 2016).

Since 2014, BHC has expanded its operations with the benefit of a joint grant program offered by SAMHSA and the Bureau of Justice Assistance, giving the program the ability to increase its case management capacity, further invest in evidence-based practices (such as trauma-informed care and Assertive Community Treatment), and offer protections of its clients against the weakening state of the local mental health system. While the outcome studies focusing on potential reduced hospitalizations, reductions in arrest and reconviction, and reductions in drug use, Miller and

Khey (2016) published the results of a thorough process evaluation to determine whether BHC was operating as proposed, with true evidence-based services in place. Overall, Miller and Khey found a strong professional orientation of the services being delivered to BHC clients, particularly those within the direct control of the court. The broad weakening of the local mental health care system, on the other hand, seemed to produce counterproductive effects on the treatment quality available to some clients. Specifically, therapeutic sessions provided by local practitioners appeared to only offer social support rather than engage in any known form of therapy, such as cognitive behavioral therapy or dialectic behavioral therapy. As a result, BHC leadership worked with its local partners to deepen its ability to offer such services to current and future clients.

Counterproductive forces to reform, such as the problems resulting from a weakened mental health care system as noted above, are likely *more* common when the target population is individuals with mental illness or with co-occurring disorders. Further, this is even more likely the case in jurisdictions that need these types of innovation the most. Anecdotally speaking, such issues may explain why the pace the expansion of other types of specialty courts have outpaced mental health courts: only 70 mental health courts are in existence today, with one formal and two informal versions in Louisiana *not* included in that total (and for a state that desperately needs relief). In addition to the growing research supporting the efficacy of mental health courts, the human stories behind the numbers can be quite astounding:

> A mental health advocate in the 22nd Judicial District BHC recalls a success story – That was [client x], case study #1. He absolutely refused to go to self-help groups, like AA. Had a strong desire to function independently and lived on his own in Abita Springs. He had a long history of difficulty with communicating, organization problems, and always seemed to have an unhealthy living situation. We found out at one point his house didn't have heat and we were able to buy him a floor heater. He also neglected his physical health, then he started doing better and got prescription glasses. [As he participated in BHC], he became a leader in the AA community and even started running groups. He even came back to BHC years later to try and help out some one he met in AA. Prior to BHC, [client x] had 37 charges from 1988 through 2012, which include simple battery, aggravated battery, resisting arrest, domestic abuse, driving with a suspended license, possession of marijuana, driving while intoxicated (over four convictions), and much more. Since he was accepted into BHC, he had no new criminal charges, became a model client, and just 'got it.' (Khey, unpublished research).

The recent policy shifts to accept Medicaid expansion in 31 states and Washington DC have aided to shield the mental health court target population from a weak local mental health systems of care. With the help from a mental health court team, clients often find themselves able to navigate the system and connect with needed services, particularly when receiving Medicaid assistance. It provides more avenues for covered treatment provision and opens up a menu of available services that can aid in healthy outcomes. For example, in the 22nd Judicial District BHC, it is estimated that just more than half of the program's participants benefited from Medicaid and Medicaid expansion. This issue becomes critical as our national leaders debate the future of Medicaid and Medicaid expansion.

7.2 Older Initiatives, Mental Health Court Precursors

Before mental health court, court intervention relating to mental illness occurred infrequently through civil commitments, competency hearings, not guilty by reason of insanity (NGBRI) pleas, or when defendants challenge criminal justice processing through their attorneys (often, public defenders) for reasons related to their mental state (at the time or during the time of the offense). Primarily due to jail overcrowding and heavy court caseloads, local criminal justice systems searched for alternatives and improvements in justice processing, largely led by the courts on criminal justice task forces across the country (BJA, 2000). Yet, court-centered innovation to serve individuals with mental illness began in the 1960s with the use of diversion (Matthews, 1970). For example, both the cities of Chicago and New York court systems heavily relied on partnerships with the mental health care system. In fact, the Chicago system maintained an embedded partnership – the Psychiatric Institute – to directly handle misdemeanor referrals from the court on site, and further, offer an in-patient facility immediately next to the jail for felony case referrals. One of the primary goals of the Institute was to offer the court alternatives to criminal justice sanctions, whenever possible (particularly when considering public safety in its calculus). The possible recommendations were much like what mental health court offers today – outpatient treatment and referrals to drug and alcohol treatment. One divergence from mental health court, however, was that this system often recommended civil commitment as a viable alternative for the court to weigh in its decision-making. Meanwhile, the New York system was set up to allow for local police to directly divert individuals with potential mental health concerns directly to local hospitals. From this point, the hospitals had a direct line of communication with the courts to continue criminal processing and assist in planning alternatives, whenever possible, for both misdemeanor and felony cases.

While these interconnected systems of care faded away with deinstitutionalization, diversion persisted in some ways. For example, in Steadman et al. (1995) profiled diversion programs for individual with mental illness and found 230 out of 685 jail systems surveyed had linkages to such diversion programs, many of which had linkages to the local courts. In fact, several key similarities to mental health emerged from the successful programs reviewed. For example, one program featured an interdisciplinary team of 10 staff members to work intensively with 100 clients at a time. This project is further aided by "key players" that include judges, a local mental health director, public defenders, district attorneys, probation officers, and a supervisor of services in the local jail.

Research on these innovations needs improvement (Schneider, 2010). While there seems to be many good ideas for court intervention, the only one with a significant (and current) evidence base remains to be mental health courts. Thus, mental health courts are seen as *the* diversion tool for the courts for this target population. In fact, the Treatment Advocacy Center released a report entitled, "Mental Health Diversion Practices: A Survey of the States," that attempts to estimate the percentage of populations served by two sources of diversion – mental health courts and crisis intervention teams (CIT, see Chap. 3; Stettin et al., 2013). Their findings can be found in Table 7.3. What we have learned from these past experiences is that a

Table 7.3 Treatment Advocacy's Center grades of states' diversion practices

State	% served by a mental health court	% served by CIT	Average % of population served	Grade	State	% served by a mental health court	% served by CIT	Average % of population served	Grade
D.C.	100%	100%	100%	A+	Virginia	6%	70%	38%	C
Utah	85%	97%	91%	A+	Texas	44%	27%	36%	C
Florida	67%	97%	82%	A	Wisconsin	11%	60%	36%	C
California	78%	79%	79%	A	Kansas	18%	49%	34%	C-
Ohio	63%	88%	76%	A	Tennessee	16%	51%	34%	C-
Connecticut	100%	37%	69%	B+	Indiana	25%	37%	31%	C-
Illinois	78%	59%	69%	B+	Maryland	30%	31%	31%	C-
Idaho	76%	58%	67%	B+	New Hampshire	40%	19%	30%	C-
Nevada	88%	37%	63%	B	North Dakota	22%	34%	28%	D
Washington	62%	63%	63%	B	Michigan	48%	3%	26%	D
Colorado	35%	86%	61%	B	Wyoming	0%	52%	26%	D
Georgia	49%	70%	60%	B	Montana	17%	30%	24%	D
Maine	34%	83%	59%	B	Louisiana	8%	38%	23%	D
New Mexico	63%	50%	57%	B	New Jersey	7%	33%	20%	D
North Carolina	24%	87%	56%	B	South Carolina	27%	10%	19%	F
Arizona	21%	84%	53%	B-	Vermont	35%	1%	18%	F
Minnesota	31%	70%	51%	B-	Alabama	34%	0%	17%	F
Delaware	100%	0%	50%	B-	South Dakota	0%	29%	15%	F
Oklahoma	59%	40%	50%	B-	Iowa	8%	13%	11%	F
Pennsylvania	60%	40%	50%	B-	Massachusetts	13%	3%	8%	F
Oregon	54%	38%	46%	C+	Mississippi	2%	13%	8%	F
Kentucky	28%	61%	45%	C+	Arkansas	10%	0%	5%	F
Missouri	51%	38%	45%	C+	West Virginia	9%	0%	5%	F
Alaska	44%	44%	44%	C	Rhode Island	0%	0%	0%	F
Hawaii	70%	12%	41%	C					
Nebraska	42%	40%	41%	C					
New York	75%	5%	40%	C	Nat'l average	48%	49%	49%	C+

team-based effort often lends to optimal results. The added value of judicial oversight often lends an enforcement mechanism for accountability, both for key stakeholders and justice-involved individuals.

7.3   Assisted Outpatient Treatment Court (AOT)

Arguably a relative of a mental health court, Assisted Outpatient Treatment court or AOT has become much more prevalent recently. AOT is court ordered treatment which includes medication and is typically for persons who have a history of non-compliance with treatment. Currently AOT courts are permitted in 47 states in the United States under specific state statutes. Each state has their own statute, many of which are named after a specific case.

Treatment Advocacy Center defines AOT as "the practice of providing community-based mental health treatment under civil court commitment, as a means of (1) motivating an adult with mental illness who struggles with voluntary treatment adherence to engage fully with their treatment plan; and (2) focusing the attention of treatment providers on the need to work diligently to keep the person engaged in effective treatment." Note that the main difference between this treatment court and others is that it is a civil process and not criminal. The court in this case is more of an ally and works with all stakeholders to ensure the overall health and wellness of individuals involved. Further, Treatment Advocacy Center (2022) shares about the research and proven success of AOT courts stating, "A substantial body of research conducted in diverse jurisdictions over more than two decades establishes the effectiveness of assisted outpatient treatment in improving treatment outcomes for its target population. Specifically, the research demonstrates that AOT reduces the risks of hospitalization, arrest, incarceration, crime, victimization, and violence. AOT also increases treatment adherence and eases the strain placed on family members or other primary caregivers."

AOT is the perfect example of the concept of harm reduction that can be applied to many of the topics discussed in this writing. Harm reduction has been mainly used in the discussion of substance use but can also be applied to the concept of AOT. SAMHSA defines harm reduction as "a proactive and evidence-based approach to reduce the negative personal and public health impacts of behavior associated with alcohol and other substance use at both the individual and community levels" (SAMHSA, 2022). While not all persons involved in AOT Court have substance use concerns, they are reducing their own negative impacts as well as those of their families, friends, and communities. SAMHSA (2020) also best explains "the primary goal of recovery through community treatment and habilitation and has historically been referred to as "the hospital without walls." It is intended for consumers with SMI (severe mental illness) who have needs that have not been effectively met by traditional approaches." In other words, AOT is the least restrictive last resort, e.g., harm reduction.

This program has received substantial buy-in through Congressional action via the twenty-first Century Cures Act. Truly, this legislation opened up a fountain of funding to support broader adoption of AOT across the country via competitive grants sponsored by SAMHSA.

7.4 A Note on Veterans Treatment Courts

One of the most recent adaptation of drug court – veterans treatment court – is also closely aligned with mental health court due to its primary focus on trauma related to military service and/or combat. This may include post-traumatic stress disorder, traumatic brain injury, and military sexual trauma. Recent data suggests that one in five veterans experiences mental health disorder symptomatology or cognitive impairment, and one in six veterans deployed in Operation Enduring Freedom and Operation Iraqi Freedom can be diagnosed with substance use disorder (RAND, 2008). Yet, the most powerful reason why to hold a unique and separate veterans treatment court aside from either drug court or mental health court lies in the story that first inspired the idea:

One day, a Vietnam veteran appeared before Judge (Robert) Russell (in drug court in.

> Buffalo, New York). He had not been making his treatment appointments, and he refused to communicate with the court team or his treatment providers. As the judge tried to engage him, he remained unresponsive, his eyes on the floor. In a moment of exasperation, Judge Russell called two members of his court to the bench. Hank and Jack were also Vietnam veterans, so the judge asked that they spend some time with the gentleman, veteran to veteran. An hour later, when Judge Russell called the case again, the man approached the front of the court-room, stood at parade rest, and looked the judge in the eye. The judge then asked him if he was ready to accept the support and treatment that were being offered to him through the court. He immediately responded, "Yes, sir." That was the spark…. (Justice for Vets, 2017).

Veterans treatment court is designed to tap into the military culture and structure to benefit its clients. It leverages military training that often instills brotherhood and strong camaraderie to support the recovery of a veteran with mental illness and/or substance use disorder. Further, expertise is brought into veteran treatment courts to aid in navigating the exclusive benefits available to veterans for their past military service through the Veterans Health Administration, Veterans Benefits Administration, the State Department of Veterans Affairs, and local veteran service organizations. For example, veterans may benefit from general health care, substance abuse treatment, group therapy, transportation, peer mentoring by a veteran in recovery, transportation services, housing services, and much more. Often, veterans treatment courts seek to offer connectivity to all of these benefits in one place with individualized case management services to ensure that no one slips through the cracks.

With almost a decade of development, veterans treatment courts are beginning to develop an evidence base of their own. Most recently, Knudsen and Wingenfeld (2016) determined that a well-run veterans treatment court significantly decreased PTSD symptoms, improved client treatment orientation, promoted sleep, aided in improved family relations, decreased substance use, reduced depression, supported emotional well-being, and helped with perceived overall energy. Only 9 of the 86 participants were rearrested in 12 months. These findings are indeed promising, yet they lack scientific rigor. To address this, the National Institute of Justice has commissioned a rigorous, multisite evaluation of veterans treatment courts with initial findings to be published in the next 2–3 years.

7.5   The Future of Mental Health Courts

While veterans treatment courts benefit from having the firm support of the Federal government through different aspects of the US Department of Veterans Affairs, mental health courts and their local partners often have to shoulder the cost of the specialty court and the requisite array of services. For example, a newly initiated veterans court in southeastern Louisiana estimates its costs as $50,000 for a case manager's salary and benefits, $40,000 per annum in treatment costs not covered by Veterans Affairs, $8000 in drug screen and confirmation to ensure compliance, and $2000 in operating costs, supplies, and incidentals, for a total of roughly $100,000 per year to comfortably operate this type of specialty court. Many jurisdictions use state-allocated funds and/or court funds generated by fees generated by adjudications to cover these costs.

We are at an interesting crossroads relating to mental health courts. In the current political climate, veterans treatment courts are well-positioned to reap both direct and indirect benefits through reinvestment in the US Department of Veterans Affairs. Yet, mental health courts are showing signs of stress. A review of media accounts offer anecdotal evidence of potential problems on the horizon: in Delaware, a panel is recommending to unify the state's specialty courts instead of keeping them separate (Reyes, 2017); in Flint, the Genesee Health System was facing a budget crises which is threatening mental health court services (Pierret, 2016); in South Dakota, the state legislature did not fund a request to create its first mental health court due to fiscal concerns (Walker, 2017). Critically, the fate of Medicaid will prove to be central to the viability of mental health courts across the country. As a relatable illustration, the GAINS Center reviewed a common issue currently faced by all specialty courts, including (and particularly) mental health courts – the impact of having public benefits terminated or suspended when a person is incarcerated. As clients are waiting to have their benefits reinstated, they often face insurmountable problems trying to make ends meet, finding timely care, gaining access to medication, and so on (GAINS Center, 1999). If Medicaid were significantly curtailed or eliminated, very real possibilities being considered by the 115th United States Congress with tacit backing of President Trump, a significant burden would be shifted to localities and states to be able to provide care to mental health clients and the wider target population.

Yet, the bipartisan twenty-first Century Cures Act takes Federal leadership on mental health (and mental health courts) in a positive direction. It reauthorizes the Comprehensive Justice and Mental Health Act to continue to provide grant funding for mental health courts and innovative research in this domain. Additionally, the legislation enables improvements in data monitoring. This will allow for us to more effectively monitor any change in policy with greater precision, which will further allow for us to seek corrective action for any political shift that has unintended consequences. There appears to be significant momentum for criminal justice reform, including for individuals with mental illness and co-occurring disorders. It seems likely, then, that progress will continue, despite countervailing forces – the result of which may produce stifled progress, but progress nonetheless.

7.6   A Key Weakness in the Court's Role: Revocation, a Case Study

In the Journal of the American Academy of Psychiatry and Law, an article titled *Mental Illness and Revocation of Restricted Probation* discusses the court case of William Burke versus the State of Montana (Kambam & Guyer, 2006). In this lawsuit, William Burke appealed the ruling set forth that he violated his probation, but instead his behavior was related to his mental health diagnosis. William Burke was sentenced to 7 years by Cascade County with the Department of Corrections after a robbery charge. He served 4 years in prison in February 2004, and then was set to serve the remaining 3 years of his term on probation. In May of 2004, Burke's probation officer "filed a Report of Violation, alleging that Burke had violated eight different conditions of his probation." Due to this, a warrant was issued for his arrest and when he appeared in court, Burke requested a mental health evaluation. "Dr. Michael Scolatti, a licensed clinical psychologist, performed an evaluation of Burke and rendered a diagnosis of antisocial personality disorder, borderline intellectual functioning, bipolar disorder with psychotic features, and attention deficit/hyperactivity disorder (ADHD). Furthermore, he reported that Burke's bipolar disorder and ADHD were 'relatively severe disorders that require medication' and illnesses that would significantly compromise his ability to conform to the law. He opined that Burke should be placed at the state hospital." A request was made by Burke's law team to have him serve the remainder of his sentence in a state psychiatric hospital to receive treatment rather than incarceration. Unfortunately, the court ruled that Burke's behavior and mental illness did not play a part in whether he was able to commit the violations that were alleged. Burke was then sent back to prison to serve out the rest of time on his original sentence.

This is a case study of court action that can occur frequently across the United States. In their final analysis, Kambam and Guyer argue: "[in] a state unimpressed by the insanity defense, [this] is not a surprising outcome; indeed, it is a near certainty that an appellate court would not find 'an abuse of discretion' when a trial judge discounted the substance of a psychological expert's opinions and remanded a probation violator to prison." In fact, a very similar scenario occurred in 2021 in Louisiana. Hector and Khey interviewed several judicial staff during their evaluation efforts of a mental health court's operations. In the latest round of interviews, several staff brought up a case where an active mental health court client (and current probationer) was facing new charges in the same jurisdiction – a proceeding that could trigger revocation of probation. This new criminal proceeding went undetected until a bailiff working in the courthouse recognized the client as this person was in the early stages of prosecution. It was this bailiff who was able to connect the client with the mental health court staff to see if they could possibly stave off a jail or prison term. After a thorough review by all stakeholders with interest in this case, the client was able to continue in the mental health court program without incarceration under new negotiated terms of probation. Yet, if this client were to be found guilty in the new criminal proceeding without intervention, it could be very likely that this client would face time, even if this client's public defender could success-fully outline the client's mental health concerns at trial.

In essence, the entire sequential intercept model must be carefully studied to determine where vulnerable persons – including those with mental illness – are susceptible to harmful outcomes.

7.7   Conclusion

Court programs have been around for a number of years, but are expanding and diversifying to better serve communities and justice-involved individuals. Luckily, with the help of dedicated individuals, some of these court programs are beginning to show signs of true success. These successes are both beneficial for those involved in the program, but also their communities and our country as a whole. These small "breaths of life" are the life support needed to resurrect a failing system. There is hope that change can happen and those in need can receive not only the services needed, but also the chance to regain their lives as productive members of society.

Two key court innovations are mental health courts (also known as behavioral health courts) and veterans treatment courts. These adaptations of drug courts (also known as specialty courts) are developing an evidence-based and a proven track record of success. While the evidence is promising, some jurisdictions struggle with funding to keep these programs running under optimal conditions or even running at all. Veterans treatment courts have an advantage in that Veterans Affairs and gov-ernment benefits due to United States veterans shoulders much of the cost (e.g., treatment cost) of the program. Thus, in the near future, veterans treatment court is likely to expand at a faster rate relative to mental health courts despite the fact that both certainly target the same symptomatology.

On a final note, much more research needs to be done in the area of court innova-tions, particularly as a resource to interventions that can occur before criminal jus-tice processing can begin. In other words, as law enforcement and community partners work to divert eligible individuals away from the criminal justice system, court players (including judges) may have an opportunity to offer resources and legitimacy that no other partner can. Specialty courts seem to be the beginning of court participation in mental health innovations, and much more development should be expected in this arena in the near future.

Discussion Questions

1. How does the establishment of a mental health court help in reducing stigma? What are the obstacles with stigma once a person completes the program? In other words, what if the community has not changed their views on mental health while this program graduate has fulfilled their obligations?
2. Drug Courts have been around for over 20 years – are they effective?
3. Why are reentry courts not more prevalent? What obstacles exist to starting and continuing this sort of alternative program?
4. What other new and innovative programs exist as alternatives to incarceration?

References

Adult Drug Court Research to Practice Initiative. (2017). URL: http://www.research2practice.org. Last accessed: 2017, June 1.

Brennan, P., Battaglia, M., & Jones, G. (Producers). (2011 – current). Last Shot with Judge Gunn. (Television Series). Fayetteville, AK: Trifecta Entertainment. See: http://lastshotjudge-gunn.com/

Bureau of Justice Assistance. (2000). Emerging judicial strategies for the mentally ill in the criminal caseload: Mental health courts in Fort Lauderdale, Seattle, San Bernardino, and Anchorage. URL: https://www.ncjrs.gov/pdffiles1/bja/182504.pdf. Last accessed: July 10, 2017.

Carey, S. M., Mackin, J. R., & Finigan, M. W. (2012). What works? The ten key components of drug court: Research-based best practices. *Drug Court Review, 8*(1), 6–42.

Council of State Governments Justice Center. (2007). Improving responses to people with mental illness: The essential elements of a mental health court. URL: https://www.bja.gov/publications/mhc_essential_elements.pdf. Last accessed: 2017, June 1.

Drug Courts Program Office. (1997). Defining drug courts: The key components. URL: https://www.ojp.gov/pdffiles1/bja/205621.pdf. Last accessed: 12 Sep 22.

Drug Policy Alliance. (2011). Drug courts are not the answer: Toward a health-centered approach to drug use. URL: https://www.drugpolicy.org/docUploads/Drug_Courts_Are_Not_the_Answer_Final2.pdf. Last accessed: 2017, June 1.

Eckholm, E. (2008). Innovative courts give some addicts chance to straighten out. The New York Times. URL: https://www.nytimes.com/2008/10/15/us/15drugs.html. Last accessed: 12 Sep 22.

Festinger, D. S., Dugosh, K. L., & Marlowe, D. (2015). Improving outcomes for low-risk/low-need drug court clients: Life in the fast lane. *Drug & Alcohol Dependence, 146*, e276.

GAINS Center. (1999). *Medicaid benefits for jail detainees with co-occurring mental health and substance use disorders.* Prepared by Sherman, R. The National GAINS Center for People with Co-Occurring Disorders in the Criminal Justice System. URL: http://www.prainc.com/gains/publications/medicaid.htm. Last accessed: 2017, June 1.

Goldkamp, J. S., & Weiland, D. (1993). *Assessing the impact of Dade County's felony drug court: Final report.* US Department of Justice, Office of Justice Programs, National Institute of Justice. URL: https://www.ncjrs.gov/pdffiles1/Digitization/144524NCJRS.pdf. Last accessed: 2017, June 1.

Gottfredson, D. C., Najaka, S. S., & Kearley, B. (2003). Effectiveness of drug treatment courts: Evidence from a randomized trial. *Criminology & Public Policy, 2*(2), 171–196.

Halper, E. (2014). Drug courts, meant to aid addicts, now a battlefield of pot politics. Los Angeles Times. URL: https://www.latimes.com/nation/la-na-drug-court-20140727-story.html. Last accessed: 12 Sep 22.

Justice for Vets. (2017). URL: https://justiceforvets.org/. Last accessed: 2017, June 1.

Kambam, P., & Guyer, M. (2006). Mental illness and revocation of restricted probation. *Journal of the American Academy of Psychiatry and the Law Online, 35*(1), 120–122.

Knudsen, K. J., & Wingenfeld, S. (2016). A specialized treatment court for veterans with trauma exposure: Implications for the field. *Community Mental Health Journal, 52*(2), 127–135.

Loong, D., Bonato, S., Barnsley, J., & Dewa, C. S. (2019). The effectiveness of mental health courts in reducing recidivism and police contact: A systematic review. *Community Mental Health Journal, 55*(7), 1073–1098.

Lowenkamp, C. T., Holsinger, A. M., & Latessa, E. J. (2005). Are drug courts effective? A meta-analytic review. *Journal of Community Corrections, Fall,* 5–28.

Marlowe, D. B. (2010). Research update on adult drug courts. URL: http://www.nadcp.org/sites/default/files/nadcp/Research%20Update%20on%20Adult%20Drug%20Courts%20-%20NADCP_1.pdf. Last accessed: 2017, June 1.

Matthews, A. R. (1970). *Mental disability and the criminal justice system.* American Bar Foundation.

McNiel, D. E., & Binder, R. L. (2007). Effectiveness of a mental health court in reducing criminal recidivism and violence. *American Journal of Psychiatry, 164*(9), 1395–1403.

Miller, J. M., & Khey, D. N. (2016). An implementation and process evaluation of the Louisiana 22nd judicial district's behavioral health court. *American Journal of Criminal Justice, 41*(1), 124–135.

Moore, M. E., & Hiday, V. A. (2006). Mental health court outcomes: A comparison of re-arrest and re-arrest severity between mental health court and traditional court participants. *Law and Human Behavior, 30*(6), 659–674.

Morse, D. S., Cerulli, C., Bedell, P., Wilson, J. L., Thomas, K., Mittal, M., Lamberti, J. S., Williams, G., Silverstein, J., Mukherjee, A., Walck, D., & Chin, N. (2014). Meeting health and psychological needs of women in drug treatment court. *Journal of substance abuse treatment, 46*(2), 150–157.

National Drug Court Resource Center. (2022). Explore. URL: https://ndcrc.org/interactive-maps/. Last accessed: 12 Sep 22.

Pierret, A. (2016). Mental health court upset with potential cuts. URL: http://www.abc12.com/content/news/Mental-Health-Court-upset-with-potential-cuts-398980391.html. Last accessed: 2017, June 1.

RAND. (2008). Invisible wounds of war: Psychological and cognitive injuries, their consequences, and services to assist recovery. URL: https://www.rand.org/pubs/monographs/MG720.html. Last accessed: 12 Sep 22.

Reyes, J. M. (2017). Drug, mental health courts merged in New Castle County. URL: http://www.delawareonline.com/story/news/local/2017/04/24/drug-mental-health-courts-merged-new-castle-county/100840368/. Last accessed: 2017, June 1.

Rossman, S. B., & Zweig, J. M. (2012). The multisite adult drug court evaluation. URL: http://www.nadcp.org/sites/default/files/nadcp/Multisite%20Adult%20Drug%20Court%20Evaluation%20-%20NADCP.pdf. Last accessed: 2017, June 1.

Schneider, R. D. (2010). Mental health courts and diversion programs: A global survey. *International Journal of Law and Psychiatry, 33*(4), 201–206.

Steadman, H. J., Morris, S. M., & Dennis, D. L. (1995). The diversion of mentally ill persons from jails to community-based services: A profile of programs. *American Journal of Public Health, 85*(12), 1630–1635.

Stettin, B., Frese, F. J., & Lamb, H. R. (2013). *Mental health diversion practices: A survey of the states.* Treatment Advocacy Center.

Substance Abuse and Mental Health Services Administration. (2020). Executive order saving lives through increased support for mental and behavioral health needs report. URL: https://www.samhsa.gov/sites/default/files/saving-lives-mental-behavioral-health-needs.pdf. Last accessed: 2022, February 7.

Substance Abuse and Mental Health Services Administration. (2022). Harm reduction. URL: https://www.samhsa.gov/find-help/harm-reduction. Last accessed: 2022, February 7.

Thompson, M., Osher, F. C., & Tomasini-Joshi, D. (2008). *Improving responses to people with mental illnesses: The essential elements of a mental health court.* Justice Center, the Council of State Governments.

Tiger, R. (2012). *Judging addicts: Drug courts and coercion in the justice system.* New York University Press.

Treatment Advocacy Center. (2022). Assisted outpatient treatment laws. URL: https://www.treatmentadvocacycenter.org/component/content/article/39. Last accessed: 2022, February 7.

Walker, M. (2017). Mental health court money left out of state budget. Argus Leader. URL: http://www.argusleader.com/story/news/crime/2017/05/02/mental-health-court-money-left-out-state-budget/101041622/. Last accessed: 2017, June 1.

Wilson, D. B., Mitchell, O., & MacKenzie, D. L. (2006). A systematic review of drug court effects on recidivism. *Journal of Experimental Criminology, 2*(4), 459–487.

Chapter 8
Prison

What we've got here is failure to communicate. Some men you just can't reach. So you get what we had here last week, which is the way he wants it. Well, he gets it. I don't like it any more than you men. – Captain, Cool Hand Luke, 1967

Prisons present a complex array of problems relating to mental health. Perhaps most notably, the prison environment is quintessentially *iatrogenic* – that is, the "treatment" for substance abuse and mental illness now comes commonly in the form of incarceration, and this treatment by incarceration is related to further sickness. In other words, the American prison environment is the antithesis of a therapeutic community. Argumentatively, this has resulted in part from a combination result of a recent "no frills" movement (Finn, 1996) and a growing scarceness of resources. Regardless, prison is often awash in contraband (e.g., alcohol and drugs) and trauma-inducing situations (e.g., physical and sexual violence, administrative segregation and isolation, and missing the death of loved ones in the free world while incarcerated). The data provided in earlier sections of this text presented the daunting statistics behind these issues: just over half of state prisoners have a mental health problem; only one third of state inmates with a mental illness receives treatment for their illness in prison; and a smaller proportion receive professional mental health therapy for their symptoms. It appears that change is occurring most slowly for prisons than any other segment of the criminal justice system, primarily due to persistent budgetary constraints dating back to at least 1998 (CASA, 1998).

8.1 Know the Role

The seminal guide on substance abuse treatment in the criminal justice system disseminated by SAMHSA offers a handy section on treatment issues specific to prison (SAMHSA, 2014). While it relates to substance use and abuse, its content easily applies to broadly treatment issues in prison (see also Guidelines for Successful Transition of People with Mental or Substance Use Disorders from Jail and Prison, SAMHSA, 2014). In its prison section, the guide spends a great deal of time discussing the issues of inmate culture. It explains that compared to jail inmates, those

© The Author(s), under exclusive license to Springer Nature Switzerland AG 2022 173
J. Hector, D. Khey, *Criminal Justice and Mental Health*,
https://doi.org/10.1007/978-3-031-15338-9_8

in prison are more likely to learn to adopt prison cultural mores as a means of survival. This path to an inmate identity is also honed by the pressures of the institution and by the common interactions between inmates with one another, and with prison staff. Of particular importance, "there are many more people who are accustomed to the setting and who take the attitude that it is 'no big deal' [in prisons, as opposed to jails]....The hardened demeanor and 'macho' attitude adopted as part of the inmate culture can discourage offenders from participating in treatment...as [it] is a sign of 'weakness.'...[For example,] inmates who enroll in treatment are often characterized by other prisoners as too weak to 'handle their drugs' in the community" (SAMHSA, 2014: 193).

Thus, there often is a unique and complex dynamic in prisons that presents countervailing forces relating to mental health: (1) the prison environment is laden with the potential to develop mental health symptoms in otherwise healthy adults, and further, puts individuals with mental health diagnoses (particularly those with co-occurring disorders) at great risk of decompensating and falling deeper into their disease; (2) the stigma of seeking help often becomes intensified in this setting, lending to a significant barrier to treatment. These forces become particularly significant when realizing that after initial intake and medical screening and assessment, follow-up typically happens only when necessary – for example, upon a mental health crisis, overdose, contraband violation, or the like. Truly, in this setting, squeaky wheels (especially the loud ones) will get attended to, yet, many prisoners become adept at hiding any signs that may raise suspicion that they need help. And further, if prison administrators sought to provide care to everyone who needs it, the cost of adequate care would quickly bankrupt all prison operations.

With this in mind, a prominent subsection in the guide is entitled "What treatment services can *reasonably* be provided in the prison setting" (emphasis added). The ideal program being advocated for is a "true" Therapeutic Community (TC) inside of the prison setting with complete segregation from the general population 24-hour, 7-days a week for optimal success. TCs feature the integration of work (and/or educational or vocational programming), professional counseling, and a healthy (e.g., pro-social) community environment. Oftentimes, prison administrators must compromise by offering as many components of the TC as possible given the resources available. In many cases, TCs are composed of individuals who remain in general population who receive a schedule of programming to attend, which features the components of a TC – counseling, education classes, group therapy sessions, and so on. Further, self-help programming has become extremely popular in this framework due to its simplicity to set up and the few resources required to sustain them. A current search of Crime Solutions rates TCs as promising overall – based on a study (Mitchell et al., 2012) that reviews 30 such programs' impact on recidivism post-release. One specific program – the Amity In-Prison Therapeutic Community – was also rated as promising upon a randomized control treatment study design revealed significant reductions of reincarceration rates (Prendergast et al., 2004). It is critical to note that many TC programs depicted a waning ability to reduce drug use among participants versus a comparison group – this should not be surprising in that best practices dictate that treatment services that begin early in incarcerated settings *which continue post-release* yield the best odds of success in reducing substance use related outcomes.

Yet, is it reasonable to assume that as long as prisons offer an array of services (such as these mentioned above) to their inmate population, regardless if they are driven to use them or not, that prisons are fulfilling their constitutional duties of inmate care? With often scarce resources and remote distancing from the community-based care system that can support jails and other forms of justice-involvement (e.g., community corrections), the answer to "what treatment services can reasonably be provided in a prison setting?" is a pressing one.

8.1.1 Reaffirming Minimal Mental Health Care: The Epicenter (California) and the New Frontier (Alabama)

In February 2015, experts at the Stanford Law School teamed up with a California State Senator to publish a study entitled "When did prisons become acceptable mental health care facilities?" (Steinberg et al., 2015). This work begins by focusing on the rapid increase of mentally ill people in the California prison system after deinstitutionalization, and then brings to light the current conditions of incarceration for individuals with mental illness, which specifically tend to result in longer sentences than those who have not been diagnosed with a mental illness. Steinberg et al. (2015) offer some glim statistics about the California State Prison System to drive their points home: as of 2015, 45 percent of inmates had been treated for *severe* mental illness in the past year (vastly more by proportion than other states as indicated by the data provided earlier in this text); the number of prison inmates with mental illness has doubled in the 15 years prior to the report's release (since 2000); and the average sentence for burglary 30 percent longer for an individual with a mental health diagnosis compared to the average sentence for defendants without mental illness who are convicted of the same crime, leading the sentencing disparities among other crime types (e.g., robbery, assault, assault with a weapon, child molestation, second degree murder, weapons charges, and drug sales – much like as seen within jails). Criminal justice reform in California was intended, in part, to ameliorate these issues – especially in light of *Coleman v. Wilson*. Yet, behavioral health disparities continue in California as evidenced by the number of inmates with mental illness gaining relief under new resentencing laws (e.g., Proposition 36) relative to inmates without mental health problems; that is, individuals with a mental health diagnosis have recently been denied resentencing relief relative to those who do not have a diagnosis.

These issues highlight the enduring nature of seeding institutional change. California has been at the forefront of a paradigm shift for prisoners with mental illness since 1994 with the formation of the California Department of Corrections and Rehabilitation Mental Health Services Delivery System (2009; see Table 7.1).

Despite years of effort, defining model policies and procedures and promulgating them throughout the prison system, and engaging in best practices, significant slippage is still commonplace. For example, in the most recent complaint in *Coleman v. Brown* (2017) – which was originally filed as *Coleman v. Wilson* as discussed earlier in this text – the Department of Corrections was found to have not provided prompt care for inmates experiencing life-threatening psychiatric crises. Small and Pickoff-White (2017) offer additional details in their expose on the facts of the case; according to their investigative journalist accounting on the matter, over 25% of individuals needing critical care for life-threatening mental health crises experienced longer than a 24-hour wait in February of 2017. Further, some inmates were placed on a waitlist, resulting in death in extreme cases. With the Federal judge in this most recent flare up of *Coleman v. Brown* deciding in favor of the defendants, as a matter of law, this means that the bar for the minimal constitutional level of care in California has been reified by the standards set forth in Table 8.1.

These revelations have disheartened many but continue drive reformers to press for possible solutions for change. While California has been consistently working in good faith toward improvements in their system, Steinberg, Mills, and Romano describe "three modest but significant proposals" to give the state some momentum to realize some *real* gains in improvement. The first step, "reform the way we sentence the mentally ill," discusses taking a different look at crimes that are non-violent and non-serious that may have been committed as a result of the person's mental illness. Rather than incarceration, a judge could then sentence the person to treatment which is much more cost-effective. Secondly, prisons must begin to provide *meaningful* treatment for inmates while they are incarcerated. Lastly, treatment should continue to the point of release, during release, and must connect with meaningful treatment in the community (Table 8.2).

To accomplish these aims, Steinberg, Mills, and Romano identify that California will still need to invest greatly in additional infrastructure, such as mental health case managers for parolees, transitional housing for inmates returning back to the community, and expanded alternatives like mental health court (see Chap. 7). These investments, it should be noted, should arguably save the public money in the long run as the cost of incarceration tends to be the most exorbitant relative to any alternative. Yet, the radical component of Steinberg, Mills, and Romano's proposition – judicial oversight of the mental health services of prison inmates – may just be the missing ingredient California needs for lasting change.

Judicial oversight is not new. Traditionally, this comes in the form of Federal consent decrees, which places prison facilities into receivership of the court – meaning that the oversight of operations rests with judges and/or the individuals they designate. This has happened with Louisiana's prisons in 1969, and with California's prisons as described above. Consent decrees have historically been wrought with political conflict and have pitted local administrators against their external overseers in a plainly adversarial approach. Steinberg, Mills, and Romano's special Mental Health Prison Oversight Court may hold a distinct advantage over consent decrees if this model can approach oversight in a non-adversarial way. That is, instead of a top-down approach to ensure oversight and compliance, a team-based approach that

Table 8.1 Summary of California Department of Corrections and Rehabilitation mental health program

Primary component	Program description
Crisis intervention	"A crisis is defined as a sudden or rapid onset or exacerbation of symptoms of mental illness, which may include suicidality or other aberrant behavior which requires immediate intervention. Crisis intervention is provided at all institutions to inmate suffering from a situational crisis or an acute episode of mental disorder. The first step in providing crisis intervention is adequate training for all institutional staff in the recognition of mental health crisis symptoms, a plan for immediate staff response, and procedures for referral to clinical staff. Custody and clinical staff cooperation is critical to ensure that an inmate in a mental health crisis is treated as soon as possible."
Comprehensive services	"The MHSDS (Mental Health Services Delivery System) offers comprehensive services and a continuum of treatment for all required levels of care. In addition to standardized screening and evaluation, all levels of care found in a county mental health system are represented in the CDCR MHSDS programs. All levels of care include treatment services provided by multiple clinical disciplines, and development and update of treatment plans by an interdisciplinary Treatment team (IDTT), which includes appropriate custody staff involvement."
Decentralized services	"Mental health services are geographically decentralized by making basic services widely available. All levels of care, except inpatient hospitalization, are available at most geographically-defined service areas. Case management and crisis intervention are provided at all institutions."
Clinical and administrative oversight	"In coordination with each institution, the CDCR Division of Correctional Health Care Services (DCHCS) and Division of Adult Institutions will continue to update standardized program policy and develop a system for monitoring delivery of program services. The CDCR shall develop an annual review schedule. A systemwide automated tracking and records system continues to evolve to support administrative and clinical oversight."
Standardized screening	"Access to mental health services is enhanced for all inmates through standardized screening of all admissions at reception centers. Standardized screening ensures that all inmates have equal and reliable access to services. The data generated by standardized screening provides the CDCR with necessary information to improve the assessment of mental health service needs. If screening reveals indicators of mental disorder, such as prior psychiatric hospitalization, current psychotropic medication, suicidality or seriously maladaptive behaviors, follow-up evaluation by a clinician shall determine the immediate treatment needs of the inmate. Early identification of an inmate's mental health needs will provide an appropriate level of treatment and promote individual functioning within the clinically least restrictive environment consistent with the safety and security needs of both the inmate-patient and the institution. Avoiding the utilization of more expensive services will aid in budget containment."
Pre-release planning	"This component of service, in conjunction with the correctional Counselor's preparation of the CDCR 611, release program study, focuses on preparing the seriously mentally disordered inmate-patient for parole. Its objective is to maximize the individual's potential for successful linkage and transition to the parole outpatient clinic, or, if required, to inpatient services in the community or the mentally disordered offender program operated at the DMH facilities. In the case of paroling inmate-patients, this includes facilitating the work of the parole and Community services Division's transitional case management program."

Table 8.2 Summary of Steinburg, Mills, and Romano's three modest, but significant proposals

Reform the way we sentence the mentally ill	Take mental health into account at sentencing. Use the *preponderance of evidence* burden of proof when determining whether a defendant's crime was likely committed as a result of his/her mental illness. If proof positive, provide non-prison/non-custodial sentences, whenever possible, for non-serious and nonviolent offenses. Note: The cost of such treatment is far less than the cost of incarceration
Provide meaningful treatment in prison	Sentencing judge should be able to order treatment in the terms and condition of an offender's incarceration. Create an oversight court (consisting of judges and mental health professionals) to review cases to ensure proper and adequate services are being rendered to each inmate. Court continues to provide meaningful oversight of treatment throughout incarceration.
Continue meaningful treatment after prison	Provide evaluation before release of potential mental health needs in the community. Refer releasees to mental health centers with full access to health and treatment records.

includes correctional, mental health, and legal professionals (all led by a judge) in shaping decision-making may prove beneficial.

While California has been at the forefront of these issues, Alabama's prisons have only begun this cycle by revealing its institutional failures to serve individuals with mental illness in the case *Braggs* et al., *v. Dunn* (2017). At the conclusion of the dramatic trial, Federal Judge Myron H. Thompson issued a 302-page ruling featuring an order for immediate and long-term relief of the violation of Eighth Amendment rights of a class comprised of mentally ill inmates and to the Alabama Disabilities Advocacy Program. Specifically, Judge Thompson found that the defendants were at fault for:

(1) Failing to identify prisoners with serious mental-health needs and to classify their needs properly; (2) Failing to provide individualized treatment plans to prisoners with serious mental-health needs; (3) Failing to provide psychotherapy by qualified and properly supervised mental-health staff and with adequate frequency and sound confidentiality; (4) Providing insufficient out-of-cell time and treatment to those who need residential treatment; and failing to provide hospital-level care to those who need it; (5) Failing to identify suicide risks adequately and providing inadequate treatment and monitoring to those who are suicidal, engaging in self-harm, or otherwise undergoing a mental-health crisis; (6) Imposing disciplinary sanctions on mentally ill prisoners for symptoms of their mental illness, and imposing disciplinary sanctions without regard for the impact of sanctions on prisoners' mental health; and (7) Placing seriously mentally ill prisoners in segregation without extenuating circumstances and for prolonged periods of time; placing prisoners with serious mental-health needs in segregation without adequate consideration of the impact on mental health; and providing inadequate treatment and monitoring in segregation.

Further, Judge Thompson carefully articulated the "abundant evidence presented in support of the Eighth Amendment claim" throughout his decision. Starting with the basics, Judge Thompson opined on the scope of the Alabama Department of Corrections population – about 19,500 men and women spread across 15 major facilities (one for women). Of this total population, evidence presented at trial suggested an approximate mental health caseload of 3400 inmates actively receiving some form of mental health treatment. A wealth of data from the Alabama Department of Corrections and its private (for-profit) mental health care provider, MHM Correctional Services, Inc., would unveil minimal resources dedicated to providing mental health care when considering this level of need. Alabama's two mental health units providing treatment for its most severely ill have 346 male residential treatment beds and 30 stabilization unit beds (for acute mental health crises), 30 female residential treatment beds, and 8 stabilization unit beds for women – suggesting that the entire Alabama prison system can professionally handle only 38 mental health crises at any given time. Further, Alabama Department of Corrections only retains one governmental employee in a leadership position with mental health expertise; all other mental health care functions reside with the contracted service provider.

MHM Correctional Services, Inc., provided the following information to the court about their current staffing across the entire system: the Alabama contract includes a medical director (psychiatrist), mid-level managers (quality improvement manager and chief psychologist), 45 full-time mental health professional counselors/social workers, four psychiatrists and eight certified registered nurse practitioners (who are qualified to diagnose, prescribe medication, and provide psychotherapy, three psychologists, and three registered nurses who supervise 40 licensed practical nurses (LPNs conduct mental health intake, monitor medication compliance and side effects). The testimony in conjunction with these scant resources led Judge Thompson to conclude that the low prevalence rates of mental illness in Alabama's prisons relative to other states was not due to high-quality mental health care in Alabama's prisons or that Alabama's prisons simply had fewer mentally ill inmates than other states. Many cases seemed to be slipping through the cracks at intake (poor supervision of minimally trained front-line staff) and evidence suggested that referrals for evaluation and treatment were often neglected. When mental illness is identified correctly, evidence suggested that follow-up care was haphazard with delays or cancellations of professional counseling largely due to a shortage of counselors or the correctional staff required to ensure safety. For inmates with severe mental illness, Judge Thompson found that the specialized mental health units operated as large segregation units with little evidence of counseling, programming, or time allotted for inmates to spend out of their cells. If hospitalization was deemed medically necessary, the Department of Corrections simply did not provide this level of care.

At trial, the Commissioner of the Alabama Department of Corrections candidly offered an explanation for these conditions – that the system is struggling with overcrowding in conjunction with understaffing. The dangerous effects of these shortcomings were on full display in court for 7 weeks. The trail began with a rousing start. A prisoner named Jamie Wallace shared painful testimony with the court, whose personal prison story was fraught with multiple suicide attempts with visible scars to show for it at trial. Mr. Wallace struggled to detail his experiences of not receiving any help from the system to the point when Judge Thompson had to order a recess and to continue testimony in chambers. After his story was detailed for the record, Judge Thompson excused Mr. Wallace and immediately ordered both sets of attorneys to provide him with a report on Mr. Wallace's mental condition and what was being done about it. In a twist, Mr. Wallace would hang himself 10 days later, thus laying bare the exact basis of the litigation at hand – the system was not just failing, it was in failure.

Highlights of the system failures that were detailed in the weeks after Mr. Wallace's testimony were jarring. For example, Judge Thompson described that correctional staff tended to "gamble" with prisoners lives as they did not have a good method of determining suicidality and had such few suicide-watch cells to work with. Further, the suicide-watch cells available were far from suicide-proof: visibility was poor for direct monitoring, cells still included places where one could tie off ligatures, and dangerous items that could easily aid in self-injury were still easily available. In fact, before the trial could conclude, another inmate (not related to the trial) had committed suicide adding to the steep uptick of prison suicides that has occurred in the last 2 years:

> [A]s explained earlier, the court had a close encounter with one of the tragic consequences of inadequate mental-health care during the trial. Over the course of the trial, two prisoners committed suicide, one of whom was named plaintiff Jamie Wallace. Prior to his suicide, defendants' expert, Dr. Patterson, concluded based on a review of Wallace's medical records that the care he received was inadequate. Dr. Haney, a correctional mental-health care expert, met Wallace months before his death, while he was housed in a residential treatment unit, and in his report expressed serious concerns about the care he was receiving. Wallace's case was emblematic of multiple systemic deficiencies. Wallace testified, and his records reflected, that mental-health staff did not provide much in the way of consistent psycho-therapeutic treatment, which is distinct from medications administered by nurses and cursory 'check ins' with staff. MHM clinicians recommended that he be transferred to a mental-health hospital, but ADOC failed to do so. His psychiatrist at the time of this death testified that the medically appropriate combination of supervised out-of-cell time and close monitoring when he was in his cell was unavailable due to a shortage of correctional officers. As a result, Wallace was left alone for days in an isolated cell in a treatment unit, where he had enough time to tie a sheet unnoticed; because his cell was not suicide-proof, he was able to find a tie-off point from which to hang himself.

From all accounts, American prison systems are often at a near- or full-crisis of mental health services, and this segment of the criminal justice system seems least able to promote change. While California has seen decades of progressive reform, many of these reforms have not been fully actualized primarily due to what has come to be a repeated mantra – resources and money. The story of the California and of Alabama will, no doubt, repeat itself in the future with other straining and failing systems – often being sparked by litigation. Each case will only serve to reinforce new standards to be promulgated across the county.

8.1.2 The Common Affront: Locking Someone in ad seg

As alluded to in the case of Alabama above, prisons often maintain controversial facilities called administrative segregation, often called "ad seg" or solitary confinement. These facilities are used in instances when an inmate is violent or has some behavioral issues as punishment, for behavior modification, or, primarily, for security reasons (e.g., an inmate is too dangerous for general population). In an article in the *National Prison Project Journal*, social psychologist Haney (2003) describes the effects of administrative segregation as "psychologically destructive," and shown to produce social withdrawal, violence, and self-mutilation behaviors and suicidal ideation, leading to what he would later term a "social death." Individuals with preexisting mental illness are, in fact, at a greater risk of negative consequences. A comprehensive review of the literature confirms this; Peter Scharff Smith (2006) finds evidence to support that solitary confinement impacts many prisoners negatively, and substantially so. These impacts are moderated by duration of confinement, environmental factors, and characteristics of the prisoner. Yet, the negative impact endures for many.

Administrative segregation often involves an inmate being locked up for, at times, 23 hours a day. Any recreational time outside of this cell is often suspended, or if it is allowed, it is often of a minimal duration. Imagine that scenario, being locked in a tiny cell for 23 hours a day for days or weeks at a time. Additionally, many of the items an inmate may have in general population are not allowed or taken away when put into administrative segregation. Until recently, California prisons were said to have used administrative segregation more so than any other state prison system – that is, until litigation forced its ways. In 2015, *Ashker v. Brown*, n.d. was settled with promises to minimize the use of solitary housing units (nearly 3000 cells at that time) and put into place policies to ensure its proper use. It now seems that Alabama may be at the brink of needing similar intervention.

What is clear is that the use of administrative segregation provides fertile ground for litigation. Of particular note, Supreme Court Justice Anthony Kennedy made clear mention of his concerns with solitary confinement in a separate opinion on a case questioning the procedural rules of a criminal trial of a death row inmate:

In response to a question, respondent's counsel advised the Court that, since being sentenced to death in 1989, Ayala has served the great majority of his more than 25 years in custody in "administrative segregation" or, as it is better known, solitary confinement....if his solitary confinement follows the usual pattern, it is likely respondent has been held for all or most of the past 20 years or more in a windowless cell no larger than a typical parking spot for 23 hours a day; and in the one hour when he leaves it, he likely is allowed little or no opportunity for conversation or interaction with anyone....It is estimated that 25,000 inmates in the United States are currently serving their sentence in whole or substantial part in solitary confinement, many regardless of their conduct in prison.

The human toll wrought by extended terms of isolation long has been understood, and questioned, by writers and commenters. Eighteenth-century British prison reformer John Howard wrote "that criminals who had affected an air of boldness during their trial, and appeared quite unconcerned at the pronouncing sentence upon them, were struck with horror and shed tears when brought to these darksome solitary abodes." In literature, Charles

Dickens recounted the toil of Dr. Manette, whose 18 years of isolation in One Hundred and Five North Tower, caused him, even years after his release, to lapse in and out of mindless state with almost no awareness or appreciation for time or his surroundings....Yet despite scholarly discussion and some commentary from other sources, the condition in which prisoners are kept simply has not been a matter of public inquiry or interest. To be sure, cases on prison procedures and conditions do reach the courts. See e.g., *Brown v. Plata*.... Sentencing judges, moreover, devote considerable time and thought to their task. There is no accepted mechanism, however, for them to take into account, when sentencing a defendant, whether the time in prison will be or should be served in solitary. So in many cases, it is as if a judge had no choice but to say: "In imposing this capital sentence, the court is well aware that during the many years you will serve in prison before your execution, the penal system has a solitary confinement regime that will bring you to the edge of madness, perhaps to madness itself." Even if the law were to condone or permit this added punishment, so stark an outcome out not to be the result of society's simple unawareness or indifference....Over 150 years ago, Dostoyevsky wrote, "The degree of civilization in a society can be judged by entering its prisons." There is truth to this in our own time. (*Davis v. Ayala, 135 S.Ct. 2187, 2205, 2015*).

Thus, administrative segregation has been vaulted to the epicenter for mental health advocacy in recent years. Expect increased litigation forcing this issue, beginning in Alabama. Earlier efforts have resulted in settlements, not a summary judgment, which lacks the authority of case law. This absence of case may soon change as keenly noted by Justice Kennedy. While the Supreme Court has yet to hear a case specific to administrative segregation, the time for its review is becoming imminent.

8.1.3   A Local Case Study: Boston

The Boston Globe published an article in late 2016 discussing the perils of the criminal justice system in Massachusetts for individuals with mental illness and substance abuse. The article uses the story of an inmate Nick Lynch to discuss the struggles experienced by an incarcerated person in Boston. The year before approximately 15,000 inmates were released from prisons and jails in Massachusetts. As with many of these stories, the problems worsen and here more than half of those released inmates had a history of addiction and more than one-third suffered from mental illness. This is not unlike many other states with inmates being released with diagnoses of one or both mental illness and/or substance abuse. Even more complicated, these diagnoses increase the likelihood of them being incarcerated again within 3 years.

The article brings up another great point stating, "The prison environment itself is a major obstacle to treatment: In a culture ruled by aggression and fear, the trust and openness required for therapy are exponentially harder to achieve." This statement is somewhat the epitome of the dilemma of crime and mental health. If prison is not the ideal environment for treatment and treatment is obviously needed, then why is the person being incarcerated? This is almost the exact same question posed by Steinberg, Mills, and Romano in California.

Further, as mentioned before, individuals are leaving prisons and jails in Massachusetts without the proper tools needed to be successful in society. Without medication, counseling, and support, those with mental illness and substance abuse issues are more likely to return to jail/prison. As one could imagine, the cost of incarceration can be expensive. Therefore, the idea of reducing recidivism would be beneficial to states and their Department of Corrections. In Massachusetts, the state would save $50,000 by lessening incarceration by just one inmate. This begs the question – what is the state doing to help released inmates? In Massachusetts, unfortunately, not much it seems. According to numbers from the state itself, more than 90 percent of the 6000 inmates who are estimated to have mental illness and released from prisons or jails received "little or no help" from the Department of Mental Health when trying to find treatment in the community.

Recently, the state has begun cutting the budget for mental health within the criminal justice system. This has largely come from reducing prescriptions provided to inmates by 35 percent between the years 2010 and 2015. The reduction of prescriptions can obviously be problematic for many reasons. The first group that was impacted was those receiving treatment for ADHD (attention deficit hyperactive disorder); many others are slated to lose access to necessary treatment in the near future if these trends continue. The politics of prisons seem to be guided by crisis, as in until mental health reaches a critical mass, many systems seem to copasetic with the minimum effort needed to remain under the radar.

8.2 Example Progressive Programming and Program Elements

A change that has developed as a result of the increasing rates of incarceration and the already overcrowded prison systems is unique prison programming. Different states have been developing new way to fight recidivism and help inmates prepare for success outside of prison. These programs can receive some skepticism and resistance; some also have not yet developed to produce conclusive results. The good news, not unlike entrepreneurship, with creativity come success. The odds are that at least some of these particular programs will result in success.

8.2.1 Pen Pals, Inc.

As discussed earlier, a diverse array of innovations and alternative programming have occurred in recent years to address mental health issues in prison settings. Many of these alternatives seek to develop vocational and life skills as well as lessen the impact of the prison setting to inspire hope. From this movement, animal care programs have emerged to help inmates in this capacity. Although many programs of this nature exist across the country (and in many others), Pen Pals was developed out of a major natural disaster – Hurricane Katrina – which caused many animals to be without care as families evacuated their devastated homes. Dixon Correctional Institute (DCI) in Louisiana is a medium-sized, medium-security prison that is first of its kind to house a full animal shelter and clinic called Pen Pals.

In addition, Pen Pals features a fully operational clinic inside of the prison. Thus, not only can the rescued animals receive care and training from trustee inmates, but they can also receive the medical care they need without having to be transported off-site. This serves to provide the trustees with an immersion experience of operating an animal shelter in the free world with the added mental health benefits of caring for animals in this capacity. Most importantly, Pen Pals continues to serve an important function for the local region as a no-kill shelter and is likely to receive more difficult cases than many shelters in the free world – an inept analogy to how some prisoners view their own lives, or at least, have done so in the past. Here is a summary of their history, as presented on their website:

> In 2005 Hurricane Katrina hit the state of Louisiana as a category 5 storm with maximum force. A conservative estimate reveals that over 50,000 animals were abandoned by their owners in New Orleans as they fled to safety. While their intentions were to return within days to retrieve their beloved pets, the animals were left trapped in homes or chained to fences, braving toxic waters, and 105 degree heat with no food or water. Hours became days as they waited to be rescued and reunited with their owners.
>
> Rescuers were understaffed and overwhelmed by the scope of the problem and the time-critical nature of their effort. But motivated by compassion, relief came in the form of these few dedicated volunteers. Along with those volunteers, the Louisiana Department of Public Safety and Corrections, Dixon Correctional Institute (DCI) assisted by housing many of these abandoned animals. A make shift animal clinic was set up, and inmates were trained in caring for animals of all types, shapes and sizes. A vision was born out of tragedy.
>
> In response to the events of this tragic and horrific situation, an agreement was made between the Human Society of the United States (HSUS), the Louisiana State University School of Veterinary Medicine and DCI, to establish a permanent and emergency temporary animal shelter on the grounds of the prison. The HSUS obtained a grant in the amount of $600,000 to fund the construction of the facilities. The permanent animal clinic (better known as Pen Pals, Inc., Dog and Cat Shelter and Adoption Center) provides comprehensive training for future veterinarians and promotes the rehabilitation of those incarcerated who are trained to assist.
>
> Our belief is that tragedies will happen, but Pen Pals Inc., will be there with food and a leash in hand (see: https://doc.louisiana.gov/public-programs-resources/pen-pals-animal-shelter/).

8.3   Pop-Culture and Prison, New Links to Awareness

In addition to celebrities and other influential people, the mainstream media has taken to discussing the criminal justice system and mental health. Podcasts, television, as well as magazines and newspapers are covering the subjects to shed light on the system, including the flaws.

One of the more popular and raw television shows is *Lockup* on MSNBC. *Lockup* brings cameras into jails and prisons across the country to show the reality behind the bars. This reality includes interviews and insight from everyone involved from the wardens, corrections officers, support staff, and even inmates. The show has traveled to different areas and levels of prisons to show how things vary at each institution. Additionally, *Lockup* has specialty episodes to tackle some unique outliers like First Timers which covers individuals who are serving their first sentence in prison or jail, Special Investigation which covers the juvenile justice system, and Women Behind Bars which follows women in the system.

Despite the somewhat negative nature of the television show, the positive consequences are also very present. Each episode digs into the stories behind the inmates that make them human, rather than just a number. Background information, history, as well as interviews from staff and inmates create an overall picture of the tragedies that brought the person to jail or prison. This knowledge can be positive in that it helps to show the truth behind incarceration. Additionally, making the individual seem human allows for the compassion and empathy needed in some cases to aid in the rehabilitation of that person.

Lockup also provides footage and insight into the lives of mentally ill inmates. In the episode entitled Inside Wabash Valley Correctional Facility, the production staff interviews an inmate by the name of Joe Carr who is serving an 8-year sentence for robbery in this facility in Indiana. In this episode, the prison's psychologist is also interviewed where she discusses "shoe" or Special Housing Unit (SHU). At other facilities this may be called Administrative Segregation. The brief interview with the psychologist and inmate paints the picture that mentally ill inmates are often put into the SHU after harming themselves. In Joe Carr's case, he swallowed ink pens in one incident and cut his leg open in another. He goes on to describe the feelings he experienced while cutting himself "when you're going through one of them phases, you don't even feel the pain...you don't even know you're doing it." Joe also describes his feelings of anger and using the acts of harming himself to "feel better." Joe was put into the SHU for hurting himself from we describes as being anti-social. After serving his time in the SHU, he was then put back into general population at the prison, but describes the repeating cycle of self-harm. After several cycles of going to the SHU for harming himself, then returning to general population with no success, Joe was then evaluated and diagnosed with Bipolar Disorder and transferred to the Residential Treatment Unit (RTU). The interview concludes with Joe's own perspective about life after prison when he states "this is all you know...you're used to what, a population of 1200 people. Then, they turn you back into society of billions of people. Are you ready for it?"

The episode of Lockup featuring Joe Carr is just one of many that feature a person in the criminal justice system who is mentally ill. On a societal level, this leads to questions and controversy. What amount of harm is done to the individual for the repeated cycle of self-harm and punishment in the SHU? For those discussing the fiscal consequences, his repeated acts of self-harm resulted in many medical exams, most of which resulted in surgeries. How much of a burden does that put on the system? How could the burden and harm on the inmate be avoided? How could the burden on the system be avoided as well?

Another example of the portrayal of the criminal justice system and mentally ill inmates involves the controversy behind the 10-episode Netflix original *Making a Murderer*. *Making a Murderer* is dubbed a "real-life thriller" by Netflix, and a true crime documentary by other sources. This series was filmed over a 10-year period following Steven Avery, a man who had been recently released from prison after serving 18 years for rape. At the beginning of the series, he had just been released after being exonerated with DNA evidence from his original 32-year charge. Despite this happy outlook, the series quickly takes a turn to Steven then being accused of murder. He, along with his nephew, Brendan Dassey were arrested for the rape and murder of Teresa Halbach and sentenced to life in prison.

The controversy infiltrates this story in many ways including police corruption, evidence tampering, and questionable ethics. As it relates here, the mental health of both men, Steven Avery and Brendan Dassey, was called into question. As this book is being written, there is still development in this case bringing to light relevant issues regarding the treatment of individuals with mental health concerns by the system. It appears that we are at a moment in which coverage of mental health issues is beginning to increase across platforms, medium, and by source.

8.4   Out of the Box Innovations

There are some positive trends in regard to prisons in other parts of the world. In recent years, The Netherlands has seen such a decline in crime that they have actually been closing their prisons. The stereotype in the United States is that prisoners serve "hard time" while in prison and they will be remorseful of the crimes they committed. For American prisons, the assumption is that the tough times of prison create a situation in which the person learns to not want to return to prison. It is somewhat of a behavior modification process. If the conditions inside prison are worse than outside or home, the idea is that a person who commits crimes would then not want to return to prison. The person would then want to do all possible to avoid another sentence, like changing their behaviors and no longer committing crime. The problem with this assumption and argument is that it just does not work in America. If this were the case, most prisons would be useless and empty at this point. The view of using prison as a form of punishment has really only led to an increase of inmates currently in prison as well as an increase in those that return for repeated offenses.

Prisons around the world are trying different approaches within their prisons to show the possibility that the alternative to "hard time" works better to combat recidivism. Rather than using a prison and sentence as punishment, other countries are working toward a prison sentence as a time for change and reform where the person can learn other skills to use after time served as well as maintain their support system with family and their mental health. In Suomenlinna Prison, often referred to as the "open prison" inmates in Finland do not see barbed wire and large fences around the grounds of the prison. The prison director Tapio Iinatti describes the thought process behind the way this prison is set up "The main idea here is to prepare the inmates for release into the community. It doesn't make sense for an inmate to be in a closed prison for, say, 6 years and to suddenly enter civilian life. We also offer rehabilitation for people who have had problems related to alcohol, drugs or mental illness. And in any case, it's not so easy to be here."

Another prison described as using a humane approach is Halden Prison in Norway. Halden Fengsel has been dubbed "the world's most humane maximum-security prison." This nickname was given for many reasons including the lack of a security fence. Halden does not have the typical razor wire, electric, or tall fence surrounding and yet prisoners have not tried to escape. Much like Finland, Norway looks at the time inside the prison as preparation for life outside and there is both no life sentences or death penalties. This is a stark contrast to most American prisons, including that the maximum sentence for crimes is 21 years. The Norwegian Correctional Service has the motto "better out than in" to say that they ensure a person leaves prison improved. In order to do this, the government uses resources to provide a social support system, a job, and housing. Additionally, Norway provides education, healthcare, and a pension for all citizens. The interesting part of this is that at the time of this article in 2015, Norway spent about $93,000 per inmate per year on incarceration as compared to $31,000 in the United States. Taking this into consideration, the United States incarcerates on average 700 people per 100,000 while Norway is about 75 per 100,000. The United States could save nearly $45 billion per year if they were to also take on this practice.

> Norway banned capital punishment for civilians in 1902, and life sentences were abolished in 1981. But Norwegian prisons operated much like their American counterparts until 1998. That was the year Norway's Ministry of Justice reassessed the Correctional Service's goals and methods, putting the explicit focus on rehabilitating prisoners through education, job training and therapy. A second wave of change in 2007 made a priority of reintegration, with a special emphasis on helping inmates find housing and work with a steady income before they are even released. Halden was the first prison built after this overhaul, and so rehabilitation became the underpinning of its design process. Every aspect of the facility was designed to ease psychological pressures, mitigate conflict and minimize interpersonal conflict.

It seems that cost is *the* impetus for change in the United States. In times of recession, the pressure to change seems to reach a tipping point. While there appear to be some radically progressive policies in countries such as Norway, it seems that there may be room to learn from other countries' willingness to spend money lavishly on rehabilitative practices. In other words, countries such as Norway may offer the United States the ability to learn which rehabilitative processes and programs are promising, for which target population, and be able to consider cost-effectiveness before investing.

8.5 More Traditional Innovation

More than likely, prison administrators will look towards innovations that have seen success in different segments of the criminal justice system that may be adopted and customized for corrections. One such innovation is customizing the Crisis Intervention Team model to fit correctional settings. A study by McNeeley and Donley (2021) reviews one such adoption of CIT by the Minnesota Department of Corrections. Back in 2011, the Minnesota Department of Corrections made CIT available to its correctional officers. Not all staff at the time of the study were trained, yielding the ability of McNeeley and Donley to focus on a random selection of prison incidents at one maximum security prison facility in the state. To determine whether CIT made any impact, they were able to compare incidents involving CIT-trained staff versus those involving untrained staff.

Upon a content analysis and deeper quantitative analyses, McNeeley and Donley revealed that critical incidents that occurred at this facility seemed not to be immediately impacted by either CIT techniques or the presence of CIT employees. Yet, they were able to decipher that subsequent resolution of these episodes and compliance with instructions were impacted by such factors, showing statistically significant increases in compliance by incarcerated persons. Perhaps more critical of their findings, McNeeley and Donley revealed that the proportion of employees with CIT training was positively correlated with mental health referrals. One troubling finding, however, is that the use of force was not in any way impacted by CIT techniques or the presence of CIT employees, leading the researchers to suggest that there was enough support for positive outcomes in their analyses, yet more work needed to be done to achieve better outcomes. Perhaps too much time had passed between initial training and the incidents included in this study – from 2011 compared to 2016–2018, when the incidents had occurred?

In addition, this study highlighted the paucity of CIT research in correctional settings – only a handful of such studies exist at the time of this writing. It is likely such efforts will continue to be expanded upon in the near future.

8.6 Conclusion

Prisons tend to get the least amount of attention in regard their mental health practices. When considering that near 95% of the American prison population will return back to the community at some point, this lack of attention is slowing changing. Currently, administrative segregation and intake are notable exceptions – there has been an array of interest in these two issues in recent years that have a growing research base. Many other facets of inmate mental health remain unclear, ill-defined with aging data, and is given tacit attention relative to jail inmate and jail inmate reentry, in particular.

While research activity and programmatic begins to grow, it seems that litigation will continue to define the critical issues that prison administrators will need to address into the near and distant future. Expect an increase in litigation in the upcoming years to continue to refine the definition of constitutionally accepted levels of care in prisons, particularly as it relates to administrative segregation.

Discussion Questions

1. What are your thoughts about judges and others with authority stepping in to demand systemic change?
2. How do you explain why offenders with mental illness serve longer prison sentences than offenders without mental health concerns? How do we begin to address this disparity?
3. What are the most powerful tools available to reform the way we sentence people with mental illness after a criminal trial?
4. How does society see incarcerated persons? What are our views of this population once they return back into our communities? What are the most common tools to change these views?
5. In what sorts of ways can being incarcerated for long periods of time impact a person's mental health? What sort of care should they receive while incarcerated and after they return to their communities?

References

Ashker v. Brown. (n.d.). 4:09-CV-05696. United States District Court, N.D. California.

Boston Globe. (2016). There may be no worse place for the mentally ill people to receive treatment than prison. URL: https://apps.bostonglobe.com/spotlight/the-desperate-and-the-dead/series/prisons/. Last accessed: 2017, June 1.

Braggs v. Dunn. (2017). 2:14CV601-MHT. United States District Court, M.D. Alabama.

California Department of Corrections and Rehabilitation. (2009). Mental health services delivery system. URL: http://www.cdcr.ca.gov/DHCS/docs/Mental%20Health%20Program%20Guide.pdf. Last accessed: 2017, June 1.

Davis v. Ayala. (2015). 135 S.Ct. 2187, 2205.

Finn, P. (1996). No-frills prisons and jails: A movement in flux. *Federal Probation, 60*(3), 35–44.

Haney, C. (2003). The psychological impact of incarceration: Implications for post-prison adjustment. *Prisoners once removed: The impact of incarceration and reentry on children, families, and communities.* URL: http://webarchive.urban.org/UploadedPDF/410624_PyschologicalImpact.pdf. Last accessed: 2017, June 1.

McNeeley, S., & Donley, C. (2021). Crisis intervention team training in a correctional setting: examining compliance, mental health referrals, and use of force. *Criminal Justice and Behavior, 48*(2), 195–214.

Mitchell, O., Wilson, D. B., & MacKenzie, D. L. (2012). The effectiveness of incarceration-based drug treatment on criminal behavior: A systematic review. *Campbell Systematic Reviews, 8*(1), 1–76.

National Center on Addiction and Substance Abuse. (1998). *Addiction treatment in prison will reduce crime, save billions of tax dollars, says CASA report.* News Briefs. www.ndsn.org/jan98/prisons1.html. Last accessed: 2017, January 3.

Prendergast, M. L., Hall, E. A., Wexler, H. K., Melnick, G., & Yan, C. (2004). Amity prison-based therapeutic community: 5-year outcomes. *Prison Journal, 84*(1), 36–60.

Small, J., & Pickoff-White, L. (2017). Judge threatens to fine California prisons for delayed mental health treatment. KQED. URL: https://ww2.kqed.org/news/2017/04/20/judge-threatens-to-fine-california-prisons-for-delayed-mental-health-treatment/. Last accessed: 2017, June 1.

Smith, P. S. (2006). The effects of solitary confinement on prison inmates: A brief history and review of the literature. *Crime and Justice, 34*(1), 441–528.

Steinberg, D., Mills, D., & Romano, M. (2015). When did prisons become acceptable mental healthcare facilities? Stanford Law School. URL: https://law.stanford.edu/wp-content/uploads/sites/default/files/publication/863745/doc/slspublic/Report_v12.pdf. Last accessed: 2022, January 30.

Substance Abuse and Mental Health Services Administration. (2014). Treatment improvement protocol 44: Substance abuse treatment for adults in the criminal justice system. URL: https://www.ncbi.nlm.nih.gov/books/NBK64137/pdf/Bookshelf_NBK64137.pdf. Last accessed: 2017, June 1.

Chapter 9
Release and Reentry

> *You may not control all the events that happen to you, but you can decide not to be reduced by them. – Maya Angelou.*

Re-entering society can be one of the most difficult obstacles a justice-involved person can face in their lifetime. All facets of one's life change instantly upon release from prison. The controlled environment of a prison facility allows an inmate to create a routine and have stability in relationships and daily activities. A person behind bars knows exactly when the next phone call to a loved one will take place, the next meal, activity time, etc. These things are no longer regular, or controllable, on the outside in society. Often times, individuals struggle in the chaos that exists outside the prison walls. The best chance for success involves planning and preparing for those changes and learning coping skills to handle them in a healthy manner. Unfortunately, this is not always realistic on many levels. The most comprehensive evaluation of prisoner (e.g., excludes jail inmate) recidivism available reveals that 30.4% of prisoners return to prison within a year, 43.3% return in 2 years, 49.7% return in 3 years, 52.9% return in 4 years, and 55.1% – over half – return in 5 years (Durose et al., 2014). If one simply looks at prisoners being arrested after release, many of which require stays in jail as arrestees await criminal justice processing, the statistics are even bleaker: 43.4% are arrested within a year, 59.5% within 2 years, 67.8% within 3 years, 73.0% in 4 years, and 76.6% in 5 years. Further, a large proportion of individuals rearrested after release from prison are drawn back into the criminal justice system (including jails and diversion programs), typically through a sanction by the court and/or by probation/parole violations and revocations. Ultimately, the plan to reduce contact with the criminal justice system exists within the transition planning before, in the moment of, and after release from incarceration, with the courts and probation/parole being key players in the reentry movement. This needs to include both jails and prisons, but importantly, it needs to include a mental health element more substantial than just attending to substance abuse treatment issues.

J. Hector, D. Khey, *Criminal Justice and Mental Health*, https://doi.org/10.1007/978-3-031-15338-9_9

9.1 They're Back! But They Aren't Poltergeist: Stigma Revisited

Think about reentry akin to many common "phases" of one's lifespan – the transition from high school to college (e.g., emerging adulthood), the transition from college to the work force (e.g., adulthood), the transition of living with a spouse and/or parenthood, etc. Now, think about how complex these transition periods would be after a significant negative stretch in a person's life. Leaving jail or prison and going back to "the real world," and even leaving a substance abuse treatment facility or mental health setting, is often daunting. All of these transitions can be wrought with anxiety provoking situations, such as the fear of the unknown, or simply, the fear of failure and of the implications of such. This time frame creates a very vulnerable space for many people – feelings of uncertainty and pressure seem omnipresent in an already unstable time.

The key problem to success is revealed when one realizes that this tricky transition period is often complicated by past and current experience of trauma. One well-done study on prevalence rates of trauma experienced by male prisoners details the extent of this issue – 44.7% inmates were exposed to physical trauma as a minor, 31.5% as an adult, and 25.1% as both a minor and as an adult. These rates exclude sexual trauma – 10.9% of inmates were exposed to sexual trauma as a minor, 4.5% as an adult, and 3.7% as both a minor and adult (Wolff & Shi, 2012). One last rate to keep in mind, those who have experienced both physical and sexual trauma – 9.6% of inmates experienced both as a minor. The prevalence rates of trauma exposure are even more staggering for incarcerated women. For both men and women, the vast majority of these experiences remain untreated, and many men remain undiagnosed to the mental illnesses these traumatic experiences can have a role in triggering. Now, imagine entering an important transitional period in your life with these confounding issues weighing on you.

The vast majority of people going to prison are non-violent and are inevitably going to come back to the community – and many do not tend to come back "better" at this time. Reentry is a *normal* event as 100 million American adults (about one-third of working age adults) are cataloged in state criminal history systems versus roughly 69 million American adults 25 and older having Bachelor's degrees; and 6.6% of Americans born in 2001 are estimated to serve time in a prison at some point in their lives (BJA, 2014; Bonczar, 2003; Moore et al., 2015; Ryan & Bauman, 2016). Many more Americans have experienced incarceration in their lifetimes, either jail or prison – the exact amount remains unknown as available jail data is unable to reveal this figure. The point is that while reentry is normal in the sense that it is common, the label of being an ex-offender remains potently stigmatic. This label potentially intensifies with complications of mental health. American criminal justice is revising its approach as a result. Yet, those with mental illness are likely to have continued problems as the capacity to deal with high-risk individuals begins to grow and expand.

Maruna and LeBel (2003) aptly discuss the role of stigma in the reentry context as the criminal justice system begins to reshape the paradigm of corrections to (re-) include social services. In this new approach they call the strengths-based paradigm, Maruna and LeBel point out that criminal justice practitioners are pushed to ask what positive contributions inmates can offer instead of the old question of what deficits people in the system may have:

> In the reentry context, the strengths *narrative* begins with the assumption that ex-convicts are stigmatized persons, and implicitly that this stigma (and not some internal dangerousness or deficit) is at the core of what makes ex-convicts likely to re-offend....[This push towards criminal involvement] is clearly based on a labeling/social exclusion story - on which, of course, the very idea of "reintegration" is also premised. Johnson (2002: 319) writes, 'released prisoners find themselves "in" but not "of" the larger society' and 'suffer from a presumption of moral contamination.' To combat this social exclusion, the strengths paradigm calls for opportunities for ex-convicts to make amends, demonstrate their value and potential, and make positive contributions to their communities. (Maruna & LeBel, 2003: 97; also quoting Johnson, 2002).

It is through these opportunities of contributing to society that can begin the de-labelling process for stigmatized people, part of what Maurna calls "making good" (Maruna, 2001). The us in the us-versus-them paradigm can begin publicly recertifying and reclassifying an individual as returning back into the group, in a very tribal sense. This reciprocal relationship can offer the stigmatized person hope while also showing the public that the ex-offender is worthy of support and investment as they reintegrate back into the community (Maruna & LeBel, 2003).

9.2   How Are We Dealing with It?

Generally speaking, there are three broad approaches to reentry: (1) jail to community reentry, (2) prison to community reentry, and (3) reentry court. Before explaining each approach, it is first important to note here that the existing literature on what works in reentry converge on this point: holistic services designed to address individual offender needs that begin prior to release and continue in an aftercare situation are most apt to be successful (Lowenkamp et al., 2006; Osher, 2006; Osher, 2007; Petersilia, 2004; Pearson & Lipton, 1999; Travis & Visher, 2005). This consistent finding is, in part, driving previously isolated and siloed pieces of the criminal justice and mental health systems to begin collaborations and seek broader partnerships. If a true continuum of care is to be devised to ensure successful reentry (e.g., not returning back to prison, encouraging pro-social and healthy lifestyles, and self-sufficiency), communication and coordination is paramount.

One of the first tasks of these emerging partnerships often becomes trying to figure out how to maximize returns on extremely limited resources. The validated risk and need screening and assessment tools described in Chap. 5 become critical to accomplish this goal. When used properly, these tools not only match which evidence-based programs and services will help each individual returning back to the community, they can help prioritize available resources – particularly the most intensive (and often the most costly) ones – to those who are at most in critical need. Yet, the goal for each approach should be to begin services as early on, as well as during the transition back to the community, and continue these services to ensure successful reintegration.

9.2.1 Jail to Community Reentry

Jail-based reentry can often be tricky due to the short amount of time jail professionals have to work with. Improvement in mental health outcomes can only be realized through an ability to track data on inmate connectivity to services, whether in jail or back in the community. Without such data, it may be impossible to detect the moments people fall through the cracks of the system, often only to inevitably return to an emergency room, the jail, or the medical examiner or coroner's office. In 2008, Jeff Mellow and colleagues authored an extensive *Toolkit for Reentry* for jail administrators, which continues to offer terrific structure for reentry for jail inmates depending on length of stay in jail and level of risk and need. These best practices have not changed much since, and many jails are striving to improve. Changes are occurring slowly as the focus on jail administrators continues to be to provide a constitutional jail – as a result, many of these improvements may be construed as above and beyond instead of standard practice at this time.

The toolkit begins by describing four discrete tracks, or paths, of jail inmates. Track one refers to the easiest swath of jail inmates, those with low needs and/or have a very short stay ahead of them in jail. These individuals should receive easy-to-use resource guide to assist them in the reentry process. Services such as help finding housing, employment, substance abuse treatment and support, legal aid, and so on should be included and presented on a basic reading level. While the ideal goal of jails should be to screen and assess everyone coming through booking, it may not be possible to do so in every case depending on timing of release, personnel available to screen and assess, and volume of individuals going through the booking process. To enhance the ability to capture individuals needing services in this track, jail administrators may provide training to their booking staff to give them a keener eye of identifying signs and symptoms of mental illness and substance abuse. Additionally, these inmates should receive information on available government benefits, especially Medicaid, as Medicaid often the primary provider of mental health and substance abuse treatment for vulnerable individuals. In a perfect world, data systems would be set up to allow each individual to be tracked from jail and into the local treatment system (and vice versa). While achieving this ideal may be daunting, it does not have to be. For example, some treatment providers in the New Orleans metropolitan area have linked up with local jails to receive an electronic roster of individuals being booked through the jail on a daily basis. While arduous, providers have tasked staff with monitoring these rosters for "frequent fliers" or known clients to be able to intervene quickly and provide transitional care as promptly as possible.

Track two is tailored to inmates with medium needs or to those who may just have a longer stay (but have not been identified as high needs). These individuals are able to be successfully screened and assessed. If they are identified as low needs, they are referred to Track one to receive helpful information and resource guides. On faith, it is assumed that these individuals have the wherewithal to guide their own path forward, often with success. At minimum, there is no (or minimal) indication of the potential barriers to successful reentry as revealed by screening and assessment. Inmates in Track two should also receive all of the helpful resource materials, but further, they should also receive an individualized reentry plan to give some structure of activities for these individuals returning back to the community. The best practice here is for jail practitioners to create these reentry plans *in collaboration with* the inmates. Together, staff and inmates can discuss issues with family relationships, housing, health care, mental health, substance abuse needs, and so on. At the end of this process, each inmate will receive an easy to follow self-guided plan to aid in their transition back into the community. Appointments with community service providers may be necessary; however, it will be up to each Track two inmate to ensure these appointments are made on their own. At times, some assistance is provided; however, follow-up by jail staff is rare as it is seen as unnecessary. Again, this is where data tools become critical in case local partnerships find that many people in Track two are not getting the services they need after they are released from jail. An ideal reentry plan should, at minimum, address the domains in Table 9.1.

Track three inmates are those whose risk and needs assessment scores place them as high needs, but not necessarily high risk. In these cases, jail staff are instructed to replicate Track two services while increasing care by coordinating services in the community and having outside partners begin to collaborate on services as early as possible after release. Here, appointments are made prior to release, and follow-ups are done to ensure connectivity to services. Track four inmates are those who are high risk and high needs; due to their obvious need for priority, jail staff and community partners often collaborate to begin services while incarcerated, as early as possible, and as intensive as possible. These individuals require immediate access to services, whenever possible with vigilant supervision to ensure compliance and the best chances of success. These individuals should receive concierge-like services to connect them with potential benefits or resources that can aid in their reentry, particularly Medicaid and health care. Further, best practices dictate that a case manager be assigned to them, at minimum, immediately upon release.

While these tracks offer guidance to jail administrators, it is important to recognize that these tracks intend to only offer broad structure to ideal concepts of handling reentry in the industry. In other words, it is intended that these tracks are modified and customized for each jail to match and meet its needs (specifically, the needs of its inmates and target populations). The *Reentry Toolkit* also offers several examples of jurisdictions that have made these customizations: Travis County, Texas, New York City, New York, Davidson County, Tennessee, Essex County, New Jersey, Montgomery County, Maryland, and so on.

Table 9.1 Domains to be addressed by written reentry plans (Mellow et al., 2008)

Domain	Description
Mental health care	Attend to the proximal and distal mental health concerns; includes substance abuse
Medical care	Attend to the proximal and distal physical health concerns; includes tuberculosis, hepatitis, and HIV screening and care
Medications	Ensure continuity of prescription drugs
Appointments	Ensure that appointments/referrals with service providers in the community are made, reminders are created, and follow-ups occur
Housing	Devise a housing plan in partnership with the returning individual, ensure its viability, and evaluate the potential stability it can offer
Employment	Connect the returning individual to an employment opportunity and/or employment services specialists; alternatively, or in addition, connect the returning individual to education/vocational development specialists
Substance/alcohol abuse	Directly connect returning individuals with resources in the community to support recovery and continued sobriety
Health care/benefits	Offer services or a referral to services that can offer health benefit enrollment assistance, primarily Medicaid
Income/benefits	Offer services or a referral to services that can offer government benefit enrollment assistance such as disability, food stamps, etc.
Food/clothing	Offer services or a referral to services that offer food pantries, free or low-cost clothing, and similar assistance
Transportation	Connect returning individuals to low-cost and no-cost transportation options in the community
Identification/driver's license	Partner with local agencies responsible for government identification and be able to provide returning individuals with an official form of ID; try to aid in restoring driver's license privileges, whenever possible
Life skills	Train returning individuals in life skills such as budgeting, parenting, etc.
Family/children	Offer aid and education in regard to child support compliance, family reunification, and so on
Emergency contacts	Arm returning individuals with a list of emergency contacts in the community in case they need emergency assistance
Referral services/ court dates	Connect returning individuals with local agencies for potential services/ care as well as inform him/her of impending court dates and obligations
Summary, jail-based services provided	Provide an easy-to-read summary of all of the services, treatment, and care given to an individual while in jail as a reference and to aid the future provision of care

9.2.1.1   An Example of an Early Adopter: Hampden County Sheriff's Department

A prime example of a multifaceted, jail-based reentry program fully integrated in a wider, comprehensive public and mental health system lies in Ludlow, Massachusetts (Solomon et al., 2008). This story of Hampden County begins in early 1990s when a concern was raised by the local health clinic professionals when they reflected on their data of missed appointments – it turns out that many patients missing appointments simply could not make it in because they were held up somewhere else. That somewhere else happened to often be the local jail ran by the Hampden County Sheriff. In the wake of these concerns, the sheriff at the time directed his staff to allow health care providers entry into the jail in order to provide care – care that was not present in any substantial capacity before this point. Coordination of efforts and justice-mental health (and public health) collaboration was initiated. Shortly after these provider partners started working in the jail, they further realized that a majority of the clients they were seeing day in and day out all were returning to four ZIP codes. With this in mind, the local partnerships sought to target these four zip codes by contracting services with the existing community centers there, thereby establishing a reliable continuity of care from incarceration into release.

In 2015, the Hampden County Sheriff's Department reported that continued development of these systems with local partners, now called the After Incarceration Support Systems (AISS), has been utilized by over 17,500 clients. Interestingly, the vast majority of individuals seen by AISS are participating in a voluntarily, well more than individuals on probation and parole – this insinuates a level of success. Beyond insinuation, local analysis shows a substantial reduction of recidivism. These results should also be attributed to the systemic changes to jail policies and procedures to optimize the opportunities of connecting inmates with the services that they need. Upon introspection, jail administration realized that about 90% of their inmates were abusing some form of substance, 87% were male, 40% were under 30 years old, 57% were minorities, 73% were unemployed when they were arrested, 48% did not have a high school diploma or its equivalent, 40% have a mental health problem(s), 55% reported that they did not have positive family support, and about 40% did not have a stable home to return to. Over the years, the jail has perfected its solution; To address these problems, the jail has built the capacity to deploy several evidence-based screening and assessment tools (e.g., Level of Service Inventory (LSI-R), Texas Christian University Drug Screen (TCUDS – a tool in the public domain), the CAGE Assessment, the Clinical Institute Withdrawal Assessment Alcohol Scale (CIWA-AR), and the Clinical Opiate Withdrawal Scale (COWS)), offer withdrawal protocols, provide treatment services for all levels of risk and need internally or via its partners, and have conceived their role differently, steeped in a public health model:

> In Hampden County (Massachusetts), the sheriff's department has developed classification matrices for violent offenders, nonviolent offenders, and those serving mandatory sentences that chart out their time at each security level by sentence length. For example, a nonviolent offender serving 18 months who complies with his reentry plan and demonstrates excellent institutional conduct will spend 10 days at medium security, 1 month at minimum security, 2 months at secure prerelease, and the balance (or less) on day reporting (living at home and reporting regularly to the day reporting center). The department's matrices are adjusted regularly on the basis of population levels at the facility and prove to be an effective tool to prevent jail overcrowding and to place individuals at security levels that will allow them to work and receive community-based treatment prior to release. Thus, the classification needs of the institution and the reentry needs of individuals are both served by this process. (Solomon et al., 2008: 31).

Further, the collaboration has led to the development of a reentry crown of the local system – the AISS One-Stop Reentry Center – perfectly located for broad community impact in the Mason Square neighborhood. At this Center, case manager aid in connecting individuals with intensive "wrap" services, all provided onsite by its community partners. These services include early recovery support, health and mental health services, psychiatric services, parenting groups for men and women, male violence interventions, targeted healthcare for homeless individuals, intensive outpatient services, job support groups, per-led support groups, writing groups (for women), food bank services and assistance with the SNAP application process, anger management, housing support, educational services, employment services, employment retention support, mentorship, resource and support group for sex offenders, support groups in spanish, and a women's only support group. All of these services, together with other sites of support such as a the Substance Abuse Unit inside of the Hampden County Jail, the substance abuse services for women at the Western Massachusetts Regional Women's Correctional Center, and the Western Massachusetts Correctional Alcohol Center (which also specializes in opioid treatment as 65% of individuals in this setting have histories of opioid abuse), individuals across the risk and needs spectrum are almost certain to receive tailored services that so critically begin during incarceration and stick with the ideal of treating an individual in the least restrictive setting, in this case, as soon as possible (Fig. 9.1).

These innovations have spread across the country: San Bernardino, Snohomish County, New York City, Suffolk County, Montgomery County, Atlantic County, Norfolk County, Douglas County (OR), Miami-Dade County (FL), Maricopa County (AZ), Westchester County (NY), and Essex County offer stellar examples of how others are finding solutions that work best for the local community.

9.2.2 Prison to Community Reentry

Due to the massive numbers of individuals already in prison of which an estimated 95% are bound to return back into the community at some point, prisons are increasing their capacity to install robust reentry programming before release as well. Prisoners may face considerably more challenges simply due to the length of their stay away from society. Pro-social relationships (e.g., family) may further be strained, financial obligations may falter (e.g., forcing a repossession of a car), debts may loom, and issues with reinstating a driver's license may grow complicated (e.g, outstanding traffic tickets may force heavy fines or further legal trouble). Additionally, inmates with health conditions may not receive optimal care behind bars and/or prison may place them at increased risk of contracting blood borne-pathogens, human immunodeficiency virus, hepatitis, syphilis, gonorrhea, chlamydia, and tuberculosis; they will, however, receive a level of care protected by the constitution (Bick, 2007).

In light of these challenges, the robust reentry processes described for inmates returning from jail must be further refined to be able to produce successful results. This can become daunting given the sheer relative volume of individuals on

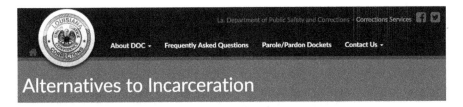

Data of Louisiana's offender population shows that offenders are most at risk of returning to prison within the first two years of release, often because they lack programs and services to achieve stability in their communities. Sometimes, they fall back into old patterns and associations. As a result, the Department has established alternatives to incarceration. P&P Officers refer probationers and parolees to a variety of programs in the community designed to address the issues they commonly face, including substance abuse treatment, mental health treatment, sex offender treatment, anger management, job training/skills programs and driving schools.

In 2014-15, the Division of Probation and Parole opened five Day Reporting Centers (DRC) in addition to the three that already existed. There are now DRC's in the following locations: Monroe, Lake Charles, Alexandria, Baton Rouge, Covington, Lafayette, New Orleans, and Shreveport. DRC's serve the local area offenders, providing life skills, job training and various treatment.

To further reduce costs while continuing to provide safety for the community, certain probation and parole non-violent, non-sex offenders that commit technical violations of supervision (i.e. they are not arrested for a new felony) are referred to the Don Francois Alternative Center. This 90-day program addresses the rehabilitation needs of the offender, including but not limited to, substance abuse treatment and anger management programs. Offenders are returned to supervision upon completion of the program.

Fig. 9.1 Infographic on day reporting Centers in Louisiana. (Courtesy of the Louisiana Department of Public Safety and Corrections)

schedule to be released across the country. Some correctional leaders are also exploring options for an enhanced, step-down release that features the removal of inmates from a prison setting and places them into other facilities that may offer the sort of reentry process installed at the Hampden County Jail. That is, with excellent conduct and lower security risk (e.g., risk and need), inmates may benefit from more independence and freedom while still incarcerated in the form of minimum security housing, work release, and perhaps even release back to the community with day reporting requirements (and, most likely, an electronic monitoring bracelet).

9.2.2.1 A Gem in the Rough: Lafayette Parish Sheriff Reentry

In Louisiana, where robust reentry programs remain quite scarce, the Lafayette Parish Sheriff's Office (2011) has been able to replicate successful reentry models in Georgia and Minnesota and customize it for the local area. At this time, many Louisiana prisoners are slated to receive 100 hours of life skills programing, be given a 90-day pre-release packet with helpful resources, and be placed on community supervision. After screening potential Department of Corrections inmates for eligibility (risk needs screening and assessment, physical and mental health assessments, security level determination, trades and skill level assessment, and verified local area resident), the Lafayette Parish Sheriff's Office Reentry Model operates in phases.

Upon admittance to the program, an inmate gets placed at the community corrections campus – a new facility solely dedicated to reentry. A case plan is developed with a case manager and Phase I begins. Services in Phase I include manualized Moral Reconation Therapy led by trained personnel, mental health services, educational services, vocational training (forklift certification and custodial management certification are available at this time), drug and alcohol treatment, group meetings, a life skills curriculum, anger management, financial planning and employment preparation, assistance with obtaining identification, and family reunification. For higher risk inmates, Phase II will be required after the completion of Phase I. This phase includes relapse prevention, Courage to Change, anger management, continued educational services, and more. For low-risk inmates, the transitional work program becomes available after the completion of Phase I and includes employment and educational services as well as aftercare (i.e., when these individuals are not working out in the community). Everyone at all security levels will enroll into a 90-day pre-release program which features housing and employment assistance, financial planning, medical referrals, family reunification, and help obtaining clothing, benefits (food, disability, health care, etc.), transportation, and help create linkages to community resources. At successful completion, each inmate is transferred to community supervision and is released.

It is the hope that individuals at all risk levels receive the services they need for success. Further, the Sheriff and the local area partnerships continue to explore gaps in care and better ways to ensure a continuum of care. Internal assessment shows improvement in short-term outcomes; yet, jail administration continues to look for improvements, particularly in available vocational training that links up with well-paying and needed jobs in the community.

9.2.3 Reentry Court

A concept attributed to Jeremy Travis (2000), Reentry Court is an intensive court-supervised program catering to the rehabilitation of persistently justice-involved offenders often with substance use disorders and mental health histories. Further, these individuals may exhibit symptoms stemming from complex trauma that may surmount in a post-traumatic stress disorder diagnosis or something similar (e.g., unspecified trauma and stressor-related disorder; Miller & Khey, 2016). Most reentry courts across the nation have been modeled off of the evidence-base and structure of specialty courts, such as adult drug court, but not always; reentry courts refer to any programming featuring release from prison with judicial oversight. This oversight has been explained as an essential feature to ensure compliance and to prevent failure (e.g., the return to prison) by constructively using sanctions to modify behavior and to intervene when those released from prison begin to go down a wrong path or relapse. Further, court supervision gives the ability to intervene and therapeutically respond to problems that arise that may be precursors to triggers, relapse, and reoffending. In particular, a large share of focus has been spent on employment as research has uncovered that success in this domain is paramount to success in the transition back to society. In 2015, Cook and his colleagues point out:

> …[O]ne potential limitation of previous efforts to improve the employment outcomes of re-entering prisoners is that they only start providing services after exiting from prison. It may be that post-release programs start too late to help ex-offenders deal effectively with the multiple challenges association with employment, family relations, substance abuse, and other aspects of re-entry. (358).

In one of the most sophisticated analyses of a comprehensive employment-oriented prisoner reentry program located in Milwaukee, Cook and his colleagues review 236 high-risk offenders with a history of violence or gang involvement who receive services in prison, yet do not receive judicial oversight into release. Their results were less than encouraging. While they did find that the services provided in prison seemed to help with the improvement of human capital of those returning back to the community, earnings continued to be quite low on average. Bleakly, these researchers concluded that legal work continues to be unimportant "in the economic lives of released prisoners."

Currently, there are 29 reentry courts operating across the United States, nine of which have been funded by the Department of Justice under the Second Chance Act as pilot projects with varying degrees of success and failure (Carey et al., 2017). In 2013, the National Institute of Justice commissioned the largest and most comprehensive evaluation of these funded reentry courts to date, the findings of which are beginning to emerge. Upon review, the NIJ-funded researchers discovered a wide array of differences across program, which allows for a broad review of what seems to work well and what practices may not be suitable for future investment. Preliminary findings suggest two reentry courts that show promising outcomes, two that show no gain in success relative to individuals returning to the community as they have in the past, and two that show worsened outcomes as more people are returning to prison after release than those who simply return to prison without the benefit of the program.

While these results may appear disheartening, researchers have been finding pockets of successes to draw from that which can seed improvements in existing and upcoming programs. For example, the evaluation of the Harlem Parole Reentry Court initially found stagnant outcomes for participants (Ayoub & Pooler, 2015). Importantly, the evaluators on the project employed a thorough process evaluation to unveil potential sources of problems that may be restricting success. An array of modifications have since been made, and with the further aid of additional Bureau of Justice Assistance funding, these modifications are being put into practice and are being modified for potential gains in outcomes.

9.2.3.1 The 22nd Judicial District Reentry Court of Louisiana

Situated north of Metropolitan New Orleans on the other side of Lake Pontchartrain (colloquially called the Northshore in Southeastern Louisiana), St. Tammany and Washington Parishes comprises the 22nd Judicial District Court. This jurisdiction has been notoriable due to its incredibly high incarceration rates; in fact, some claim them to be the highest in the modern world (Galofaro, 2012). The State of Louisiana has generally led the nation in its incarceration rate, currently at 776 per 100,000 incarcerated in prison relative to 385 per 100,000 nationally (Carson & Anderson, 2016). Recent estimates of the 22nd Judicial District's recidivism are even higher, at 811 per 100,000 residents incarcerated (or 1 in 86 adults), with St. Tammany further elevated at 954 inmates per 100,000 adult residents. The punitiveness St. Tammany parish has resulted in a local nickname – "St. Slammany" – and, at times, this moniker has been used with pride by local law enforcement and the district attorney. These times are changing.

The District's incarceration problem seems to have been fueled by a persistent drugs-crime connection that has remained unabated and is destined to drive increased problems without intervention. In particular, the District also leads the state in substance abuse treatment admissions at 771 per 100,000 adult residents relative to 610 per 100,000 state residents. The moment was ripe for intervention, and one standout approach has been led by a District Court Judge, Judge William "Rusty" Knight, and the team he assembled to constructively address this unyield-ing problem. The solution was a customized reentry court that is informed by research and steeped in evidence-based programming.

The original Louisiana Reentry Court program was, in fact, established at the New Orleans Criminal Court in collaboration with the Louisiana Department of Public Safety and Corrections. This collaboration resulted in a new and unique part-nership between local courts and state corrections. First, new sentencing legislation (LA Revised Statute 13:5401) was devised and lobbied to the state legislature to give judges more autonomy with reentry programming. Second, and more impor-tantly, it established a comprehensive in-reach program at the Louisiana State Penitentiary at Angola. This in-reach program provides intensive programming to participants for 24 months to qualifying inmates who are sentenced under this newly devised statute. At this time, services include substance abuse education, social skills training, mentoring by trustee lifers, and substantial vocational training that leads to national and international certifications. It also features evidence-based training, such as Moral Reconation Training, and has further been outfitted with Medication-Assisted Treatment (i.e., Vivitrol®).

The mentors are often seen as the glue of the program of the inside. Many are graduates of the New Orleans Baptist Theological Seminary Bible College housed on site at Angola. These men offer peer-based drug education, fatherhood skills, anger management training, soft skills and personal finance education, and much more. Mentors see themselves as assisting mentees with the development or retool-ing of their moral compasses, and as a living and breathing model of what could happen if participants cannot change their hearts and minds – spending long years (prime years) behind bars.

Intensive services continue at the moment of release through reintegration into the community with the 22nd Judicial District Reentry Court. Further, case manag-ers and Judge Knight remain in constant contact with participants sentenced to the in-reach program, a feature that is very unique. A part of what makes this program different is his level of caring and empathy Judge Knight has for his program par-ticipants. For example, using the drug court model, each program participant is referred to as a "client" or "participant" rather than "inmate" or "justice-involved person." In fact, the Judge often knows each client by name and makes it a point to hold status meetings (e.g., check-ins with District participants) on prison grounds quarterly, at minimum. The simple change in speech appears to mitigate the stigma and allow a person to overcome any a negative label. It begins a positive outlook, even before release from prison. The speech adjustment creates a thought adjustment. The clients are seen as a person rather than as a charge or a number as they are in prison. Prisoner #0947548 now becomes John, or Chris, or Tom, and is treated accordingly. He now has an identity, an opinion, and a choice in his life path. The empowerment and ownership is also extremely important for the mental health and self-esteem of a person. Upon release from prison, a person then is allowed to take back ownership for decisions in their own life and are no longer subject to those of a corrections officer, institution, or the state/federal government. On the other hand, this new found ownership can be extremely anxiety provoking and overwhelming. Consider the amount of time a person has been incarcerated and the amount of time to change that control-less thought pattern.

This is where Reentry Court, a modified adult drug court, comes into play. The modifications made at inception were designed to accommodate men with a long history of substance use disorder (or substance abuse patterns) in addition to longer criminal histories that typically make them ineligible for drug court. Additionally, many men who qualify for Reentry Court often have charges that are eligible to be treated under the multiple offender bill in the state, which may result in substantially longer prison sentences if not for the benefit of the program. By law, this sentencing feature is kept intact as a participant progresses through the program, with the possibility of being later filed should someone fail to comply with the program and complete either the inreach or outreach portion. This feature was designed to minimize the risk of new crimes and new victims. Before release, participants must establish employment and a housing plan (with the assistance of case management, trustee mentors, and prison staff) to ensure success on the outside. The Reentry Court outreach features a four-phase approach that span 5 years of intensive probation supervision, designed to step down services as prosocial behaviors thrive and self-sufficiency ensues. Each phase includes treatment, random drug testing, 12-step meetings, close case management, and status hearings with Judge Knight and the Reentry Court team (e.g., state attorney, defense attorney, treatment representative, and probation officer, led by the judge) – beginning with weekly status meetings, at minimum two drug tests per week, individualized treatment, and two 12-step meetings per week.

To date, only three men of 47 that have returned to prison yield a very promising recidivism rate. As this program continues to grow, comprehensive evaluation will be able to determine if these reductions in the return to prison are sustained. One key feature that appears to be driving the success of the program is that the vocational education is yielding meaningful and well-paying jobs for participants. In fact, the supervising probation officer of Reentry Court often jokes that the participants often get paid more than the probation officers that supervise them. Yet, it should be stressed here that this program has been able to develop a continuous continuum of treatment and programming that begins *before* entering prison, during incarceration, and through up to 5 years of intensive supervision. This level of programming seems to be extremely successful at breaking the cycle of substance use, crime participation, and antisocial behavior.

9.3   Known Gaps and Barriers

As reentry programs are shaping up across the country, literature on the known gaps preventing successful reentry are surfacing. Many of these gaps were mentioned earlier in this text and include connectivity to health care, especially Medicaid, access to evidence-based services, availability of transportation to reach these services and engage in prosocial activities like work and healthy recreation, ability to find gainful employment, and so on. This section addresses some of the less-thought of gaps and barriers to success. As Miller and Khey (2016) note:

> Even though the vast majority of individuals (95%) sent to prison will return to their communities, the outlook for most remains bleak in that employment is often unattainable (Bushway & Apel, 2012; Stafford, 2006), personal networks are either criminogenic or broken due to incarceration (Berg & Huebner, 2011; Travis & Waul, 2003), and substance use and mental health disorders too often remain unaddressed (Binswanger et al., 2012; Mallik-Kane & Visher, 2008). Increasingly, offender reentry programs are being delivered to a wider range of targeted populations to address various combinations of offender needs and transition issues, but only a fraction include formal program evaluation. (575).

The literature is growing in this area, and the following sections highlight a range of topics important in the current discussions of reentry, including promising programs with rigorous evaluations.

9.3.1   Technology as a Barrier

Technology can often create hurdles for individuals returning to the community. Smartphones, the Internet, and the state-of-the-art technology used by the modern workforce can all pose significant learning curve for someone previously incarcerated. A new version of a phone comes out each year or an upgrade to an application or program happens quickly, so keeping up, even just after a couple years, can be difficult. This, coupled with the stigma, can be intense and difficult. Practically no one wants to be judged for being out of date, particularly for embarrassing reasons.

On a positive note, an increasing amount of prisons are offering education programs within the walls of the prison. While technology can pose a significant security risk for facilities, some forward-thinking administrators are finding ways to circumvent the risk by removing the ability of inmates to access the Internet and communicate freely with the outside world while retaining the ability to learn technology and new skills effectively. These programs can be a great deterrent of negative behaviors for inmates while providing practical experience for future employment post-incarceration.

One example of the use of technology is with the Philadelphia Prison System. The city of Philadelphia has teamed up with two different startups to work with the prison on educating inmates. The lack of space, monitoring capacity for the technology, and funding have typically been major obstacles for adding and using technology in prisons and jails systems.

One of these startups is Chicago-based Jail Education Solutions (JES). JES, in conjunction with the city of Philadelphia, created a program to equip inmates with special, customized tablets that allow the prison to determine how they are used (Rawlins, 2014). These tablets "will offer everything from literacy classes and college coursework to vocational training and financial literacy seminars." JES used data from a RAND report citing (see: Davis et al., 2013), "inmates who received education while in prison were 43% less likely to become repeat offenders." The founder of JES, Ben Hill, discussed the use of the tablets, stating "If someone took the tablet and tried to use it outside the jail, it would be absolutely worthless."

As with most programs, a major issue is costs and funding. Initially, this program will allow both female and male inmates to have tablets, with the total being 100. To offset costs, the tablets will one day be rented for $2 a day since the beginning startup funds were only $30,000 provided by the city.

Reentry is major priority of the Philadelphia Prison System, "there are an average of 8,300 people in the Philadelphia Prison System - and over 50% of them return to prison within three years." In order to work towards successful reentry, a secondary startup, Textizen has joined in the project. Textizen created the ability for mass text messages via a web platform. Philadelphia's Office of Reintegration Services (RISE) is hopeful for the use of the platform to better serve their caseloads of ex-offenders. The system created by Textizen will allow for better communication for all clients with such large numbers allotted to only a few case managers. The benefits of the platform span past just communication between those in the community post-incarceration with their caseworkers for check-ins, but also with alerts for events and appointment reminders. Even further, program participants can use the platform to send required information like pay stubs to parole officers.

The startups involved in this pilot project were part of a competition to create adaptations and change for public safety. These are just some of the ways change can be made through technology within different areas of the criminal justice system.

9.3.2   Disenfranchisement (Felons Can't Vote)

Stigma breeds negativity in many ways for both mentally ill and incarcerated individuals. Specifically, for those involved in the criminal justice system, after receiving a felony, a person is no longer allowed to vote. While this can be a symbolic gesture, *voter disenfranchisement* is one real example of the effect of the stigmatic label "ex-felon" or "ex-convict." Under certain circumstances, the right to vote can be regained, but not always. Voting rights allow for a person to be directly connected with their community. Especially in current times, where changes to health care and potential criminal justice reform have become highly politicized, the ability to vote on these matters can be essential to the mental health of an individual. Imagine the impact on the well-being of ex-offenders to have the ability to decide (or at least have the perception of deciding) on matters that can have an impact on whether or not to eliminate mandatory sentences for drug related crimes, or to abolish the death penalty in states. Also, voting at the local level can truly change the treatment of many when there may be a proposed millage for use for local treatment services and improved reentry resources.

The other side of the voting rights argument is that by committing a crime which led to the felony, the individual violated his or her social contract with the community and deserve to have some civil rights rescinded. Although this can be true for some cases, murder being the most obvious case that most people across the political spectrum can agree upon, it may not be true, or beneficial, for all. Take, for example, a person who may have been diagnosed with an anxiety disorder and prescribed some anti-anxiety medications to use as needed. What if this person then becomes addicted to these same anti-anxiety medications? Then, the addiction progresses and self-medication ensues; long story short, they then begin buying pills on the street to feed their addiction. If at some point they are arrested with non-prescribed pills, a potential felony drug conviction may be a real possibility. Think, this scenario began with a mental illness and ended in a criminal felony charge. Does that person need treatment or incarceration or both? This question is one that has been on the forefront of criminal justice and treatment professionals, as well as researchers since the turn of the millennium. Working together to form an overall outlook can be the best course of action to help those in need and potentially stop the problem before it becomes a criminal justice issue.

9.3.3   Facing Employers

There is no question that felons have trouble finding work. This book has discussed the vulnerability of the transition period both post-treatment and post-incarceration. Part of the struggle in the transition period includes money, plain and simple. How is a person supposed to rehabilitate and recover without resources? How does one acquire these resources without sufficient funds? Without the ability to obtain legal employment due to a felony charge, where does one turn? The answer is that often a person turns back to their negative habits. This is true for individuals both with or without a mental health diagnosis, as the Cook and colleagues study poignantly points out that legal work remains unimportant in the lives of those returning from prison. This desperately needs to change.

Working brings back, again, to the topic of stigma. Finding employment can be a significant barrier for those released from prison. A criminal record, disclosing said record, and stigma and shame involved can be beyond overwhelming when attempting to rehabilitate and become a productive member of society. Most job applications ask the applicant if they have been convicted of a felony in their past. Additionally, the applicant is asked to describe the charge and sentence served. Imagine discussing past mistakes and currently being judged for those mistakes even after completing the punishment attached. This can be frustrating and significantly discouraging for former inmates.

9.3.4 Facing Relationships

Relationships can also be a struggle for a person leaving prison after a significant amount of time. Resources to maintain relationships within an institution are limited, often to only letters, phone calls, and possibly occasional in-person visits. With this in mind, it is understandable the level of difficulty in maintaining positive relationships with friends and family while incarcerated. Specifically, with regard to the type of crime committed, some friends and family may choose to no longer associate with the incarcerated person or hold a grudge. This leads to the incarcerated person mourning the loss of that relationship. Further complicated this delicate situation can be reentry of that person to society. The lost relationship may never be repaired and bring up past issues again.

After speaking with several former inmates, many have discussed struggling with family dynamics after returning home. Catching up with everyone after being away for quite some time can be a struggle. Additionally, repeating conversations regarding incarceration and prison surrounding that negative experience can hinder a person's forward progress.

9.3.5 Collateral Consequences

According to the Council of State Governments Justice Center, "collateral consequences are the legal and regulatory sanctions and restrictions that limit or prohibit people with criminal records from accessing employment, occupational licensing, housing, voting, education, and other opportunities" (Council of State Governments Justice Center, 2017). Since 2009, the Justice Center has developed and maintained an inventory of these consequences in its National Inventory of Collateral Consequences of Conviction. The Inventory currently features an easy-to-use map to zero in on any jurisdiction to better understand all of the restrictions put into place by statute or ordinance. For example, selecting Louisiana reveals over 1494 legal restrictions on ex-offenders depending on triggering offense (e.g., felony, violent felony, and so on), 920 of which are listed as mandatory and automatic. Some examples of these mandatory Louisiana restrictions include the ineligibility to possess firearms (LA RS 14:95.1, any felony, crime of violence and person offenses, weapons offenses, controlled substances offenses, and sex offenses), ineligibility to serve as a chairman or vice chairman of petition for a neighborhood crime prevention and security district (LA RS 18:1300.31, any felony), ineligibility to receive a citation in lieu of arrest (LA C Cr P Art 211, any felony or misdemeanor), and even the ineligibility to wear a hood, mask, or disguise to conceal identity during Halloween, Mardi Gras, Easter, Christmas, or other holidays (LA RS 14:313, crimes of violence, including person offenses and sex offenses). Many reentry programs are building the capacity to assist individuals returning back into the community in navigating these daunting regulations to ensure compliance, and at times, appeal to the courts to receive special dispensation from the courts, if possible, to aid in successful reentry. These appeals typically revolve around barriers to work. For example, any worker who requires access to secure areas of ports, vessels, offshore facilities, and similar maritime work environments requires a Transportation Worker Identification Credential (TWIC) – a felony can prevent an individual from obtaining a TWIC card. Almost always, initial applications for a TWIC are routinely denied and require appeal. This is one of many headaches facing ex-offenders as they reintegrate into society.

Additionally, a lot of "clean-up" work needs to be done simply due to the unintended consequences of being incarcerated, particularly as the incarceration period increases. While these issues may not traditionally be known as collateral consequences, they are being increasingly being addressed as if they were. Imagine if you were not around to handle your affairs, such as make car payments, resolve traffic citations or parking tickets, continue mortgage or child support payments, and so on. Driver's licenses may be suspended, outstanding traffic warrants may need to be resolved, outstanding debts may need to be addressed, and even years of missing tax filings may need to be rectified before new problems steamroll those fresh from incarceration. Fortunately, many new programs and services are being created to address these issues. For example, the Internal Revenue Service (IRS) has started its own Prisoner Re-entry Program (see Fig. 9.2).

9.4 How Do We Break the Cycle?

The following sections address different perspectives on how to alter the path of hyper-incarceration on which America finds itself. In particular, it discusses how everyday people can contribute to a solution. As referenced throughout this text, the American criminal justice system has failed to provide this solution on its own, and looking beyond criminal justice seems to offer an answer. As these multifaceted solutions avail themselves across the country, it will be interesting to note whether mental health takes a prominent role as part of these solutions or if it will remain an afterthought.

FACT SHEET
Prisoner Re-entry Tax Education Program

Key Points

What it is?
Get Right with Your Taxes – an educational package –information that individuals need to know about their tax responsibilities.

Who can use it?
- Prison Officials
- Halfway Houses
- Community Organizations

Who benefits from the information in this package?
As taxpayers, everyone can benefit from this information. While it is geared to a specific "prisoner" population, the content is on tax compliance and could be used for other outreach opportunities.

How to request copies of the Get Right with Your Taxes Educational Package?
- 800-TAX-FORM
- irs.gov/formspubs/index.html
- partner@irs.gov
- Relationship Managers

Why Use It?
Re-entry presents a major opportunity to educate and improve tax compliance.

Prisoner Statistics *
- 95% will be released back to the community
- >700,000 annual releases from state and federal prisons
- >9 Million cycle through local jails each year

* Source- Federal Interagency Re-entry Council

Background
Nationwide
The Administration has made prisoner re-entry a priority. At the national level, federal agencies are working together to identify and address barriers that impact access to resources necessary for successful transition of offenders back to their communities. Additionally, they are working with federal, state, and local correctional systems to implement educational programs for returning offenders pertaining to these areas.

IRS Service-wide
The IRS formed a service-wide team as a result of the IRS Prisoner Tax Compliance Summit held in August 2010. The overall mission of this team is to achieve increased prisoner tax compliance, reduce erroneous refunds and increase effectiveness for the management of prisoner tax returns. The Prisoner Tax Compliance Strategic Plan has five focus areas: Data Exchange, Compliance, Outreach, MOU Initiative and Legislative. The IRS Prisoner Outreach Initiative Team was established as an IRS team to address one of the focus areas.

Outreach
Stakeholder Partnerships, Education and Communication (SPEC), is charged with leading the Outreach Team. The goal of this team is to educate prisoners on their filing responsibilities upon re-entry. The team recognized the needs of this population, identified opportunities for tax education, and created a plan for delivery.

Opportunity Statement
SPEC is taking a progressive approach by extending outreach to prisoners in an effort to improve prisoner tax compliance. SPEC will leverage the collaborations formed through the Attorney General's Federal Re-entry Council Interagency Working Group and the Federal Offender Re-entry Group (FORGe) to reach out to the various entities involved in providing educational opportunities for returning offenders within the criminal justice system to deliver this program. The stand-alone lesson is intended to be a part of the nationwide re-entry educational and training programs targeting offenders prior to release.

The network of partners consists of: Department of Justice – Federal Bureau of Prisons, Bureau of Justice Assistance, National Institute of Corrections; Administrative Office of the U.S. Courts – Office of Probation and Pretrial Services, Federal Judicial Center; Department of Education; Department of Labor; Department of Veterans Affairs; Department of Housing and Urban Development; Department of Health and Human Services; Department of the Treasury - Internal Revenue Service; American Correctional Association; Department of Agriculture; Equal Employment Opportunity Commission; Social Security Administration; Office of Management and Budget; White House Office of Faith-based and Neighborhood Partnerships; Legal Action Center/National HIRE Network, and more.

Next Steps
The SPEC organization conducted two successful pilot programs using materials and educational products to address basic tax filing and tax compliance issues that directly affected this target population. As a result of the programs, SPEC created the Get Right with Your Taxes Educational Program to be used by prison officials engaged in re-entry preparation. The Outreach Team will leverage partner networks formed from these collaborations to ensure that local, state, and federal correctional facilities include these stand-alone educational products as an additional topic for their re-entry preparation. A facilitator does not need to have a tax law background to present this re-entry tax education program.

Last updated October 2011

Fig. 9.2 Internal Revenue Service, reentry resources. (Found: https://www.irs.gov/individuals/prisoner-re-entry-program)

9.4.1 The Role of Employers

Among employers, there exists a reluctance and often times fear to hire someone with a criminal record. The risk of another criminal act, or a person leaving again due to incarceration can be greater than most employers are willing to bear.

Management also considers the potential liability of hiring someone they know to have a criminal record. For example, it may make an employer very uncomfortable hiring someone with a burglary conviction as an HVAC repair and serviceperson knowing that he or she will go into customer's homes several times per day. If something were to turn up missing and the customer were to catch wind of the employee's criminal past, is there any liability on that employer? Luckily, programs exist to help defray the costs and fears for employers, as well as explore how to mitigate this issue of liability.

For example, tax incentives exist for employers who hire justice-involved employees or individuals returning to their communities from incarceration. Progressive changes have also been made to state statutes to eliminate civil liability for employers in many circumstances should they hire an individual returning from prison. In Louisiana, recent legislative changes add that "any employer, general contractor, premises owner, or third party shall not be subject to a cause of action for negligent hiring of or failing to adequately supervise an offender *certified to be employed* due to damages or injury caused by that employee or independent contractor solely because that employee or independent contractor has been previously convicted of a criminal offense" (LA R.S. 23:291.1, emphasis added). Specifically, certain reentry program participants (who receive comprehensive programming) are eligible to receive a certification of employment from the Department of Public Safety and Corrections. These types of actions aid to address the collateral consequences of the label of "felon" and a criminal history.

Unfortunately, the stigma of mental illness, substance abuse, and incarceration do exist and prevent former inmates from being successful in their new-found futures. For example, if a person was incarcerated for a drug charge, it is often difficult for society to see that person as anything more than a "drug addict" or "drug dealer." This thought process does nothing to help someone reclaim their life and change for the better. This type of thinking only promotes an individual to return to the negative, criminal behaviors from their past. As a society, we discuss high incarceration rates, high recidivism rates, and high crime as significant negative impacts on communities, yet we do nothing to help people overcome past mistakes and regain their freedom on a permanent basis.

Luckily, in recent years, there has been an influx of opportunities for federal grant funding to create programming to help aid justice-involved individuals re-enter society and remain positive and successful. This change begins inside the prison and must continue post-incarceration. Public education and awareness are essential in lessening stigma and promoting the positive welfare of these individuals. Once we accept the reality that people can change and become successful despite past convictions, things will then begin to change. This acceptance needs to come from all members of society, involved in the criminal justice system or not. Judges, lawyers, counselors, employers, loved ones, etc. can be a catalyst to change.

9.4.2 Ban the Box: Does It Work?

The Fair Chance Act aka "Ban the Box" is a law that was put into effect in New York City on October 27, 2015. The Fair Chance Act "bans job ads that say things like 'no felonies' or 'must pass background check,' bans any questions about criminal history on job applications bans any questions about criminal history during job interviews, and an employer can check your criminal record history only after a conditional job offer." Then, if a person is denied a position due to their criminal record, an explanation from the employer is required in writing to explain the denial. Further, a connection between the potential employee's criminal history to the job duties must be made and show "unreasonable risk." Finally, in order to allow for discussion between the potential employee and employer in case of an issue, the job has to be held open for 3 days. President Obama changed the federal employee job applications and "banned the box." Additionally, by December 2015, 24 states adopted the policy as well.

Keep in mind, as explained above, this law does not prevent employers from learning about a potential employee's criminal background. What the law does is allow a person to be evaluated for a position on somewhat of an even playing field. The Fair Chance Act has just a couple stories about persons whose lives have changed because of the passing of this law. In one example, a woman describes being a victim of human trafficking and while in captive, she was arrested many times for various sexual and drug-related crimes forced by her captors. In many ways, this is an easy argument for "Ban the Box" in that her future employment should not be impacted on past crimes while being held captive.

On the other hand, there are some instances that produce controversy for the public and employers, much like any other law. The "gray area" in many situations can vary wildly from side to side and in an argument, both political and professional, not all is black or white. Unfortunately, the dark side of "Ban the box" is that one study has shown broader discrimination occurring. According to an article in the National Bureau of Economic Research written by Jennifer L. Doleac from the University of Virginia and Benjamin Hansen from the University of Oregon (2016), young Hispanic and black men are less likely to be hired due to the general discrimination of potential employers. This concern again begs the idea of ensuring education is linked to these types of policies. As with many other topics, especially those within this book, having a direct or personal experience usually lessens negativity and stigma. For example, having a family member, who was incarcerated and then released with the hopes of a better future, usually helps to have a compassion and empathetic sense as a business owner or employer.

As of June 2017, Louisiana became the first state to "Ban the Box" on college applications. Louisiana Governor, John Bel Edwards signed House Bill 688 which will go into effect in Fall 2017. This bill would not allow post-secondary public institutions from asking about criminal history during the admissions process. This would allow individuals with a criminal background to attend or re-enroll in a college or university with the hopes of furthering their education and leading to a better career. The law, however, does come with some exceptions in that institutions can ask about criminal history after admissions for both financial aid and housing.

9.5   Conclusion

The lack of funding and increase of incarceration has forced professionals to "think outside of the box." One brainchild has been reentry programs. These programs are changing the way society views justice-involved individuals. Additionally, these programs are helping to create a supportive environment for the success of those in need. As with any treatment, support is essential. Luckily, these programs are helping to create a safe space to begin change. The hope is that this change will lead to greater success overall. If individuals can find the means to complete programs like reentry successfully, they can become role models for others.

The other issue taking center stage in the discussion of reentry has been the collateral consequences caused by imprisonment, systemic processing, and the stigma involved with being a criminal/drug abusers/mentally ill. For everyday people, dealing with problems like having a suspended driver's license, being in arrears on child support, missing a court date, or preparing for a successful job interview may be daunting. Yet if you step into the shoes of someone with a criminal record who may be experiencing one, or most likely many of these issues all at once, visualizing and attaining success can feel like an insurmountable feat.

The vast majority of the innovations discussed in this section are yet to be fully evaluated, but some do indicate a reason to be hopeful. To be certain, we do not know if Ban the Box has been successful, or if the available tax incentives offer enough of a carrot to employers to begin to hire some more perceptively "risky" individuals. However, there appears to be a push to "change the script" or rework the narrative of hiring and helping justice-involved persons. For example, Judge Rusty Knight prefers to send this message to potential employers who may hire reentry court participants: would you rather hire a perfect stranger from off of the street after reviewing his or her resume and interviewing them, or would you rather hire someone who has the full backing of a diverse array of professionals with likely better qualifications onto your team who also benefits from his judicial oversight? Who is more likely to fail a drug test? Who is more likely to be responsible? Indeed, it seems for many employers, after they experience their first success with a reentry client, they are likely to change their scripts and practices into the future.

Discussion Questions

1. How do fines and fees levied by the criminal justice system impact individuals returning to society from prison?
2. What are some of the collateral consequences for someone returning to "normal" life after release from jail or prison? Consider practical, everyday things we may take for granted – such as our relationships.
3. Imagine returning to society after a period of incarceration starting in 2000. What sorts of things would you have to acclimate to in order to be successful?

References

Ayoub, L. H., & Pooler, T. (2015). *Coming home to Harlem: A randomized controlled trial of the Harlem Parole Reentry Court*. Center for Court Innovation.

Berg, M. T., & Huebner, B. M. (2011). Reentry and the ties that bind: An examination of social ties, employment, and recidivism. *Justice Quarterly. 28*(2), 382-410.

Bick, J. A. (2007). Infection control in jails and prisons. *Clinical Infectious Diseases, 45*(8), 1047–1055.

Binswanger, I. A., Nowels, C., Corsi, K. F., Glanz, J., Long, J., Booth, R. E., & Steiner, J. F. (2012). Return to drug use and overdose after release from prison: a qualitative study of risk and protective factors. *Addiction Science & Clinical Practice, 7*(1), 1–9.

Bonczar, T. P. (2003). *Prevalence of imprisonment in the U.S. population, 1974–2001*. Bureau of Justice Statistics. URL: https://www.bjs.gov/content/pub/pdf/piusp01.pdf. Last accessed: 2017, July 10.

Bureau of Justice Statistics. (2014). Survey of state criminal history information systems, 2012. URL: https://www.ncjrs.gov/pdffiles1/bjs/grants/244563.pdf. Last accessed: 2017, July 10.

Bushway, S. D., & Apel, R. (2012). *A signaling perspective on employment-based reentry programming: Training completion as a desistance signal*. Criminology & public policy, 11(1), 21-50.

Carey, S., Rempel, M., Lindquist, C., Cissner, A., Hassoun Ayoub, L., Kralstein, D., & Malsch, A. (2017). *Reentry court research: Overview of findings from the National Institute of Justice's multi-site evaluation*. (Unpublished, preliminary evaluation report; submitted to National Institute of Justice, Office of Justice Programs, U.S. Department of Justice in February 2017).

Carson, E. A., & Anderson, E. (2016). Prisoners in 2015. Bureau of Justice Statistics. URL: https://www.bjs.gov/content/pub/pdf/p15.pdf. Last accessed: 2017, July 2.

Cook, P. J., Kang, S., Braga, A. A., Ludwig, J., & O'Brien, M. E. (2015). An experimental evaluation of a comprehensive employment-oriented prisoner re-entry program. *Journal of Quantitative Criminology, 31*(3), 355–382.

Council of State Governments Justice Center. (2017). National inventory of the collateral consequences of conviction. URL: https://niccc.csgjusticecenter.org/. Last accessed: 2017, July 2.

Davis, L. M., Bozick, R., Steele, J. L., Saunders, J., & Miles, J. N. V. (2013). *Evaluating the effectiveness of correctional education: A meta-analysis of programs that provide education to incarcerated adults*. Rand Corporation. URL: http://www.rand.org/pubs/research_reports/RR266.html. Last accessed: 2017, June 1.

Doleac, J. L., & Hansen, B. (2016). Does "ban the box" help low-skilled workers?: Statistical discrimination and employment outcomes when criminal histories are hidden. *Research Briefs in Economic Policy* (62). URL: https://www.cato.org/publications/research-briefs-economic-policy/does-ban-box-help-or-hurt-low-skilled-workers. Last accessed: 2017, July 2.

Durose, M. R. Cooper, A. D., & Snyder, H. N. (2014) *Recidivism of prisoners released in 30 states in 2005: Patterns from 2005 to 2010*. Bureau of Justice Statistics. URL: https://www.bjs.gov/content/pub/pdf/rprts05p0510.pdf. Last accessed: 2017, June 1.

Galofaro, C. (2012). St. Tammany courts give parish nickname of 'St. Slammany.' *The Times Picayune*. URL: http://www.nola.com/crime/index.ssf/2012/03/st_tammany_courts_give_parish.html. Last accessed: 2017, June 25.

Hampden County Sheriff's Office. (2015). Presentation: Special commission on substance abuse addiction treatment in the criminal justice system. URL: http://www.mass.gov/courts/docs/specialty-courts/specialty-courts-hampden-sheriff.pdf. Last accessed: 2017, June 1.

Johnson, R. (2002). *Hard time* (3rd ed.). Wadsworth.

Lafayette Parish Sheriff's Office. (2011). Reentry survival manual. URL: https://www.lafayettesheriff.com/uploads/ReentrySkillsSurvivalManual62811.pdf. Last accessed: 2017, June 1.

Lowenkamp, C. T., Latessa, E. J., & Holsinger, A. M. (2006). The risk principle in action: What have we learned from 13,676 offenders and 97 correctional programs? *Crime & Delinquency, 52*(1), 77–93.

Mallik-Kane, K., & Visher, C. A. (2008). *Health and prisoner reentry: How physical, mental, and substance abuse conditions shape the process of reintegration* (p. 82). Washington, DC: Urban Institute Justice Policy Center.

Maruna, S. (2001). *Making good: How ex-convicts reform and rebuild their lives*. American Psychological Association.

Maruna, S., & LeBel, T. P. (2003). Welcome home-examining the reentry court concept from a strengths-based perspective. *Western Criminology Review, 4*(2), 91–107.

Mellow, J., Mukamal, D. A., LoBuglio, S. F., Solomon, A. L., & Osborne, J. W. (2008). *The jail administrator's toolkit for reentry*. Urban Institute.

Miller, J. M., & Khey, D. N. (2016). Fighting America's highest incarceration rates with offender programming: Process evaluation implications from the Louisiana 22nd Judicial District Reentry Court. *American Journal of Criminal Justice*. URL: https://link.springer.com/article/10.1007/s12103-016-9372-4. Last accessed: 2017, July 2.

Moore, K. E., Stuewig, J. B., & Tangney, J. P. (2015). The effect of stigma on criminal offenders' functioning: A longitudinal mediational model. *Deviant Behavior, 37*(2), 196–218.

Osher, F. C. (2006). *Integrating mental health and substance abuse services for justice-involved persons with co-occurring disorders*. National GAINS Center.

Osher, F. C. (2007, January/February). Short-term strategies to improve reentry of jail populations. *American Jails*, 9–18.

Pearson, F. S., & Lipton, D. S. (1999). A meta-analytic review of the effectiveness of corrections-based treatments for drug abuse. *Prison Journal, 79*(4), 384–410.

Petersilia, J. (2004). What works in prisoner reentry-reviewing and questioning the evidence. *Federal Probation, 68*(2), 4–8.

Rawlins, A. (2014). Philadelphia's prisons are embracing technology. URL: http://money.cnn.com/2014/10/07/smallbusiness/philadelphia-technology-prison/index.html. Last accessed: 2017, June 1.

Ryan, C. L., & Bauman, K. (2016). Educational attainment in the United States: 2015. U.S. Census. : https://www.census.gov/content/dam/Census/library/publications/2016/demo/p20-578.pdf. Last accessed: 2017, June 1.

Solomon, A. L., Osborne, J. W., LoBuglio, S. F., Mellow, J., & Mukamal, D. A. (2008). *Life after lockup: Improving reentry from jail to the community*.

Stafford, C. (2006). Finding work: How to approach the intersection of prisoner reentry, employment, and recidivism. *Georgetown Journal on Poverty Law & Policy, 13*, 261.

Travis, J. (2000). *But they all come back: Rethinking prisoner reentry*. US Department of Justice, Office of Justice Programs, National Institute of Justice.

Travis, J., & Visher, C. (Eds.). (2005). *Prisoner reentry and crime in America*. Cambridge University Press.

Travis, J., & Waul, M. (Eds.). (2003) *Prisoners once removed: The impact of incarceration and reentry on children, families, and communities*. The Urban Institute.

Wolff, N., & Shi, J. (2012). Childhood and adult trauma experiences of incarcerated persons and their relationship to adult behavioral health problems and treatment. *International Journal of Environmental Research and Public Health, 9*(5), 1908–1926.

Chapter 10
Community-Based and Grassroots Programs

> *Mental illness, it's a bit like drugs, it doesn't give a shit who you are. And you know what's worse? The stigma doesn't give a shit who you are. – Sinead O'Connor, 2017.*

Community members can aid in making changes in mental health awareness, improving the system of care, and reentry. In fact, there appears to be substantial growth in nonprofit organizations of all sizes to affect such change, as well as the volunteer hours needed to sustain this momentum. In 2015, the Urban Institute released their annual *Nonprofit Sector in Brief*, which supports this claim (McKeever, 2015). This report reveals that the number of 501(c)(3) public charities grew 19.5% from 2003 to 2013, and 25.3 percent of American adults had volunteered for a nonprofit organization in 2014. While this proportion of adults who volunteer at least once per year is on a slightly downward trend, the number of total volunteer hours in any given year is at the highest ever recorded at 8.7 billion hours in 2014 – valued at $179.2 billion. This volunteerism is consistently concentrated in social service and care activities, including food preparation, clean-ups, food, goods, and clothing collection and delivery, direct care and/or services, teaching, mentoring, and counseling. Five years later, the Urban Institute's *Brief* (2020) depicted continued growth – registered non-profits grew 4.5% from 2006 to 2016 and 25.1% of American adults had volunteered for a nonprofit in 2017, producing 8.8 billion hours of volunteerism.

In the cases of local mental health care system improvements and criminal justice reform (e.g., reentry), this momentum has been buttressed by grant opportunities through the Substance Abuse and Mental Health Services Administration, the Bureau of Justice Assistance, and other Federal government funding agencies specifically tailored to support public-non-profit collaborations. For example, the Bureau of Justice Assistance Second Chance Act Comprehensive Community-Based Adult Reentry Program is specifically geared for community-based non-profits who engage in reentry activities such as mentoring support, treatment services, legal aid, and more. These opportunities also seem to be on the rise; however, it is uncertain how the current pandemic will shape or modulate these trends in the upcoming years. With momentum in Congress and local governments for justice

J. Hector, D. Khey, *Criminal Justice and Mental Health*,
https://doi.org/10.1007/978-3-031-15338-9_10

and mental health reform, it appears that the trajectory of improvements will continue to some degree. This chapter focuses on promising non-profit activity led by icons, world leaders, and everyday people to give readers some orientation of the rigorous activity that is affecting changes in mental health and justice.

10.1   Know the Role

Non-profits have embraced the challenges facing individuals with mental illness, those who are experiencing mental health crises, and those reentering society from periods of incarceration, treatment, and hospitalization. As noted earlier, episodes of each of these can be the most volatile and difficult struggles in people's lives – and they most often occur in our communities, on our city streets, and in the countryside. The risk of overdose and relapse is assuredly higher when individuals are confronted with their triggers, or being close to bars and hangouts, passing the abandoned house turned into a drug den, seeing or hearing from those acquaintances or sexual partners who engage in drug use and deviance, and so on. In the case of reentry, the stress of returning home, dealing with substance use/abuse/misuse, income and work, and family relationships can be overwhelming. Family members and loved ones may not always be supportive after a person has been incarcerated. In fact, some may be full of anger, mistrust, and spite, which may require counseling in order to heal the damage done from "losing" their loved ones to the system for acts that they may feel are the fault of the person coming back into their lives after long periods of absence.

Many people involved in the non-profit sector serving mentally ill and justice-involved populations have been directly or indirectly touched by problems addressed in this text. Some are parents of a daughter or son with mental illness and/or those that have served time – or other family members. Some individuals with mental illness and/or previous justice-involvement become peer supports for others who become involved with the justice system. One perfect example can be found with an even-keeled, insightful, and mild-mannered Maryland man named Eddie Ellis. In the years after his release, Mr. Ellis has been speaking about his story of incarceration after serving 22 years in prison for shooting and killing a man when he was 16 years old (Ellis, 2016). Now Mr. Ellis serves as a mentor and advocate for others with shared experiences, including being held in solitary confinement for long periods of time because of his violent conviction and not due to his prison behavior. His motivation and hard work post-release has culminated in a vibrant 501(c)(3) non-profit organization named One by 1, which Mr. Ellis serves as Chief Executive (One by 1 Inc., 2017).

At a recent speaking event at the National Association of Drug Court Professionals, Mr. Ellis was joined by his mother to share their points of view on the effect of incarceration in their lives with justice professionals engaged in reentry work (Cherry & Ellis, 2017). Their accounts were impassioned and full of lingering signs of pain from their experiences and allowed the audience a window into the common problems returning prisoners and their families will face upon release. As the conversation progressed, Ms. Cherry voiced her concern that family members often lack support to help them process their feelings. This point in particular began a lively question and answer session about how professionals can best aid families at a vulnerable time in their lives.

Everyday people turned on to "giving back" or to be a change agent – like Mr. Ellis and Ms. Cherry – are at the heart of the grassroots effort in American communities. Peer support specialists, for example, are becoming critical – if not mandatory – for the care of individuals with mental illness, substance use disorder, and/or who are experiencing a mental health crisis. Thus, at this point, any comprehensive solution to the broken mental health system of care and justice reform almost requires grassroots, community support. The following sections highlight some of the most innovative endeavors of recent years.

10.2 Facing the Stigma Head On: Heroin Walks Like Cancer Walks

In reducing stigma and viewing mental health like physical health, changing thought processes and views about funding raising is also important. In regard to "physical health," for example, there are many activities in the month of October for Breast Cancer Awareness in most communities across the United States each year. These activities include fund raising walks, charitable donations from major corporations (think Yoplait yogurt with the pink tops), and even the National Football League players wearing pink accessories while they play in a dedicated week to the cause. These activities do not only raise money for different organizations that research breast cancer in hopes of a cure, they also are critical in raising awareness of the disease and need for preventative screening and regular health checks.

In this vein, mental health-related events and campaigns happen throughout the year, with peak activity during the official "Mental Health Week" (the first full week of October as recognized by Congress; not to be confused with mental health month – May – established by NAMI and its partners). For example, the local NAMI affiliates often sponsor 5 K events each year, called NAMIWalks (2022), which raises money for each local branch. In the most recent year (2020), there are more than 25,000 participants of walks around the country, raising over $7.2 million in the United States.

In more recent times, this concept has been expanded to focus on current emerging issues, such as the opioid epidemic. Starting in 2017, the Addiction Prevention Coalition in Birmingham, Alabama, hosted an "End Heroin Bham" walk, free to everyone, with the intent to bring awareness of the recent surge in opioid-related problems and deaths occurring in the greater Birmingham area and in the state of Alabama. Likewise, the Coalition utilized a broad array of media exposure of the event to aid in its message, even if locals did not end up attending the event. Awareness and social marketing campaigns seem to be one of the primary tools of the grassroots movement in terms of relevance and sustained funding. For example, the latest End Heroin Bham campaign raised $42,414 in 2021 and is estimated to engage 3000–4000 people in the Birmingham community (Addiction Prevention Coalition, 2021).

10.3   Partners 4 Strong Minds (Strong 365) and One Mind Care Connect

Partners 4 Strong Minds (P4SM) was a non-profit organization created as a result of founder Chantel Garrett's long advocacy of her brother's schizophrenia diagnosis. With a background in marketing for corporations, Ms. Garrett spearheaded a modern campaign of advocacy and personal storytelling to change the way everyday people think about brain health and access to care. In particular, the organization began with a focus on creating awareness regarding the first/early onset of psychosis with the notion that addressing the psychosis early on and quickly after the first onset can aid in better results for long-term success in recovery. P4SM's use of messaging from friends, families, and loved ones often was found at the core of the organization's awareness campaigns and events, many of which were concentrated on the West coast of the United States where P4SM was founded.

The mission of P4SM aligned with an emerging science pointing to promising results of early intervention and by being proactive. In fact, mental illness disease processes seem to be more easily managed – and possibly in some cases, symptoms can be lessened – when early intervention occurs. It often allows for the individual to live a much more productive and stable life. Further, a person can learn their triggers and be more aware of symptoms and issues before they arise, thus empowering those with mental illness.

Similarly, Shari and Garen Staglin's experiences of advocating for their son Brandon and his schizophrenia diagnosis drove them to organize and develop the One Mind Institute. Since 1995, the Staglins focused their efforts on grantsmaking in the domain of brain health research. In 2014, Ms. Garrett and the Staglins joined forces to create the One Mind Care Connect initiative: "the combined effort expands P4SM's nationwide advocacy and personal storytelling platform under the One Mind Institute brand, and complements its grassroots approach with translational research that will help us learn more about how to best evolve and scale early psychosis treatment in the United States" (One Mind Institute, 2017). One of the current programs of One Mind Care Connect is Strong 365. Strong 365 has many facets to help families in their search for help with psychosis, specifically the early stages. A treatment tracker is maintained on the Strong 365 website, which lists programs throughout the country that provide treatment after a first episode of psychosis. The information on the website makes clear that early intervention treatment, medication management, counseling (including the whole family), brain training, and other activities are shown to aid in recovery.

10.4   Heads Together

Often, on health-related topics, a "champion" is discussed when having a celebrity or spokesperson for a campaign. As mental health emerges as a mainstream topic (again), celebrities are (re-)emerging to bring the conversation of mental health awareness to the forefront. Further, with social media, these messages are easily able to quickly reach large audiences. Some celebrities are also opening up to discuss their own personal struggles with mental illness or substance abuse (particularly with the latter). For example, Sinead O'Connor recently shared her raw feelings regarding her own mental health and suicidal thoughts with a self-shot video on her Facebook account. In her emotional 12-minute clip, O'Connor explains: "I hope that this video is somehow helpful. Not to me, but the fact that I know that I am only one of millions and millions and millions of people who are just like me, actually, that don't necessarily have the resources that I have in my heart and in my purse." Often, positive messages about mental illness and treatment are used to open conversation to happen to affect change, particularly when these messages are associated with non-profit organizations. Having these "champions" can begin to help overcome stigma and obstacles to ensure everyone receives the treatment needed.

One example of champion-led messaging comes with the Royal Foundation of the Duke and Duchess of Cambridge and Prince Harry and its project entitled Heads Together. In particular, the Heads Together project adjoins the Royal Foundation "in partnership with inspiring charities that are tackling stigma, raising awareness, and providing vital help for people with mental health challenges" (Royal Foundation, 2017). Having world leaders, such as Prince William, Duchess Kate, and Prince Harry, speak on mental health is providing legitimacy to the cause. It can further bring hope to all affected. As such, the Heads Together program is a potent awareness campaign that unites existing organizations and elevates their cause through celebrity power – partners including Best Beginnings, the Campaign Against Living Miserably, Contact (mental health coalition for the military), Mind, Place2Be, The Mix, YoungMinds, and the Anna Freud Centre. It also includes star power from across the pond in the United States with Born This Way.

10.5 Born this Way

The Born This Way Foundation founded by musician, Lady Gaga, with its slogan "empowering youth and inspiring bravery." The Foundation features different programming and advice based on research as well as tips and direct links for seeking help when needed. Lady Gaga uses her own personal experience with post-traumatic stress disorder to dispel the concept of stigma and promote a positive community.

> I have wrestled for some time about when, how and if I should reveal my diagnosis of Post-Traumatic Stress Disorder (PTSD). After five years of searching for the answers to my chronic pain and the change I have felt in my brain, I am finally well enough to tell you. There is a lot of shame attached to mental illness, but it's important that you know that there is hope and a chance for recovery. (Born This Way Foundation, 2017).

Her organization provides user-friendly information in a manner geared toward youth and helping them to create "kind communities and enhance mental wellness." Areas on the website currently focus on topics such as kindness, positive environments, mental wellness, and research and resources, and further features a Born Brave blog featuring voices and stories from across the country.

The website includes a section entitled Hack Harassment which works to combat online harassment for youth. Hack Harassment assembles its partners – Intel, Vox Media, and Recode – to work behind the scenes to find innovative ways to help keep online spaces free of harassment. Hack Harassment also includes section for users featuring an anti-harassment pledge and an application for college-aged students to become campus ambassadors at their college or university. The idea of a campus ambassador is nothing new and has been used by many different organizations to promote education and information within the college campus community. Yet, the star power of Lady Gaga can further elevate campus messaging and give help to its legitimacy.

In 2017, Lady Gaga and Prince William opened to one another about their experiences with mental illness via a FaceTime call shared with the world with the hashtag #okaytosay (a Heads Together awareness tool). For Prince William, he shared personal details about his brother Harry's need to seek counseling to help with his struggles after the death of his mother.

Lady Gaga: …The beautiful videos of the Heads Together campaign…told beautiful stories and it reminded me how much my mental health changing changed my life.

Prince William: [Most of our charitable work] seemed to stand back to mental health issues, and you know, I read your open letter you wrote the other day and I thought it was incredibly moving and very brave of you to write down such personal feelings. I wanted to ask you very much how you found speaking out and how it made you feel?

Lady Gaga: It made me very nervous at first. For me, waking up everyday and feeling sad and going on stage, is something that is something very hard to describe. There's a lot of shame attached to mental illness. You feel like something's wrong with you. And, in my life, I go "oh my goodness look at all this beautiful, wonderful things that I have. And I should be so happy." But you can't help it that if in the morning when you wake up, you are so tired, you are so sad, you are so full of anxiety and the shakes that you can barely think. But, it was like saying, this was a part of me and it was okay.

Prince William: …for me, the little bits that I have learned about mental health so far is that it's okay to have this conversation. It's really important to have this conversation, you won't be judged. It's so important to break open that fear and taboo which is only going to lead to more problems down the line.

Lady Gaga: Yes, it can make a huge difference. I feel like we are not hiding anymore; we're starting to talk and that's what we need to do really.

Prince William: Absolutely. It's time that everyone speaks up and feels very normal about mental health. It's the same as physical. Everyone has mental health and that we shouldn't be ashamed of it. Just having a conversation with a friend or family member can make such a difference.

Lady Gaga: Even though it was hard, it was the best thing that could come out of my mental illness – was to share it with other people and let our generation as well as other generations know that if you are feeling not well in your mind, that you are not alone. And that people that you think would never have a problem do. (Transcript from video posted on headstogether.org.uk, available here: https://

www.headstogether.org.uk/prince-william-and-lady-gaga-get-their-heads-together-on-mental-health-to-help-show-young-people-that-its-ok-to-say/).

This collaboration will pick up again in October when Prince William plans to meet up with Lady Gaga to take the next steps in this conversation and create some action out of it. Along with this example, there are many other celebrity champions who have surfaced in recent years to bring to light issues related to mental health.

10.6 The Boris Lawrence Henson Foundation

An actor, Taraji P Henson, founded the Boris Lawrence Henson Foundation (BLHF) (2022) in 2018 and named after her father. She created this organization in light of her own mental health challenges, which she felt she had no support for in her younger years. The vision of the organization "is to eradicate the stigma around mental health issues in the African-American community" and raising trust among communities of color by linking people in these communities with cultural and language appropriate services. The efforts of the foundation are broad: the organization provides (1) information and referrals to treatment, specifically to trusted partners; (2) education and literature about wellness; (3) cultural competency training for professionals to broaden their network of trusted partners; (4) scholarships to invest in culturally informed and person-centered mental health professionals of the future; (5) mental health services to underserved schools and youth in underserved communities; and (6) supportive reentry resources for individuals returning from incarceration back to their communities. Of note, BLHF has developed an immersive experience – The Unspoken Curriculum – that promises to engage learners in a deep conversation about the lived experiences of people of color at primary and secondary schools across the United States. Specifically, it targets young people of color in this conversation to shape "how youth view themselves – and each other – in society." In essence, this programming helps learners better understand how stigma operates to shape behavior in communities of color.

10.7 Brands

In line with discussions on mental health awareness in previous chapters, more companies are raising awareness to not only discuss the topic, but also provide funding for a variety of mental health-related efforts. Therefore, conscious consumers can choose to spend their money with companies working toward change. A Google search for brands that donate to mental health awareness or related campaigns will now result in seemingly limitless results. Similarly, reading the "About Us" section of brand's website can inform the consumer or potential consumer on the story of the company.

These brands, whether with the purchase of a specific item, collaboration with another company or their entire line, allow the consumer the ability to give back in a way. A person purchasing these products can do so with the intention that some money will go to different charitable organizations helping to lessen stigma, support awareness, or even offer access for mental health.

Further, in 2016 NAMI launched StigmaFree Company which is an initiative to "highlight and cultivate a company culture of caring and enhanced engagement around mental health." NAMI describes a StigmaFree Company using specific steps to change employee health. These steps are "create company policies regarding mental health, show support to employees, provide management training, and decrease stigma in the workplace." Beyond these steps, the partnership between the company and NAMI encourages "Corporate Social Responsibility (CSR), or business practices that take responsibility for a company's impact on social well-being. This initiative combines CSR with employee engagement activities available in our StigmaFree Company Welcome Kit. The kit equips companies with the resources, assets and information they need to promote mental health awareness in the workplace and to encourage acceptance and understanding."

Notable StigmaFree Company (2022), Brand Partners include:

- Starbucks.
- Bank of America.
- Boeing.
- Delta Airlines.
- Fox Sports.
- Macy's.
- Kaiser Permanente.
- Showtime.

10.7.1   Clothing Brands

Many clothing brands have emerged with pieces geared toward lessening stigma with uplifting messages. Often the founders of these brands have a story about themselves or a friend or family member that led to the creation of their products.

- Wear Your Label was a Canadian based clothing company created by two friends "to spark conversations about mental health" (Wear Your Label, 2017). Both of the co-founders have suffered from mental illness and wanted to let others know that "it's okay not to be okay," and the importance of self-care. Their shirts feature sayings like "stigma free" and "i am enough" and come in unisex sizing to be inclusive to all gender and gender fluid individuals. Wear Your Label had expanded to also include jewelry with a bracelet series that not only provides awareness for different mental health diagnoses, but also included information on those disorders and where to seek help if needed. Even though this effort has come to an end in 2018, it continues to serve as a model for other advocates to expand in this space. – *NAMI StigmaFree Company* (since removed after closure).

- Kenneth Cole – *NAMI StigmaFree Company.*
- To Write Love on Her Arms started as a fundraiser to help cover the costs of treatment for a friend. Later, founder Jamie Tworkowski decided to convert his idea into a nonprofit aimed at helping others with depression, substance use disorder, self-injurious behaviors, and thoughts of suicide.
- You Are Enough Co. – 100% of the net proceeds of their apparel line featuring uplifting messages goes to mental health awareness and research.
- Social Goods – offers hats, t-shirts, and other items in support of the mental health coalition.

10.7.2 Beauty Brands

A number of beauty brands have begun campaigns or collaborations with the focus of mental health awareness and access to treatment in mind.

- Philosophy – the company with their Hope & Grace Initiative. Since 2014, the company has donated $5.4 million to "support community-based mental health efforts." *NAMI StigmaFree Company.*
- Bubble – the skincare brand donates a portion of their proceeds to youth mental health organizations, offers a discount for the therapy app BetterHelp on their website, as well as lists a number of mental health resources on their site for ease of access to anyone.
- Clove + Hallow – beauty brand that works with Mental Health America of Georgia combat stigma.

10.7.3 Others

- Ban.do – the Feeling Feelings Card Deck is not only great for use for self-care, but also a portion of proceeds are donated to The Loveland Foundation.
- Awareness Coffee Company – their mission is to use bag designs to create awareness. They donate a portion of the proceeds of their Mental Health blend to groups like NAMI an Active Minds.

Some brands offer limited edition collections or collaborations (check your favorite ones!).

10.8 Active Minds

Active Minds was created by a woman named Alison Malmon following the suicide of her older brother, Brian. As both were college students at the time, Ms. Malmon was struck by the dearth of discussion of mental health issues on her campus. After a few years of activism, she incorporated the Active Minds non-profit in late 2003; the organization works as a student-led group on college campuses across the United States to bring awareness to mental health issues at these campuses. In almost 15 years, Active Minds has grown to over 400 chapters with thousands of student members at universities across the nation. Additionally, there is now a national conference where members of different groups can come together annually at a forum to help growth, understanding, and awareness. The organization offers many different, turnkey-style programs that can run independently at each campus (e.g., individual-led efforts) as well as group-based efforts such as Active Minds' signature Send Silence Packing® event (Active Minds, 2017).

Send Silence Packing® gives passersby a visual representation of suicide among college-aged students. To do so, a traveling tour of donated backpacks are brought to each site to be laid out in a high traffic area on campus, like outside of the student union or main campus "quads." As a visual representation, the backpacks symbolize the number of college students who take their lives each year; signage is placed near the backpacks with statistics, ways to seek help, and other helpful information. In 2017, the Send Since Packing® campaign has reached over 15 campuses, including the University of North Alabama, Alcorn State University, the University of North Texas, The University of Denver, Colorado State University, Mt. San Jacinto College, and Occidental College.

10.9 SLIDDE, University of Louisiana at Lafayette

Further, on a direct community level, universities themselves have made awareness efforts on their own. One great example of programming is at the University of Louisiana at Lafayette. There, a student organization called SLIDDE, School Leaders Involved in Drinking and Drug Education, has been created. The program was started within the Counseling and Testing Center to provide education, awareness, and prevention on campus for drinking and drug use. It has now grown to be an official student-led organization and is involved in many different activities on campus throughout the academic year, such as an annual 5 k run that occurs in the Spring. These events are often coordinated with popular campus events to ensure wide visibility and maximum exposure. In fact, most modern colleges and universities offer such programming through a division or office of student health. Therefore, it should not be surprising to see mental health programming becoming more prominent in such messaging in some capacity. For the time being, grassroots organizations such as Active Minds are filling the voids on campuses across the country, as are campus-based NAMI organizations. Much more activity is expected in the upcoming years in this arena (University of Louisiana Counseling and Testing Center, 2017).

10.10   Dave's Killer Bread

Created in 2005 as part of a family bakery, Dave's Killer Bread has grown to become *the* top-rated organic bread in the United States. The story of the Dahl brothers, Dave and Glenn, is a testament to community partnerships working to help solve some of the nation's struggles. Dave served 15 years in prison and was given a job by his brother to work in their family bakery after his release. Their dream was to create bread that was both organic and non-GMO, and they succeeded. Now, the company has more than 300 employees with distribution in all 50 US states, Canada, and Mexico (thanks to the distribution power of Flowers Foods who acquired Dave's Killer Bread; products currently reach 85% of Americans). Even further, 1 in 3 of their employees at the original bakery has a criminal background. As a company, they are working to reduce the struggles of stigma and recidivism in the United States.

Additionally, Dave's Killer Bread Foundation has been created to aid in education and implementation of Second Chance Employment. The Foundation has created a Second Chance Playbook which features all topics related to understanding how and why hiring individuals and providing them with a "second chance" is beneficial to the community and their organization. Organizations can join the community and have access to the Playbook, and even attend the Second Chance Summits held across the country. The Second Chance Playbook not only provides guides, but also video modules covering topics such as "risk mitigation and insurance, legal compliance and the use of criminal background checks, financial incentives for hiring Second Chance candidates, organizational culture and values, the hiring and staffing process, successful onboarding and orientation, and more" (Dave's Killer Bread Foundation, 2017).

10.11   Conclusion

Many of these organizations mentioned above both reduce stigma and raise awareness about mental health and the criminal justice system. More importantly, their efforts are part of the steps in making a change for their communities and society as a whole. Support and positivity can manage to spark change in many ways. Persons suffering from mental illness that have a criminal background can also find solace in partnering with these, and many other, organizations to tell their stories. Education to the public is an essential component in success for all involved.

Part of the importance of the awareness campaigns mentioned in this chapter is to aid students and professionals to understand the normality of mental health issues in our society. If we can begin educating students and arm them with the information in these campaigns, this can drastically impact the careers of these individuals or professionals already working in these careers – which can thus have an impact on justice-involved individuals and those with mental health concerns (most likely, both).

Discussion Questions

1. In your opinion, which celebrity campaign is the most promising in changing public attitudes regarding mental illness?
2. How can being a conscientious consumer serve to amplify positive mental health messages?

References

Active Minds. (2017). About us. URL: http://www.activeminds.org/about. Last accessed: 2017, October 30.
Addiction Prevention Coalition. (2021). End heroin Bham. URL: https://ehbc.swell.gives/. Last accessed: 2022, February 5.
Boris Lawrence Henson Foundation. (2022). BLHF. URL: https://borislhensonfoundation.org/. Last accessed: 2022, February 7.
Born This Way Foundation. (2017). Born this way. URL: https://bornthisway.foundation/. Last accessed: 2017, October 30.
Cherry, S., & Ellis, E. (2017). *Speaking at the national association of drug court professionals.* NADCP.
Dave's Killer Bread Foundation. (2017). About us. URL: https://www.dkbfoundation.org/about/. Last accessed: 2017, October 30.
Ellis, E. (2016). I am one of the success stories from D.C.'s second-chance law for young offenders. URL: https://www.washingtonpost.com/opinions/i-am-one-of-the-success-stories-from-dcs-second-chance-law-for-young-offenders/2016/12/16/f1f2c9a4-c211-11e6-8422-eac61c0ef74d_story.html?utm_term=.ae7c13f61e28. Last accessed: 2017, October 30.
McKeever, B. (2015). The nonprofit sector in brief 2015: Public charities, giving, and volunteering. URL: https://www.urban.org/research/publication/nonprofit-sector-brief-2015-public-charities-giving-and-volunteering. Last accessed: 2017, October 30.
NAMI. (2022). StigmaFree company brands. URL: https://nami.org/About-NAMI/Who-We-Are/Meet-Our-Partners/StigmaFree-Company-Brand-Partners. Last accessed: 2022, February 7.
NAMIWalks. (2022). NAMIWalks your way. URL: https://www.namiwalks.org/. Last accessed: 2022, February 5.
One by 1 Inc. (2017). Welcome to one by 1. URL: http://www.onebylinc.org/. Last accessed: 2017, October 30.
One Mind Institute. (2017). About one mind institute. URL: https://www.onemindinstitute.org/about-one-mind-institute. Last accessed: 2017, October 30.
Royal Foundation. (2017) About our foundation. URL: http://www.royalfoundation.com/about-our-foundation/. Last accessed: 2017, October 30.
University of Louisiana Counseling and Testing Center. (2017). School leaders involved in drinking and drug education (SLIDDE). URL: https://counselingandtesting.louisiana.edu/content/slidde/school-leaders-involved-drinking-and-drug-education-slidde. Last accessed: 2017, October 30.
Urban Institute. (2020). The nonprofit sector in brief 2019. URL: https://nccs.urban.org/publication/nonprofit-sector-brief-2019. Last accessed: 2022, February 5.
Wear Your Label. (2017). Wear your label. URL: https://wearyourlabel.com/. Last accessed: 2017, October 30.

Chapter 11
Self-Care for Professionals

At the root of this dilemma is the way we view mental health in this country. Whether an illness affects your heart, your leg, or your brain, it's still an illness, and there should be no distinction. – Michelle Obama.

The idea of burnout exists in many different professions, especially those related to both mental health and criminal justice. No matter the political stance or outlook, most would agree that the job of police officers is a difficult one. For the most part, when police are involved in an incident it is a negative one. Police patrol for traffic stops or speeding on highways, respond to emergency calls, and escort inmates when transferred or appearing in court. Often traffic stops and speeding result in tickets, and emergency calls can result in arrests and/or involvement of medical personnel. All of these are negative, again, much of the job of police. Now, consider repeating this scenario daily for years. Tough thoughts, right? This is the reality for most that serve on the "frontline," yet, this sentiment can be widespread throughout the entire system coming into contact with individuals with mental illness.

11.1 What No One Talks About: Our Own Mental Health

In previous chapters, many topics were discussed as it relates to treatment for those with a mental health diagnosis as well as how those individuals interact with law enforcement, emergency medical services, and probation and parole. It is critical to take into account how these interactions impact the overall well-being of those frontline professionals. With their jobs being stressful, straining, and high-intensity, there can and often will be, adverse reactions. The irony is that often first responders, mental health professionals, and other law enforcement personnel spend much of their time helping others to a point where they begin neglecting themselves. Self-care for professionals working in these fields is not only essential for their wellness, but also for their loved ones and those they are helping in the community.

Job strain and stress can influence anyone, both in the short and long terms. Repeating the same tasks over and over and receiving a similar result each time is frustrating no matter the context. Combine this frustration with encountering people

J. Hector, D. Khey, *Criminal Justice and Mental Health*,
https://doi.org/10.1007/978-3-031-15338-9_11

(typically) in very negative and seemingly repetitive situations, and one quickly realizes how overwhelming this can become. Stigma is also a concept that comes into play for professionals and self-care. Often, many professionals do not want to admit that they are in need of help. The idea of seeming "weak" in a profession like law enforcement can be detrimental to a career.

Burnout and compassion fatigue are two common consequences of an occupation working directly with individuals in crisis and related both to mental health and the criminal justice system. Both can touch many occupations that reach beyond first responders. Additionally, doctors, nurses, mental health professionals, case workers, and even judges and lawyers can feel the effects of burnout and compassion fatigue. Further, the impact of burnout can vary depending on many factors. At times, a simple break or vacation can be enough to refuel and reconnect with one's work. Unfortunately, in the American work culture, taking time off or for vacation is not often celebrated. In fact, many people allow their leave time to go unused.

Many professionals benefit from attending conferences and training sessions throughout their careers. No matter the length of time in a career, there are always new and innovative techniques and programs being developed. Learning from pioneers in the industry and even peers can be valuable. Additionally, interacting with others who work in the same industry and experience a similar daily life and schedule can aid in understanding processes. Commiserating with those who lead a related professional life can often take away stress and burden. This is not unlike unwinding after a class or day of work with friends to vent. The benefits of having professional friends can be immense.

Realistically, it is impossible *not* to be impacted by the job within these occupations. The better focus and idea is to find a balance and maintain a level of positivity and happiness outside of work. Often, these occupations require long hours and days outside of the typical "9–5" and work week. Working "odd hours" can prohibit a person from finding activities and hobbies of interest to maintain a work/life balance. These challenges can be taxing on a person, no matter the nature of their occupation.

11.1.1   Burnout, Compassion Fatigue, and Vicarious Trauma: Working with People in Crisis

The literature on work burnout is continuing to become more relevant in the workplace in the twenty-first century – with mental health professionals and beyond. The concept of designing workplaces to aid in the promotional of both physical and mental wellness certainly has gained momentum; for example, the heavyweights of Silicon Valley seem to compete on designing work campuses that include such things as food courts with healthy options, gardens, creative spaces, and so on. At times, popular culture seems to highlight how some employers have taken this concept to an extreme. For example, in what has become one of the more infamous of these campuses, the Googleplex features a hair salon, on-site medical care, various cafeterias with free food, bicycles to use (free), childcare (again, free), a full-service laundry room, massage therapy, and pet-friendly spaces to take advantage of the allowance of dogs on campus (Ulanoff, 2009). While the pandemic is ongoing, these are the same sorts of organizations that are leading the way to supporting work from home options or blended work options to maximize both employee well-being and productivity. Mental health professionals seem to be more mindful of burnout than their colleagues in criminal justice due to the nature of their training; yet, both are at risk of two special factors that can complicate burnout – compassion fatigue and vicarious trauma (also known as secondary trauma).

Each of these terms – burnout, compassion fatigue, and secondary traumatic stress – are often conflated by various sources both professional and lay. While the three are intertwined, they are quite distinct. Burnout generally refers to feelings of exhaustion directly because of one's work. This burnout can come in the form of physical and/or emotional exhaustion and feeling drained, which can lead to low job satisfaction, interpersonal problems, sickness, substance use/misuse/abuse, and so on. For example, odds of experiencing burnout will almost always increase as one increases their work hours – if an employee consistently puts in 80, 90, or 100 hours per week, burnout is almost guaranteed. While a 100-hour work week may seem impossible, it can be very likely for most American medical residents as they prepare to launch into careers in medicine. The latest standards published by the Accreditation Council for Graduate Medical Education requires accredited programs to abide by the following rules: (1) "Duty hours must be limited to 80 hours per week, *averaged over a four-week period*, inclusive of all in-house call activities and all moonlighting"; (2) "...up to 10% or a maximum of 88 hours to individual programs based on a sound educational rationale"; (3) "Residents must be scheduled for a minimum of one day free of duty every week (when averaged over four weeks" (ACGME, 2017). Of the 1515 studies on duty-hour limits identified by Philibert, Nasca, Brigham, and Shapiro in 2013, these researchers assessed 83 of the highest-quality ones to review the impact of limiting the work hours of medical residents. Not surprisingly, limitations on hours had a benefit on burnout and overall mood, with some evidence to support that these limitations also improved patient safety. Note that these findings have direct consequences for the quality of mental health services, particularly in teaching hospitals (e.g., where significantly more poor and uninsured patients receive their care), as young psychiatrists push themselves to meet their work demands. Evidence bears that burnout can be problematic for the employee as well as any others impacted by their work.

To investigate burnout in depth, Maslach developed an instrument – called the Maslach Burnout Inventory (MBI) – to assess what he postulated were the three dimensions of burnout (Maslach et al., 2006). The first dimension is emotional exhaustion caused by one's overwhelming work demands, which saps one perceived energy. The second dimension is depersonalization and cynicism, which results in feelings of detachment from one's job. The third and last dimension is feelings of inefficacy, which one perceives themselves as ineffective, not growing or learning, and stuck in a rut. The MBI was developed in a way to gauge varying levels of burnout as Maslach felt it was not an all-or-none concept. As such, burnout is a dynamic concept that has been shown to have impacts in any vocation. It can be mitigated in various ways, such as the notorious concept of "loving what you do." However, even those who are passionate about their work can experience burnout.

Compassion fatigue is a concept developed by Charles Figley (2002), which adapts the concept of burnout to individuals who serve to care for others, such as nurses, doctors, counselors, case workers, and so on (also known as caretakers and helpers, whether professional or lay, such as in a case of an adult child taking care of their aging parent(s)). These concepts align very closely; however, the effects of compassion fatigue tend to predominately result in desensitization, depression and anxiety disorders, disconnection with family and close friends, and social isolation (Mathieu, 2012). A common popular culture example of compassion fatigue lies with adult children having to take on caretaking duties of their ailing parents. Day, Anderson, and Davis explored this issue in a 2014 article in *Issues in Mental Health Nursing* among 12 adult daughters turned caregivers of a parent with dementia. Using semi-structured interviews, these researchers discovered four overarching themes that seemed to predict risk of developing compassion fatigue in these caregivers: uncertainty (mostly over the seemingly unpredictable sickness and what the future brings), doubt (mostly that the caregivers doubted their ability to take care of their parent in a manner they deserve), attachment (noting a close attachment with the parent), and strain (due to juggling the demands of life with the added responsibilities of caregiving). The interviews in the study gave striking life to the potential results of compassion fatigue – helplessness, hopelessness, diminishing empathy, and isolation. "When [my parent walked away from the house], it's just been a constant in the back of my mind. What could happen next time?", "Not feeling that I'm able to take care of her the way I should be able to take care of her.", "That kind of has my rest broken, and when I get to work the next day, I'm just no good, I'll sleep all day.", "Juggling my time, taking care of the house, and my house there, and my job and friends and family. It's just hard to juggle sometimes.", "I think I had reached a point where I felt resentful toward her. I used to love the weekends. I dread Fridays because that means that I don't have any relief at all. All Friday night...Saturdays...Sunday.", "You can't stop" (Day et al., 2014).

Vicarious trauma layers on the potential complications that can arise in professionals or laypersons caused by caring for an individual(s) experiencing significant trauma in their lives. In a very real sense, the trauma that touches people's lives rubs off on the individuals that seek to help in the recovery process. The most salient recent examples of this lie in first responders of 9/11, the Boston Marathon bombing, Hurricane Katrina, and so on. However, horrendous images of physical trauma are certainly not necessary to trigger vicarious trauma. Professionals who aid sexual assault victims, children in child welfare cases, and so on are certainly at risk for being exposed to vicarious trauma. If this exposure goes unabated, it may develop into clinical diagnoses, such as post-traumatic stress disorder. Specifically, the Diagnostic and Statistical Manual V (American Psychiatric Association, 2013) included new criteria for post-traumatic stress disorder (italics emphasize modifications):

A. Exposure to actual or threatened death, serious injury, or sexual violence in one (or more) of the following ways:

1. Directly experiencing the traumatic event(s).
2. Witnessing, in person, the event(s) as it occurred to others.
3. Learning that the traumatic event(s) occurred to a close family member or close friend. In cases of actual or threatened death of a family member of friend, the event(s) must have been violent or accidental.
4. *Experiencing repeated or extreme exposure to aversive details of the traumatic event(s) (e.g., first responders collecting human remains; police officers repeated exposed to details of child abuse).*

Note: Criterion A4 does not apply to exposure through electronic media, television, movies, or pictures, unless this exposure is work related.

As Levin et al. (2014) point out, no clear data exists on how the addition of A4 results in differences in PTSD incidence and prevalence, or other potential impacts. Much more research needs to be done in this area. In fact, the literature on first responder physical and mental health after vicarious trauma exposure is at its nascent stage, with primary focus on line officer police and emergency medical services personnel at this point. Further, research has yet to delve into the civilian and sworn staff who work traumatic crime scenes (Rivera Waugh, 2016). In 2012, an extensive international search for extant literature uncovered 28 high-quality, peer-reviewed studies on PTSD prevalence among "rescue workers" through 2008 (Berger et al., 2012). On average, the "going rate" regarding prevalence of PTSD among first responders was found to be 10 percent. Not only is this figure alarming; Berger and his colleagues' overall search for literature did not pick up on a large array of interest in the topic before 2008, reinforcing the idea that this area is fertile ground for much needed research.

11.2 Traumatic Experiences and Fatigue: What We Know

Across occupations, especially in jobs which entail interfacing with people in difficult and traumatic situations, the symptoms of burnout are strikingly similar: emotional exhaustion, depersonalization, decreased empathy, isolation, depression, anxiety, cynicism, losing a sense of self-worth (particularly when related to job performance and ability), and so on (Walsh et al., 2012). Research has shown that when police officers are under stress and have negative coping strategies, it can lead to problem drinking (Swatt et al., 2007). Specifically, researchers who studied Baltimore police officers found a strong relationship between stress on the job and drinking, with problematic drinking being mediated through anxiety and depression. In other words, officers who were stressed tended to drink; yet, if they were stressed and anxious/depressed, they tended to be at higher risk of problem drinking. This research echoes findings from other occupations; yet, perhaps not many other occupations experience acute stress as do first responders.

It should not be a surprise to learn, then, that a growing array of research and treatment efforts has been invested into coping skills for professionals, whereas, before the turn of the century, there was not much information to inform us (Anshel, 2000). Despite years of progress in research, there is not one particular evidence-based coping skills training program that is in regular use. Beyond just finding positive ways to cope, the development of a robust self-care program has become a best practice in public service. While programming may not be as generous as the offerings at the Googleplex, the increasingly more prominent role of self-care programming seems to be a sustained pattern into the twenty-first century.

11.3 Self-Care: Why Is It Important

The 2016 National Survey on EMS Mental Health Services shows the importance of self-care in sharp relief (National Association of Emergency Medical Technicians, 2017). In this most recent edition of the survey, 58% of respondents (including paramedics, EMTs, EMS training coordinators, and medical and EMS directors and managers) either disagreed or strongly disagreed when asked if they are satisfied with the mental health services provided by their agency to their employees; 52% of respondents reported that their agency did not even have such mental health services (37%) or were not aware of these services if they were available (15%); only 26% of respondents claimed that their agency had programs available to help employees with substance use and dependence issues; 42% of respondents reported that their agency does not offer health and wellness services; and 41% of respondents reported that they disagree or strongly disagree when asked if they know where to go for help within their agency. The qualitative feedback is even more damning:

- Initiating mental health services through the [employee assistance program] is an invitation for mandatory competency evaluation, grounds for dismissal.
- Most of the people in my organization do not feel comfortable using any service provided by the organization for fear that the information will come back and be used against them in the future.
- [Employee assistance program] provided for three sessions per incident. I do not believe that to be adequate for someone seeking help.
- Currently, acute emotional injuries and mental health are not considered to be work-related by worker's comp.
- I was seeing a mental health professional for PTSD after an ambulance accident that resulted in the death of the driver in the other…Worker's comp denied my claim…leaving me stuck with the bills.
- The agency I work for sees mental health as a weakness. If you ask for help you become verbally abused by co-workers, supervisors and station managers. I

needed help and was told, "that's why women don't belong in EMS. They're overly emotional...."
- Mental health is a joke to management. They still operate on the philosophy that if you can't handle it, you're in the wrong line of work.
- Attitude at our department is, if you can't handle it, get out, sissy.
- I strongly believe that in the workplace mental health is viewed as taboo, not to be talked about and if found out, viewed as a weakness.
- In seeking help you are shamed, made fun of by superiors, and told to suck it up, it's part of the job.
- There is absolutely no concern for the mental or physical health of employees at my agency.
- Rural agencies that operate off monies strictly derived by billing simply cannot afford to offer these types of services to their employees.

Surveys like these are important yet are relatively uncommon among first responders. As we begin to address these issues outlined above with EMS personnel, it is important to remember that they are likely occurring with regularity among all types of first responders. Much more research is direly needed to monitor these issues, particularly as we devise ways to offer improvement in self-care among our first responders.

11.4 Examples of Self-Care Programming

At this time, there appears to be a limited array of programming tailored to meet the needs of first responders. Such programs include Addiction and Trauma Recovery Integration Model (ATRIUM), Essence of Being Real, Risking Connection®, Sanctuary Model®, Seeking Safety, Trauma, Addiction, Mental Health, and Recovery (TAMAR), Trauma Affect Regulation: Guide for Education and Therapy (TARGET), and Trauma Recovery and Empowerment Model (TREM and M-TREM). Many of these programs generally target trauma exposure and are customized to first responders by those who adopt them and/or whose creators offer some guidance on such customizations for professionals themselves. A minority of these, such as ATRIUM, Essence of Being Real, and Risking Connection®, have been formulated for specifically professionals. Regardless, the industry standard for any of these trauma-informed approaches must garner the following key principles for the best result: (1) safety (e.g., the physical setting feels safe and human interactions promote a sense of safety), (2) trustworthiness and transparency (e.g., any decisions by the organization or leadership is transparent), (3) peer support (e.g., support involves similarly situated individuals who have been exposed to trauma), (4) collaboration and mutuality (e.g., eliminating the perception of power differences between administrators and professional staff in regard to trauma-informed care/services/support), (5) empowerment, voice, and choice (e.g., ensuring the organization supports trauma-informed care throughout its organizational structure), and (6) cultural, historical, and gender issues (e.g., the organization offers services that are responsive to gender, cultural, and historical issues; SAMHSA, 2014, 2017).

For example, Risking Connection® offers organizational consulting to aid in establishing a proprietary system that equates to a turn-key solution for self-care. As with many solutions discussed throughout this book, Risking Connection® was borne as a response to litigation and developed with the mitigation of litigation risk in mind. The program offers an advantage in that it is grounded in theory (constructivist self-development theory, relational psychoanalytic theory, developmental psychopathology, and cognitive schemas) and offers the ability for professionals to enroll in "train-the-trainer" courses to ensure sustainability within an organization after launch. See Table 11.1 for a summary of Rising Connection® to get an idea of the overall programmatic approach. The other programs named above use similar approaches to ensure that an organization develops and maintains a culture that is trauma-informed and trauma-responsive.

Table 11.1 Risking Connection® summary of model, program goals, and expected outcomes

Emphasis	Programmatic goals	Expected measurable outcomes
A framework for understanding common trauma symptoms A common inclusive language Relationships as the primary agent of change Respect for, and care of, both the client and the service provider (vicarious traumatization) as critical to healing Strategies and tools to support adoption of the model in clinical, social, and organizational processes	Utilize the proprietary risking connection framework to respond to the impact of traumatic life events Frame common symptoms and behaviors as adaptations to traumatic life events Respond to survivors of traumatic experiences from a strengths-based approach Demonstrate collaborative crisis management that reduces the risk of re-traumatization Demonstrate increased self-awareness of their reactions to individual clients Integrate knowledge of the impact of vicarious traumatization in the formulation of organizational and individual self-care plans Create trauma-responsive cultures including policies, processes, and people systems	Knowledge of content and models essential to risking connection Shift in beliefs favorable to trauma-informed care Demonstration of behaviors aligned with trauma-informed care Changes in professional quality of life including an increase in compassion satisfaction, decrease in burn out, and a decrease in secondary (or vicarious) traumatic stress Responses that reduce the use of restraints and seclusion at organizations Decreases in staff turnover, staff injuries from client management, increase in staff satisfaction with job Increases in foster parent retention and decrease in foster placement disruptions

Adapted from the California Evidence-Based Clearinghouse for Child Welfare (2017) resources

11.5   Conclusion

With the growth in incarcerated and justice-involved individuals, the demand on professionals has also increased. For first responders responding to a crisis, as well as those providing treatment during and after incarceration, strong anecdotal evidence documents the impact on these professionals from increasingly difficult encounters. Our system is overflowing, and those with the care and desire to help resolve it are being pushed to the limit. The importance of self-care should be evident, yet administrators of first responders have been slow to ratchet up support. Treatment is *essential* not only for the target population discussed throughout this book who seem to be in frequent contact with the criminal justice system, but also for the people who spend their days helping this population. Our society needs to support and shelter those in need and ensure that all have the same access and ability to seek out and receive the treatment and care they deserve – including first responders.

For the little information that we have on the topic regarding the perceptions of mental health among first responders, coping skills, and the perception of first responder culture of being unfriendly to those who need help, there certainly is more than enough evidence to support a dire need for broader adoption of self-care programming. Remember, investing in our professionals is also investing in individuals with mental health concerns.

Discussion Questions
1. What community supports (programs, groups, etc.) are there to help first responders and law enforcement be successful in their jobs? Do these programs exist in your area?
2. How can we reduce the barriers for first responders to seek mental health help?
3. How can the community come together to facilitate a positive relationship with law enforcement? How can this be accomplished with communities of color?
4. Are certain cities/communities/states/countries doing a good job managing police-community relationships? What models exist?
5. What are some types of self-care activities, programs, or services for university students? Are there any available on campuses in the state you reside?

References

Accreditation Council for Graduate Medical Education. (2017). Common program requirements. URL: http://www.acgme.org/Portals/0/PFAssets/ProgramRequirements/CPRs_2017-07-01. pdf. Last accessed: 2017, October 30.

American Psychiatric Association. (2013). *Diagnostic and statistical manual of mental disorders* (5th ed.). American Psychiatric Publishing.

Anshel, M. H. (2000). A conceptual model and implications for coping with stressful events in police work. *Criminal Justice and Behavior, 27*(3), 375–400.

Berger, W., Coutinho, E. S. F., Figueira, I., Marques-Portella, C., Luz, M. P., Neylan, T. C., et al. (2012). Rescuers at risk: A systematic review and meta-regression analysis of the worldwide current prevalence and correlates of PTSD in rescue workers. *Social Psychiatry and Psychiatric Epidemiology, 47*(6), 1001–1011.

California Evidence-Based Clearinghouse for Child Welfare. (2017). Risking connection®. URL: http://www.cebc4cw.org/program/risking-connection/detailed. Last accessed: 2017, October 31.

Day, J. R., Anderson, R. A., & Davis, L. L. (2014). Compassion fatigue in adult daughter caregivers of a parent with dementia. *Issues in Mental Health Nursing, 35*(10), 796–804.

Figley, C. R. (Ed.). (2002). *Treating compassion fatigue.* Routledge.

Levin, A. P., Kleinman, S. B., & Adler, J. S. (2014). DSM-5 and posttraumatic stress disorder. *Journal of the American Academy of Psychiatry and the Law Online, 42*(2), 146–158.

Maslach, C., Jackson, S. E., & Leiter, M. P. (2006). *Maslach burnout inventory* (3rd ed.). Consulting Psychologists Press.

Mathieu, F. (2012). *The compassion fatigue workbook: Creative tools for transforming compassion fatigue and vicarious traumatization.* Routledge.

National Association of Emergency Medical Technicians. (2017). 2016 national survey on EMS mental health services. URL: http://www.naemt.org/docs/default-source/ems-health-and-safety-documents/mental-health-grid/2016-naemt-mental-health-report-8-14-16.pdf?status=Temp&sfvrsn=0.9606132567905388. Last accessed: 2017, October 30.

Philibert, I., Nasca, T., Brigham, T., & Shapiro, J. (2013). Duty-hour limits and patient care and resident outcomes: Can high-quality studies offer insight into complex relationships? *Annual Review of Medicine, 64*, 467–483.

Rivera Waugh, J. (2016). *Crime scene investigators and traumatic event-related stress: A quantitative study.* SAGE.

Substance Abuse and Mental Health Services Administration. (2014) SAMHSA's concept of trauma and guidance for a trauma-informed approach. URL: https://store.samhsa.gov/shin/content/SMA14-4884/SMA14-4884.pdf. Last accessed: 2017, October 31.

Substance Abuse and Mental Health Services Administration. (2017). Trauma-informed approach and trauma-specific interventions. URL: https://www.samhsa.gov/nctic/trauma-interventions. Last accessed: 2017, October 31.

Swatt, M. L., Gibson, C. L., & Piquero, N. L. (2007). Exploring the utility of general strain theory in explaining problematic alcohol consumption by police officers. *Journal of Criminal Justice, 35*(6), 596–611.

Ulanoff, L. (2009). The Googleplex: Everything you've heard is true. *PC Magazine.* URL: https://www.pcmag.com/article2/0,2817,2344010,00.asp. Last accessed: 2017, October 30.

Walsh, M., Taylor, M., & Hastings, V. (2012). Burnout and post traumatic stress disorder in the police: Educating officers with the Stilwell TRiM approach. *Policing: A Journal of Policy and Practice, 7*(2), 167–177.

Chapter 12
What Works, What's Promising, and Lessons from the Pandemic

It's been a long time coming. But I know, a change is gonna come. – Sam Cooke.

This book came about through the collective experience of both authors. Jada and Dave, independently and together on various projects, have seen a need to bring crime and mental health to the forefront of many conversations. Not only in the professional realm, but also in working with students. As it stands today, students graduating in criminal justice will more than likely encounter justice-involved individuals with mental health concerns. It is important that those students, turned professionals, understand the obstacles and cracks in the system that individuals face. This book is just a starting point for many conversations to come on these topics. The hope is that beginning the discussion can also begin the solution.

12.1   Looking Forward

Society is slowly beginning to raise awareness on criminal justice system reform, mental health stigma, and substance use needs. Hopefully, these positive strides continue and bring more access to care, programming, and treatment needed for those involved in the justice system as well as preventative measures with mental health concerns.

Prevention for mental health, substance use, and crime all have common ground. Programs exist at the federal, state, and local levels to implement prevention framework for behavioral health, and public health topics. Integration with these programs is essential for individuals in need, specifically within substance use and criminal justice.

Prevention thought processes can be important for changing stigma and being proactive about concerns within society. For example, proactive preventative measures can inform the public about risks and potential problems a person can

J. Hector, D. Khey, *Criminal Justice and Mental Health*,
https://doi.org/10.1007/978-3-031-15338-9_12

experience. Even further, being part of a certain group can increase those risks. Whether it be a specific racial or ethnic group, gender, socioeconomic status, or even just a specific neighborhood can affect the risk of someone's potential to experience negative impact. Education and awareness about crime risks, drug addiction risks, and mental health symptoms can help to create an informed individual. Additionally, this also lessens the stigma associated with each and creates an open dialogue to begin discussing these topics in a healthy manner.

Continuing to have conversations regarding mental health and overall behavioral health are important to keep the topic relevant. These conversations allow for education and information to be exchanged. As with any important topic, positive message creates positive outlooks.

12.1.1 Legislative Progress

State legislatures often address bills related to both mental health and criminal justice, especially when there is a change in administration. These bills can themselves be solely about addressing issues within either of these areas, or there may be amendments hidden within another bill related to a completely different topic.

Every few years, NAMI provides a state mental health policy trends report to help shed some light on gains, stagnation, and losses in mental health policy/programming in each state. This report helps to shed light on both positive approaches states are taking in mental health, as well as those that are lacking in improvements. In 2015, the report breaks down information by subjects including criminal justice, suicide prevention, and inpatient and crisis care. Each section provides a summary of the bill as well as links to the state-related bills within that area of focus. It also includes a general sense of trends in mental health-related expenditures by state (see Table 12.1). In 2019, the policy report takes a different tact by focusing on exemplar policy options from around the country and provides some context as to the lessons learned along the way in shaping these policy decisions resulting in state legislation and forward progress.

A notable mention from the 2015 report features innovation in criminal justice practices. In Utah, the state legislature introduced a bill to work toward positive criminal justice reform, including mental health initiatives. The 2015 bill HB 348 entitled Criminal Justice Programs "amends Utah Code provisions regarding corrections, sentencing, probation and parole, controlled substance offenses, substance abuse and mental health treatment, vehicle offenses, and related provisions to modify penalties and sentencing guidelines, treatment programs for persons in the criminal justice system, and probation and parole compliance and violations to address recidivism."

Highlights of Utah's HB 348 incorporate the state's Division of Mental Health and Department of Corrections to work together to establish performance goals and outcome measures for treatment programs. Then, these departments are to collect data and evaluate those performance goals and outcome measures and supply the

Table 12.1 Summary of findings from the NAMI State Mental Health Legislation Report

State	2013	2014	2015	State	2013	2014	2015
Alabama	Maintain	Increase	Maintain	Montana	Increase	Maintain	Increase
Alaska	Decrease	Decrease	Decrease	Nebraska	Decrease	Decrease	Increase
Arizona	Increase	Increase	Increase	Nevada	Increase	Maintain	Decrease
Arkansas	Increase	Decrease	Decrease	New Hampshire	Increase	Increase	Increase
California	Increase	Increase	Maintain	New Jersey	Increase	Increase	Increase
Colorado	Increase	Increase	Increase	New Mexico	Maintain	Increase	Increase
Connecticut	Increase	Increase	Increase	New York	Maintain	Increase	Increase
Delaware	Increase	Increase	Increase	North Carolina	Decrease	Decrease	Decrease
District of Columbia	Increase	Increase	Decrease	North Dakota	Maintain	Maintain	Decrease
Florida	Maintain	Increase	Increase	Ohio	Increase	Increase	Decrease
Georgia	Increase	Maintain	Increase	Oklahoma	Increase	Increase	Maintain
Hawaii	Increase	Decrease	Maintain	Oregon	Increase	Maintain	Increase
Idaho	Increase	Increase	Increase	Pennsylvania	Maintain	Increase	Pending
Illinois	Increase	Maintain	Pending	Rhode Island	Increase	Decrease	Maintain
Indiana	Maintain	Maintain	Increase	South Carolina	Increase	Increase	Increase
Iowa	Increase	Increase	Decrease	South Dakota	Increase	Increase	Increase
Kansas	Increase	Increase	Decrease	Tennessee	Increase	Maintain	Maintain
Kentucky	Increase	Decrease	Decrease	Texas	Increase	Maintain	Increase
Louisiana	Decrease	Decrease	Maintain	Utah	Increase	Increase	Maintain
Maine	Decrease	Increase	Increase	Vermont	Increase	Increase	Maintain
Maryland	Increase	Increase	Maintain	Virginia	Increase	Increase	Increase
Massachusetts	Increase	Maintain	Increase	Washington	Increase	Increase	Increase
Michigan	Increase	Decrease	Maintain	West Virginia	Maintain	Increase	Increase
Minnesota	Increase	Increase	Increase	Wisconsin	Increase	Increase	Maintain
Mississippi	Increase	Maintain	Maintain	Wyoming	Decrease	Decrease	Decrease
Missouri	Increase	Increase	Maintain				

results to the public. These policies are to not only increase awareness for the populous of Utah, but also begin the process of working toward treating those in need and reducing recidivism. Further, HB 348 requires the Department of Corrections of Utah to establish and implement standards for treatment programs in county jails as well.

This bill is one of many in the steps toward positive change for both persons with a mental illness in the criminal justice system. Other positive notes in the 2015 NAMI State Mental Health Legislation report surround topics previously discussed in this book. For example, CIT or Crisis Intervention Training for Law Enforcement has been added in different ways to Indiana, Illinois, and Maryland. Illinois is requiring a standard certified training program, while similarly, Maryland is mandating a program for Baltimore city and county police officers. Additionally, Indiana is creating a CIT Technical Assistance Center (TAC) to create an advisory committee to oversee all CIT related activities within the state. States are also looking into creating other specialty courts as well. South Carolina and Arizona have put bills in place to create mental health courts. The 2019 report highlights notable improvements in prioritizing several legislative efforts, such as investing and embedding mental health and suicide prevention programming into public education, protecting Medicaid coverage for mental health services and preventing cuts to funding, initiating private insurance reform to improve broader compliance with the Mental Health Parity and Addition Equity Act of 2008 (which mandates that insurance companies cover mental and substance use disorder treatments *to not be more restrictive* than coverage for other medical conditions), and broader legislative requirements mandating alternative responses to crises in lieu of primarily relying on law enforcement.

As a society, working together, change can be done to better the health of everyone. Using history and current data, there appears to be hope in small organizations or movements to work toward positive, health change.

12.2   Change Is Taking Place, Slowly

Often, when changes are attempted in states and local communities, mental health is shot down because of misinformation, lack of education, and stigma. Health departments are making cuts due to losses in federal funding. Those cuts often come from mental health programming since other areas are viewed as more urgent needs as it relates to health.

A quick Google search of any combination of the words "mental illness," "jail" or "prison," and "death" will bring forth some truly eye-opening results. Change can begin with a conversation, continued awareness campaigns, and increasing collaborations where they previously did not exist. It appears that some of the most successful changes are occurring at the local level with partnerships that span from the courts to professionals to persons of faith to laypersons.

12.3   Change Agents

A positive resource for many partnerships and the organization they represent can be grant writing. Grants can range from thousands of dollars to millions and cover varying aspects of topics related to both crime and mental health. These grants can be offered from both private organizations and the federal government. For example, in some instances the specialty courts mentioned in previous chapters were initially funded by a federal grant.

Organizations like SAMHSA and BJA offer grants on a yearly cycle. State and local governments and nonprofit organizations can submit an application to receive

Table 12.2 Recent grant programs targeting mental health, substance use disorder, and reentry issues (2017)

Grant program	Program description
Adult Drug Court Discretionary Grant Program (BJA)	Supports specialty courts and their key partnerships; current categories include implementation (e.g., start-up capital), expansion (e.g., offer broader treatment modalities, expand to target special populations, etc.), and statewide enhancement
Second Chance Act Reentry Program for Adults with Co-Occurring Substance Use and Mental Disorders (BJA)	Targets adults with co-occurring disorders as they return to communities after a period of incarceration; supports units of government or tribal government
Justice and Mental Health Collaboration Program (BJA)	Supports broad collaboration to improve outcomes for individuals with mental illness and co-occurring disorders; geared for county and parish governmental units to take lead on collaborative partnerships with its key stakeholders in the community *or* law enforcement agencies to serve as lead partner in this type of project
Grants to Expand Substance Abuse Treatment Capacity in Adult Treatment Drug Courts and Adult Tribal Healing to Wellness Courts	Supports specialty courts needing to beef up their evidence-based treatment provisioning, particularly medication-assisted treatment

the funding. These grant opportunities allow communities that would not otherwise have the funding available to show proof of concept for their ideas, implement them, evaluate their results, and refine their knowledge of the problems they are attempting to solve. If these awards can provide proof of success with evidence and support, the hope would be continued funding to allow for the sustainability of these program to continue positive change (and to replicate these models elsewhere throughout the country).

As highlighted throughout this book, the change agents involve partnerships among mental health and criminal justice professionals, lawyers, faith leaders, congregants, employers, researchers, legislators and policy-makers, non-profits, and community resource liaisons, among many others. Many of these grant opportunities (see Table 12.2) force the issue of having these key stakeholders come together to be eligible for funding. It matters less on what brings these players together rather than the outcomes they can create when they get on the same page. These changes are occurring throughout the country thanks to Federal leadership on mental health and criminal justice reinvestment and reform over the two decades.

12.4 Theoretical Considerations

Many theorists have opined on the critical nature of theory to structure our understanding of human behavior. As such, pouring over theory and testing their hypotheses and practicality in the real world can give us insight on how to intervene on behalf of those who are suffering from mental illness and/or substance use disorder. For example, if we know that selecting and prioritizing social relationships with individuals who like to use drugs and get themselves into criminal trouble increases the risk one engages in the same behavior, we can act to disconnect those ties as best as we can. Perhaps, more likely, if we assist in helping someone connect with pro-social ties and assist in making these relationships a priority for this same individual, the risk of getting into trouble is greatly diminished even if bad influences remain in the background (Akers, 1990). Theory can help vet practical solutions, test these ideas, refine them, and provide a scientific process on solving the problems facing us.

12.4.1   Restorative Justice and Relevant Theory

According to classic labeling theory, societies are hardwired to use social control to regulate behavior – particularly to correct behavior that break social norms. An easy example of this process can be found in the concept of the "outlaw" in the American Old West. Outlaws were the worst of men, formally casted off from good society with a complete loss of legal rights. Labels exist in many forms: criminal, bad, bandit, robber, druggie, and so on; these also serve to reify those on the normative side and reinforce good behavior ("don't be like 'them'"). According to theory, these efforts of social control routinely backfire. In other words, efforts to punish bad or wrong behavior may drive vulnerable people, particularly the young and impressionable, toward a criminal lifestyle or deeper into mental illness.

This idea originated with Frank Tannenbaum (1938) who observed that official reactions to social behavior (e.g., by the criminal justice system or its parts – or, by the mental health care system) can change a person's self-concept (e.g, their identity) in two ways. First, when a label such as "criminal," "convict," "delinquent," "incorrigible," "insane," or "mentally ill" is applied to a person by the system, these individuals are often subsequently immersed into an environment (jails/prisons) rich with learning opportunities from others who have been similarly labeled. Second, labeled individuals are frequently subjected to social admonishment by everyday people ("informal" sources, such as family, school, potential employers, etc.), which erects barriers to any hope of getting on the "right" path – a crime-free or healthy life. This second effect of a label is called secondary deviance (Lemert, 1951, 1972). At some point in the lives of labeled people, the labels are gradually accepted until they "stick." Over time, these individuals align their lifestyles and their behaviors to suit their altered "primary status" – a concept called "the self-fulfilling prophesy."

These twentieth-century concepts witnessed a renaissance in criminology and criminal justice when the restorative justice movement come about, yet have remained relevant in circles of mental health researchers for their obvious ties to the effects of stigma on individuals. For newcomer theorists in the restorative justice movement, there was a missing element in older renditions of labeling when applying it to crime. In some cases, these theorists saw shame as *good*, and healthy, for offenders and victims alike. When done in a certain way, shame can bring reconciliation and healing. John Braithwaite calls this reintegrative shaming; the theory of reintegrative shaming focuses on *the manner* by which the formal systems apply shame by punishment and admonishment. Namely, if the system can correct behavior holistically, it can be rehabilitative – shame must be accompanied by general forgiveness, acceptance, and reintegration to be transformative.

Shame is normal and natural. It is a reaction to social behaviors that fall outside of social and/or legal norms. For example, a disapproving mother may react to a son's bad attitude and signs of disrespect. This condemnation could be reinforced by others close by – for example, neighbors, family members, or church members – depending on a localized cultural values. Shame works primarily to elicit feelings of remorse and drive recompense. A kid caught stealing an expensive graphing calculator at school may be admonished by a teacher and disciplined by the principal. Quickly thereafter, the principal may call the child's family, starting this cycle of shaming at home. According to reintegrative shaming, the goal would be to make sure the student quickly reconnects with pro-social ties at school, at home, and even in the community through apology, forgiveness, and acceptance. The calculator goes back to the victim, the victim makes peace with the offender, and surrounding players help to heal everyone accordingly. Braithwaite (1989) warns that shaming can be stigmatizing, and this can possibly amplify deviance – as seen with traditional labeling theory. If this calculator-stealing kid were sent to detention with all the other bad kids, kicked out of Advanced Placement calculus, and left to pick up the pieces, his shame may put him on a darker future path.

Each modern society seems to have its own brand of shaming. For example, Japanese culture has promulgated a pure type of reintegrative shaming in each generation for many centuries. In fact, Japanese offenders are expected to enter a ritual that begins with an apology to which the victim is compelled to help bring the offender back into the fold. If either offender or victim violates these cultural mores, it can bring shame and scrutiny. Any observer of American culture can note the departure this Japanese ritual has with similar interactions in the United States. Thus, reintegrative shaming can be considered a paradigm shift – much like what is going on with criminal justice reform at this time.

12.4.2   Reintegrative Shaming in Action

According to a stream of new literature, the concept of reintegrative shaming can easily guide the practices of a model mental health court for optimal results – at least theoretically. In fact, sociologists Ray et al. (2011) picked up on this notion and attempted to determine whether observed court proceedings of model mental health courts promulgated feelings of respect and forgiveness while tamping down feelings of disapproval when compared to traditional court proceedings. To scientifically accomplish this task, Ray, Dollar, and Thames used an observation instrument that was designed to measure these constructs in action, called the Global Observational Ratings Instrument. Specifically, this instrument taps into the following:

- How much reintegrative shaming was expressed?
- How much stigmatizing shaming was expressed?
- How much support was the offender given during the court proceedings?
- How much approval of the offender as a person was expressed?
- How much respect for the offender was expressed?
- How much disappointment in the offender was expressed?
- To what extent was the offender treated as a criminal?
- How often were stigmatizing names and labels used to describe the offender?
- How much disapproval of the offender as a person was expressed?
- How clearly was it communicated to the offender that they could put their actions behind them?
- How much forgiveness of the offender was expressed?

To ensure to minimize any bias in applying a score to each of the items to be observed above, the study uses three observers to ensure interrater reliability. If mental health courts operate as intended, the researchers should find substantial differences between the mental health court process compared to the traditional court process in these domains – and this research supports this hypothesis. Yet, while these findings are hopeful (pun intended), they did not seem to translate into reductions in recidivism. In this vein, the researchers did not holistically observe the fidelity of the observed mental health courts to other important components required for the optimal success of these programs (Miller & Khey, 2017). In other words, while court proceedings could elicit feelings of reintegrative shaming and forgiveness, adequate treatment protocols may have not been followed, or if followed, may not have employed evidence-based practices proven to work within this target population. In a recent follow-up study, Dollar and Ray (2015) strengthen their original work by continuing to follow the court for 3 years. In all, the conclusions remain the same – client disapproval by the judge and mental health court personnel was done in a way that was respectful, relationships among participants and court personnel showed evidence of respect and caring, disapproval tended to focus on the behavior and not on any individual, everyone on the mental health court team avoided stigmatizing words and labels, and so on.

By now, it should be easy to see how theory can inform practice; yet, in this case, and for this target population, reintegrative shaming does not offer a complete solution. It certainly optimizes the chances for success and eliminates significant barriers (if not *the* most significant barrier – stigma) that prevent ultimate success. Importantly, the fundamentals of evidence-based mental health treatment are paramount. These findings certainly inform future research and evaluations of the mental health court model. In particular, it underscores the importance of process evaluations. In other words, it is important to not only ensure that the mental health court process is working as intended and as guided by the principles of reintegrative shaming, evaluations also need to probe the treatment protocols to determine if these are modeled after practices already proven to work in the field (Miller & Khey, 2017).

12.4.3   The Future of Reintegrative Shaming in Research

The interest in the practicality of reintegrative shaming in the United States has waned since a peak of interest in the late 1990s and early 2000s (as determined by Federal funding specifically to explore reintegrative shaming in theory as well as in practice). Mental health courts seem to be the exception. In fact, funding for these programs continues to grow as well as the interest in establishing new courts across the country. Further, interest in the topic remains strong in academia and in research organizations – the online library of the Centre for Justice and Reconciliation holds over 12,800 citations and abstracts for scholarly work and technical "white papers" on restorative justice. In fact, the Centre continues to add about 1000 entries in each year (Khey, 2014). Even with all of this positive activity, some of these entries warn proponents of the impediments that exist to stymie future development of programming based on restorative justice principles (e.g., Riley, 2017). Reintegrative shaming may not be *the* solution, but certainly holds promise of optimizing the results of evidence-based programming discussed throughout this book.

One of the missing pieces of current research seems to align with one of the greatest barriers to justice reinvestment – being able to specify a target population known to respond to particular treatment to result in crime reduction. Over the years, researchers have found success in changing offenders' perceptions after being exposed to reintegrative shaming processes. As a whole, research shows that these differences translate into reductions in recidivism for only some individuals, not a majority or all. Future research will need to give better clarity as to why this is occurring. This research should also consider blending in the literature of the reentry and criminal justice reform movements – again, reintegrative shaming may help optimize the power of programming that has come about. Programs that offer after-care to help people returning back to their communities that connect them to employment, mental health and substance abuse treatment, counseling, housing, transportation, education, and vocational training may need to seek out opportunities to apply reintegrative shaming techniques. This appears to be the advantage of reentry court relative to other programs of the sort; just like we have seen with mental health court in providing the structure for reintegrative shaming to occur, reentry court offers the same potential. Future research will need to explore whether this reintegrative shaming is complete in reentry courts in that it can translate into tangible things like gainful employment, family reunification, and pro-social relationships.

With the growth spurt of both mental health and reentry courts, it appears that the reintegrative shaming principles will continue to flourish and guide continued success of criminal justice reform programming. Much more research needs to be done – for example, at what point must reintegrative shaming principles be applied to work properly in the reentry process? Is it possible to start this process before release? If so, does it help? In the community, what is the earliest point criminal justice professionals can apply these principles in the sequential intercept model? Essentially, all of these questions seem to ask, at what point in time is it reasonable to start the healing process and welcome offenders back into the fold.

12.5   Pandemic Considerations

The primary tool mental health care systems around the world have utilized to ensure access to care during the COVID-19 pandemic has been and continues to be telemedicine. Innovations in virtualized meetings have promulgated throughout the justice system as well, keeping the justice-involved population connected to services with varying degrees of success (yet to be studied). At the time of this writing, the literature offers an array of pandemic-related modifications to operations with scant evidence to better understand levels of success based on these shifts. Even if such evidence were to exist, caution would need to be used when interpreting any findings due to pandemic-related interruptions and ever-constant shifting conditions that continue to this day. One such report by Burton et al. (2021) reviews how the psychiatric services at San Quentin State Prison modified the provision of care to fit the broader changes make to the general operation of the prison – even noting that San Quentin had a historical record of modifying operations that dates to the 1918 flu pandemic. Remarkably, the general operation guidance was similar. In 1918, the prison had responded to a pandemic generations ago by eliminating large gatherings, dispensing cloth masks, minimizing close contact of any persons, and developing a quarantine system for new arrivals. In 2020, the system responded to this generation's pandemic by similarly instituting a quarantine system and moved to reduce the density in prisons by selectively releasing a proportion of non-violent incarcerated persons. In addition, visitation was modified, court and other official hearings (e.g., parole) were shifted to tele- or videoconference, and masks were distributed throughout the facility. For mental health services, one of the major adaptations Burton, Morris, and Hirschtritt describe was directly due to the fact that correctional administrators stopped all transfers between facilities – thus, any one at San Quentin that required inpatient care would need to remain at the prison. To address this, staff created temporary mental health facilities at the prison and reassigned staff to ensure coverage to provide oversight of this new temporary unit. Tele- and videoconferencing was essential to ensure continued legal hearings and access to psychiatric services that were previously performed exclusively in-person. This report extensively discusses the barriers that needed to be overcome in order to make tele- or videoconferencing ubiquitous, particularly as corrections administrators had consider the tools to access such technology (cell phones, computers or other personal devices, and Internet access) as contraband. In the end, San Quentin was able to deploy nine telepsychiatry stations in various housing units throughout the prison with quick speed. In fact, the researchers reveal that 60% of psychiatric appointments were handled via telehealth by March 2020.

These innovations have provided a wealth of opportunities for underserved systems and those vulnerable people embedded in them. For example, Krider and Parker (2021) note that tele-mental health services have been expanded in rural prison settings. In interviews with correctional professionals in five rural US jurisdictions, Krider and Parker were able to find that there was a general sense of appreciation for the rapid adoption of such tools given a broader expectation that telemedicine would be difficult or impossible to deploy. Even more, they found high levels of user satisfaction with these new options, which may open the possibility of continued use beyond the pandemic which may impact positive outcomes in rural areas across the country.

12.6   Concluding Remarks

Treatment for mental illness can help in many ways, particularly with reducing the chances of individuals to not become justice-involved or – more likely – reduce the chances of not returning to the criminal justice system. Data suggests that there is, on average, an 8-year delay from the onset of mental health symptomatology to first indications of treatment. This delay is due to a complex array of barriers to treatment, of which stigma tends to be the most potent. All too often, the criminal justice system becomes an entry point to mental health services. This is not to say that jails and prisons are illegitimate entry points; yet these institutions have long been beleaguered with the lack of resources to engage this target population with the care they need. Likely, jail and prison administrators and their staff are unaware of specific mental health diagnoses among their inmates as there are far too many gaps in even the detection of these issues in incarcerated populations.

The aging data on mental health – and, generally speaking, the lack of data in many areas – inhibits progress, particularly among justice-involved populations. It is also important to invest in broader epidemiological surveillance systems as we do with other diseases and conditions. Doing so will allow for professionals to better monitor progress, change, incidence of new and emerging issues, and so on. As twenty-first Century Cures Act begins to shape the infrastructure of change, it is important for professionals to understand their role in mental health awareness and how the organizations they belong can fill a gap of information that is all too common in this domain.

This book is not meant to be negative in nature, but rather bring to light the issues surrounding crime and mental health – particularly on how crime and mental health intersect all too often. The first steps to change involved acknowledging and understanding the issues at hand. As a society and community, the cracks in the system need to be viewed, reviewed, assessed, and reassessed in order to move forward with solutions. This will take some time and effort, but it can be done.

References

Akers, R. L. (1990). Rational choice, deterrence, and social learning theory in criminology: The path not taken. *Journal of Criminal Law & Criminology, 81*(3), 653–676.

Braithwaite, J. (1989). *Crime, shame, and reintegration.* Cambridge University Press.

Burton, P. R., Morris, N. P., & Hirschtritt, M. E. (2021). Mental health services in a US prison during the COVID-19 pandemic. *Psychiatric Services, 72*(4), 458–460.

Center for Justice and Reconciliation. (2012). http://www.restorativejustice.org. Last accessed: 2012, May 16.

Dollar, C. B., & Ray, B. (2015). The practice of reintegrative shaming in mental health court. *Criminal Justice Policy Review, 26*(1), 29–44.

Khey, D. N. (2014). Reintegrative shaming. *The Encyclopedia of Theoretical Criminology*, 1–5.

Krider, A. E., & Parker, T. W. (2021). COVID-19 tele-mental health: Innovative use in rural behavioral health and criminal justice settings. *Journal of Rural Mental Health, 45*(2), 86–94.

Lemert, E. M. (1951). *Social pathology: A systematic approach to the theory of sociopathic behavior.* The Free Press.

Lemert, E. M. (1972). *Human deviance, social problems, and social control* (2nd ed.). Prentice Hall.

Miller, J. M., & Khey, D. N. (2017). Fighting America's highest incarceration rates with offender programming: Process evaluation implications from the Louisiana 22nd Judicial District reentry court. *American Journal of Criminal Justice, 42*(3), 574–588.

Ray, B., Dollar, C. B., & Thames, K. M. (2011). Observations of reintegrative shaming in a mental court. *International Journal of Law and Psychiatry, 34*(1), 49–55.

Riley, K. (2017). Empowering justice: An intersectional feminist perspective on restorative justice in the sex trade. *American Journal of Economics and Sociology, 76*(5), 1157–1190.

Tannenbaum, F. (1938). *Crime and the community.* Columbia University Press.

Index

Printed in the USA
CPSIA information can be obtained
at www.ICGtesting.com
LVHW050721080823
754622LV00005B/162

9 783031 153372